GENERAL SURGERY

GENERAL SURGERY

C J Mieny

Academica

Published by Academica,
a division of Van Schaik Publishers,
1064 Arcadia Street, Hatfield 0083 Pretoria

First edition 1992
Second impression 1998
Third impression 2001

ISBN 0 86874 416 6

Typeset in 9 on 11 pt Times rom by Kohler Carton & Print, Pinetown
Printed and bound by Interpak, 22 Willowton Road, Pietermaritzburg

Preface

The success of this text in Afrikaans has led to the publication of a revised English edition.

The book, although mainly aimed at undergraduate students, can also be read by junior registrars as an overview of the subject at the start of their surgical training. It is a useful text for general practitioners as a reference work in their daily practice and during preparation for continuing medical education programmes.

To fulfil these multiple aims, each chapter is structured to begin with a series of questions relating to day-to-day clinical practice. This is followed by a classification of relevant diseases.

After dealing with the clinical picture and the differential diagnosis, special investigations and treatment options are discussed in some detail.

The specialty subjects like urology, orthopaedics, neurosurgery and cardio-thoracic surgery are not covered except in so far as it is related to the management of the severely injured patient.

CJ Mieny
Pretoria

Alisha Rai

Contents

Head and neck 1

SALIVARY GLANDS

How does the patient present?

- With a mass in the anatomical region of the salivary glands; at the angle of the mandible, in the submandibular triangle, or on the palate.
- With a visible mass at the angle of the mandible, which often lifts the earlobe and is sometimes bilateral.
- With pain and a mass. The pain can be a dull ache, or very acute. Sometimes it is exacerbated by eating.
- With a discrete mass in one or more of the salivary glands.
- With diffuse enlargement of one or both parotid glands, or of one or both submandibular glands.
- With enlargement of all the salivary glands and the lacrimal glands.

What must the clinician consider?

- A painless mass in the region of the salivary glands:
  Differential:
  - Pleomorphic adenoma (mixed salivary gland tumour) – 70% of tumours
  - Adenolymphoma (Warthin tumour) – 10% of tumours
  - Muco-epidermoid tumour – 5% of tumours
- Mass associated with a dull, aching pain:
  Carcinoma. Various types together make up 15% of tumours.
- Multiple masses in the salivary glands and lacrimal glands:
  Mickulicz-Sjögren disease
- Bilateral enlargement of the salivary glands associated with vague pain in children:
  Idiopathic sialadenitis of childhood
- Painful enlarged salivary glands:
  Bilateral in children: mumps
- Unilateral or bilateral enlargement, post-operatively in the elderly:
  Bacterial parotitis
- Painful enlargement of a submandibular gland exacerbated by meals:
  Stone in Wharton's duct.

What else does the clinician wish to ascertain from the history?

- How long has the mass been present? A short history is suggestive of malignancy.
- Are a dry mouth and dry eyes associated with multiple gland enlargements? This suggests Mickulicz–Sjögren disease.

What does the clinician find on examination?

The mass

- Is it a discrete mass, in the gland, with clearly defined edges, hard, rubberlike and smoothly lobular? If so, there is a 90% chance that it is a pleomorphic adenoma.
- Is it a discrete mass, soft and cystic? – Highly likely that it is an adenolymphoma, but a cyst must also be considered.

- Is the hard, poorly defined mass, with an irregular surface? Consider a carcinoma.
- If it infiltrates surrounding tissues, the masseter muscle or the skin, it is a malignant tumour.
- Is the salivary gland diffusely enlarged? – consider inflammatory conditions.

The facial nerve function

If paresis or paralysis presents in the distribution of the branches of the facial nerve, carcinoma can be diagnosed. It is important to test nerve supply to the corner of the mouth by asking the patient to show his teeth. Also test innervation of the ocular muscles by asking the patient to close his eyes tightly.

The salivary ducts

Palpate the duct bimanually, with one finger inside the mouth. Stones are especially common in the Wharton duct and are sometimes palpable. Inspect the openings of the ducts. The Stensen duct opens into the cheek opposite the second molar. The Wharton duct opens on *diaphragma oris* just lateral to the frenulum of the tongue. Note the following:

- Are the openings normal?
- Is normal sputum being excreted?
- Does the opening look oedematous?
- Is there a purulent discharge?

Lymph nodes

Feel for enlarged lymph nodes in the preauricular region and in the neck. Their presence suggests malignancy.

Special investigations

1. **Bacterial cultures from the salivary ducts:** Milk out the contents of the ducts and culture.
2. **X-rays:** Ordinary X-rays of the *diaphragma oris* usually demonstrate stones in the Wharton duct, since all stones contain calcium.
3. **Sialogram:** Lipiodol is injected into the Stensen- or Wharton duct and anteroposterior and lateral X-ray views are taken. A sialogram may show a dilated duct proximal to an area of stenosis, a stone (which shows up as a filling defect), or generalized dilation of the ducts and acini (sialectasis or sialadenitis).

   A sialogram may show a filling defect in the secondary ductal system. Ducts which are displaced around a filling defect, suggest a benign tumour. Destruction of the ducts is indicative of a carcinoma. Infiltration instead of displacement of the ducts also indicates carcinoma.
4. **Computer tomography (CT):** A mass at the angle of the mandible or in the submandibular triangle can be identified as a salivary gland tumour with the aid of CT. It can also be performed as an adjunct to sialography, further accentuating the appearance of the tumour.
5. **Biopsy:** This is one of the pitfalls in the management of salivary gland tumours. **Never perform an open biopsy on a mass at the angle of the mandible, even though it may appear to be superficial.** In 90% of cases it will be a salivary gland tumour. The danger lies in potential spread of the tumour or injury to the facial nerve.

   The majority of salivary gland tumours (more than 80%) are benign and can be excised without a preceding biopsy. If there are signs suggestive of malignancy, a needle biopsy must be performed first. The needle tract must be positioned so that it can be surgically removed along with the mass. The biopsy must be taken only by the surgeon who intends to perform the operation.

Tumours

Pleomorphic adenoma

This benign tumour is found mainly in the parotid gland (90%). The remainder are found in the submandibular gland and in minor salivary glands on the palate.

It is a clearly defined, slowly growing tumour. However, it does have a tendency to form protrusions through the capsule. The majority are found in the superficial lobe of the parotid gland. On a cross section, soft, yellowish-white, fleshy areas, areas of myxoid to gelatinlike tissue and areas of very firm cartilaginous tissue are seen.

Histologically, the tissue consists mainly of epithelial and mucoepithelial cells, which form ductules, acini and microcysts. Myxoid areas, which closely resemble cartilage, are also present. A small percentage (5%) may undergo malignant change. The old theory that every time a pleomorphic adenoma recurs after incomplete excision it is more malignant, is no longer accepted.

It is more likely that the more malignant forms of the tumour are more inclined to recur. If there are no signs of malignancy with a well-encapsulated tumour, the facial nerve is intact and no palpable lymph nodes are present, a biopsy is not performed. The management is a superficial parotidectomy.

The incision is made from a point anterior to the ear, forward towards the neck, curving two fingerbreadths below the ramus of the mandible to avoid the mandibular branch of the facial nerve. The main trunk of the facial nerve is situated in the space between the mandible and the mastoid process, a fingerbreadth below and deep to the bony external meatus of the ear, which is clearly palpable. Dissection is thus carried out superficial to the nerve until the superficial lobe of the parotid gland has been removed. The tumour is usually found in the superficial lobe. If the tumour is situated in the deep lobe, the superficial lobe must be removed formally before the deep lobe is dissected out, with preservation of the facial nerve and its branches, all of which must be carefully lifted and protected by ligatures. The wound is then closed, with suction drainage.

Adenolymphoma (Warthin tumour)

These soft swellings are found mainly in males and almost always in the parotid duct. They are bilateral in 10% of cases. There is some doubt as to whether this tumour is really a neoplasm. It may be a hamartoma and epithelial tissue may be sequestered in the lymph nodes inside the capsule of the parotid gland. Histologically, it comprises a double layer of epithelial cells covered by superficial eosinophils. The deep layer is polygonal and often flattened. The epithelium can occur in lymph node clefts, with underlying germinal centres. It is usually managed in the same way as a mixed salivary gland tumour; and the diagnosis is made postoperatively on histological grounds.

Malignant tumours

Malignant tumours of the salivary glands occur either in the ductal system or the acini. About a third of malignant tumours arise from the acini and are adenocarcinomas. A third arise from the ductal system and are epidermoid tumours and a further third are anaplastic or malignant mixed salivary gland tumours. 75% of all malignant tumours are found in the parotid. However, only 25% of parotid tumours are malignant. 50% or submandibular and minor salivary gland tumours of the mouth are malignant.

Muco-epidermoid tumours

This is the third most common type of parotid tumour. Cystic clefts containing mucuslike material are seen on section. Three main cell types are found, namely squamous cells, cells with PAS positive material in their vacuoles, and mucus cells. The tumour is graded for malignancy according to histological appearance. The more mucus found in the sections, the more benign the tumour's course. 75% of tumours have a slow progression and are curable by surgical excision. The other 25% spread to lymph nodes and also via the bloodstream.

Some of these tumours have a predominantly squamous pattern with anaplasia.

Adenocarcinomas

Adenocystic carcinoma (cylindroma)

These tumours consist of small dark cells containing little cytoplasm. There are cystic spaces filled with mucus and hyalin between the cells. They colour positively with carmine dyes, indicating mucin. These tumours are less aggressive, but spread to lymph nodes in about 30% of cases.

Adenocystic carcinoma has a tendency to spread locally, especially perineurally. They are also inclined to recur after excision.

Acinar cell adenocarcinoma

These tumours consist of acinar cells with a dark, eccentric nucleus and a granular, basophilic cytoplasm which forms primitive acini. These tumours have a low malignant potential but spread to lymph nodes and via the bloodstream. Such metastases may present only ten to twelve years later. Metastases in the lungs can sometimes remain static for years.

Anaplastic adenocarcinoma

They have a trabecular pattern, exhibit aggressive local infiltration, spread to lymph nodes and via the bloodstream and have a poor prognosis.

Malignant mixed salivary gland tumours

These tumours have an underlying mixed salivary gland appearance with squamous- and adenocarcinoma elements. They can develop in longstanding pleomorphic adenomas or *de novo*. They can follow a malignant course, with metastases to lymph nodes and via the bloodstream.

Management of carcinoma of the salivary glands

If malignancy is not suspected preoperatively, a superficial parotidectomy is performed. Histological diagnosis is made on frozen section. If it confirms one of the lower grade malignancies, such as muco-epidermoid tumour, adenocystic carcinoma or acinar cell carcinoma, the deep lobe of the gland is also removed, with preservation of the seventh nerve. If the histological diagnosis confirms one of the more malignant tumours, such as squamous cell carcinoma, anaplastic carcinoma or mixed salivary gland malignant tumour, the seventh nerve is removed along with the deep lobe and a nerve transplant is performed, using the greater auricular nerve. Surgery is followed by irradiation. If malignancy is suspected preoperatively, because of facial nerve palsy or enlarged lymph nodes, a needle biopsy is done to confirm the diagnosis and a total parotidectomy is performed, including sacrifice of the seventh nerve, nerve transplantation and followup irradiation. A block dissection is performed if lymph nodes are palpably enlarged. If there is local infiltration outside the parotid capsule, an extracapsular radical excision is performed, if this is practically possible and if there are no signs of distal metastases. The extracapsular excision includes the masseter muscle, a part of the ramus of the mandible, the mastoid process and the bony external meatus of the ear, en bloc. *This operation is also followed by irradiation.*

If the extent of spread makes the radical operation impossible, or if there are distal metastases, a biopsy diagnosis is followed by irradiation and chemotherapy.

Prognosis

The five year survival rate of patients with muco-epidermoid tumours, adenocystic carcinoma and mixed salivary gland malignant tumours is higher than 80%. The ten year survival rate drops to around 60%. Anaplastic carcinomas have a very poor prognosis.

Inflammatory conditions of the salivary glands

Bacterial parotitis sometimes occurs in the aged following major surgery. The underlying aetiology is dehydration and poor oral hygiene, which causes thick, viscous saliva. Patients often have nasogastric tubes *in situ* and breathe through their mouths. The opening of the Stensen duct dries out and swells closed, with build-up of debris on the mucous membranes. It is thus a result of unsatisfactory postoperative care, with dehydration and poor hygiene of the oral mucous membranes.

The parotid is surrounded by a thick capsule; and swelling of the gland causes severe pain. Sometimes the pressure within the parotid capsule rises so high that ischaemia of the seventh nerve results, causing paresis or even palsy.

Management

- *Correct the patient's hydration with appropriate intravenous fluid administration.*
- *Perform a meatotomy under local anaesthetic, place a sound in the duct and open the meatus.*
- *Take a pus swab. Usually either staphylococcus aureus, streptococcus, or sometimes pneumococcus is the causative organism.*
- *Administer the appropriate antibiotic, usually penicillin.*
- *Massage the parotid hourly in the direction of the opening of the Stensen duct.*

Usually the condition resolves with conservative treatment. If there is no improvement, it may be necessary to open the parotid. Make a formal incision, as for a parotidectomy, avoiding the mandibular branch of the facial nerve. Split the capsule of the parotid gland to relieve pressure. The pain usually improves rapidly. It is very seldom necessary to perform this operation.

Chronic inflammation of the salivary glands

This condition is usually secondary to a stenosis of the main ducts or of the meatus of the ducts. A sialogram showing sialoadenitis with dilated ducts and acini confirms the diagnosis. Sometimes bacteria are cultured in the saliva from these ducts.

Sialectasis in childhood

Sometimes children present with painful, swollen parotid glands. No bacteria can be cultured and a sialogram shows sialectasis. This condition resolves spontaneously in time.

Stones in the salivary ducts

Stones are most commonly found in the Wharton duct. The saliva from the submandibular gland is more viscous and the drainage of its duct is not as effective as that of the parotid gland. For these reasons, stones occur almost exclusively in the submandibular gland duct. The stones contain calcium and are thus visible on ordinary X-rays. Sialography shows a filling defect in the ductal system. Secondary infection arises in the gland due to stasis. If the stone is palpable in *diaphragma oris* near the meatus, it can sometimes be squeezed out after a meatotomy. If it is situated deeper in the duct, it can be removed by the following procedure:

- A good light source, a good asssistant, good suction and local anaesthetic are prerequisites.
- Place a suture around the duct to prevent the stone from slipping back into the gland.
- Make an incision that overlies the stone and squeeze it out.
- Remember that the lingual nerve crosses the duct further back and may be injured.

If the stone is situated in the gland, the gland must be excised. The incision must be made two fingerbreadths below the ramus of the mandible to avoid the mandibular branch of the facial nerve. The gland has a superficial and a deep part, which winds round the posterior edge of the myelohyoid muscle. Avoid the hypoglossal nerve in this area. The facial nerve and artery run through the gland and must be ligated. The Wharton duct runs forward from the deep part of the gland and is crossed by the lingual nerve, which must be avoided when the duct is excised.

Mickulicz–Sjögren disease

- There is a diffuse enlargement of all four salivary glands and of the lacrimal glands.
- A dry mouth, conjunctivitis, keratitis and arthritis are associated.
- The disease is characterized by a diffuse lymphoid infiltrate.
- It is probably an auto-immune disease.

NECK SWELLINGS

How does the patient present?

- With a single swelling.
- With multiple swellings.
- The swellings can be painless.
- If pain is present, it may be vague, or severe and continuous.
- Is the pain influenced by meals?
- The patient may present with malaise and fever, and a swelling in the neck may be a chance finding.

What else does the clinician wish to ascertain from the history?

- Was there any contact with infectious diseases?
- Is there pain in the throat or in the mouth?
- Is there dysphagia, or are there voice changes or problems with respiration?
- Are any ulcers present in the mouth or on the skin of the head or neck?

What must the clinician consider?

- If the mass is in the midline, and moves with swallowing, it is a thyroid mass.
- If the masses are multiple, they are lymph nodes.
- If they are lymph nodes, they can be divided into:

Infective

- Non-specific
  Nodes which drain an infection in the head and neck area, eg tonsillitis
- Specific
  Tuberculosis
  Glandular fever (infectious mononucleosis)
  Catscratch disease

Tumours

- Primary
  Hodgkin disease
  Non-Hodgkin lymphoma
  Salivary gland tumours
  Chemodectoma
- Metastases
  Head and neck region
  Thorax
  Abdomen

Other conditions

- Sarcoidoses
- Is it a single mass?
- Where is it situated anatomically?
  In the anterior triangle formed by the mandible, the sternomastoid muscle and the imaginary anterior midline.
- If it moves when the tongue is protruded, it is a thyroglossal cyst.

The mass lies in relation to the anterior border of the sternocleidomastoid muscle and is deep to the muscle

- Solid
  A lymph node metastasis
  Carotid body tumour
  Salivary gland tumour
- Cystic
  Branchial cyst
  A tubercular cold abcess
  A cystic hygroma
- Pulsatile mass
  Unfolded carotid (medical student's aneurysm)
  Carotid aneurysm

The mass is in the posterior triangle formed by the sternocleidomastoid muscle, the trapezius muscle and the clavicle

- Solid
  Lymph node (metastasis)
  Cervical rib
- Cystic
  Cystic hygroma
  Pharyngeal diverticulum
- Pulsatile mass
  Aneurysm of the subclavian artery – usually associated with a cervical rib.

Important statistics to bear in mind if the patient is older than forty-five

- *About half of all neck masses arise from the thyroid*
- *About a third are metastases in lymph nodes, with a primary tumour that can be clinically demonstrated*
- *All the other conditions together form about a fifth of all masses in the neck*

If thyroid swellings are not taken into consideration:

- *Two-thirds (60%) of the neck swellings are metastases to lymph nodes*
  10% are primary lymphomas
- *10% are congenital lesions (branchial cysts)*
- *10% are salivary gland swellings*
- *Remember that in children and teenagers the profile differs radically and the emphasis shifts to inflammatory nodes*
- *In young adults aged between thirty and forty-five, primary lymphoma becomes more important.*

Common conditions

Enlarged lymph nodes

Metastases

On thorough clinical examination, the primary lesion can be found in 90% of cases. The most common primary lesions are found in the oral cavity (squamous carcinoma) or on the skin of the head and neck (squamous carcinoma and melanoma).

A further 5% of primary lesions can be found by using special methods and the help of an ear-, nose- and throat surgeon, who can perform indirect laryngoscopy and a thorough examination of the nasopharynx. Examination of the larynx, nasopharynx and oesophagus under anaesthetic may be necessary. If the lymph nodes in the posterior triangle are situated just superior to the clavicle, the primary tumour is usually found in the lung, stomach or pancreas.

In about 3% of cases the primary lesion is never found, despite repeated examinations. The approach to these cryptogenic primary lesions is as follows:

Never resort to an open biopsy immediately. It may adversely affect the eventual optimal management of the total lesion, primary and metastases. First look very carefully for the primary, using the following special investigations:

- *Chest X-rays*
- *Lateral X-rays of the neck*
- *X-rays of the sinuses*
- *Barium meal*
- *Thyroid radio-isotope scan*
- *Laryngoscopy under anaesthetic with biopsy of the nasopharynx and base of the tongue*
- *Oesophagogastroscopy*
- *Bronchoscopy with cytology*
- *Aspiration cytology of the gland*

The cytology can give an indication as to where to look for the primary. If it is an adenocarcinoma, search the abdominal cavity thoroughly for the primary.

Mammography is also sometimes helpful.

If no primary lesion can be found after all these investigations, an open biopsy of the lymph node with frozen section histology must be performed. The histological diagnosis usually confirms a squamous cell carcinoma, an adenocarcinoma, a melanoma or a lymphoma.

Squamous cell carcinoma

Submandibular or central lymph node

A modified radical block dissection with retention of the sternocleidomastoid muscle is the treatment of choice. The patient must be followed up and if the primary lesion is found (usually posterior tongue or larynx), this must be treated on its own merits.

Supraclavicular lymph nodes

The primary is usually situated in the oesophagus. Block dissection is not indicated.

Melanoma

A modified block dissection must be performed.

Lymphoma

A modified block dissection is indicated if no other signs of spread of the disease are evident. These patients may later need multimodality treatment.

Adenocarcinoma

If the submandibular gland is involved, the carcinoma may be of salivary gland origin. A modified block dissection is then indicated. A modified block dissection is not indicated when the tumour occurs elsewhere in the neck, since this will not influence the further course of the disease at all.

Primary lymph node tumours

Patients present with enlarged cervical lymph nodes without any other associated symptoms or with symptoms of systemic illness, such as generalized weakness, loss of weight, pallor, pruritis and fever. There is sometimes a history of bone pain or abdominal pain after alcohol consumption. The nodes are rubberlike, hard, discrete and smooth; they are not tender. On general examination, the patient may appear anaemic. The liver and spleen may be enlarged. The diagnosis is confirmed by a lymph node biopsy, which is carried out as follows:

- *The pathologist must be present in theatre.*
- *A wide exposure is necessary and the lymph node itself must not be handled.*
- *Put stay sutures through the node.*
- *Dissect, with the help of traction applied to the stay sutures.*
- *The pathologist receives the node and performs the following procedures:*

1. *Makes impressions after the node has been split, to identify T- and B-cell markers.*
2. *Prepares cryosections to identify T-cell markers.*
3. *Prepares sections fixed in plastic.*
4. *Places a section of the gland in glutaraldehyde for electron microscopy.*

5. Prepares a cell suspension for cell culture.

- *In a nonacademic setting, the lymph node must be fixed in 4% neutral formalin-salt solution.*
- *Remember that inguinal lymph nodes are often enlarged due to infections in the foot. A lymph node from another area is preferable for diagnostic biopsy.*

Aetiology of lymphomas

In animals, lymphomas are caused by viruses. In humans, the Burkett lymphoma is caused by the Epstein-Barr virus. Lymphomas are relatively common in immunocompromised patients, especially if they have also received organ transplants. It would thus appear that these patients have an abnormality of their immune systems, especially immune stimulation with unsuccessful regulation by T-suppressor cells.

Hodgkin disease

Although this disease is fortunately quite rare and comprises only 2% of all tumours, it becomes significant in children and young adults, where it is one of the most common malignancies found. During the last decade the prognosis of this illness has improved notably, through advancements in radiotherapy and chemotherapy. Although the surgeon's role has become less important, there are still some basic surgical principles to be remembered in the treatment of this disease.

Classification of Hodgkin disease

- Lymphocyte-predominant
- Mixed cellularity
- Lymphocyte-depleted
- Nodular sclerosis

Lymphocyte-predominant Hodgkin disease

The histological picture resembles that of normal lymphocytes. Often multiple sections must be examined to identify Reed-Sternberg cells. The disease is more often found in young people and has a good prognosis.

Mixed cell type

In this condition fewer lymphocytes are seen, but there are plenty of eosinophils, plasma cells and histiocytes present. There are also many Reed-Sternberg cells. This disease is more common in men and its prognosis is worse than lymphocyte-predominant, and better than lymphocyte-depleted, Hodgkin disease.

Lymphocyte-depleted Hodgkin disease

Lymphocytes are rare and the lesions consist of Reed-Sternberg cells or their pleomorphic variants. Fibrosis and necrosis are present. The disease is found in older patients and their prognosis is poor, because the disease is usually widespread when it presents.

Nodular sclerosis

The main cell type is the lacunar cell, a variant of the Reed-Sternberg cell. These cells are large and have a single hyperlobulated nucleus. The cytoplasm undergoes retraction when fixed with formalin, giving the impression that the cells lie in empty spaces or "lacunae". Another characteristic is collagen bounding, which divides the tissues clearly into nodules. This illness presents in young adults and has a good prognosis.

Classification of non-Hodgkin lymphoma

The following classifications are used:

- The Rappoport classification, which is based on the growth pattern and cytological appearance of the tumour.
- The Luke-Collins classification, where the disease is classified according to cell origin into B-cell, T-cell, histiocyte and unknown cell types, using immunological and cytochemical methods.
- The classification most often used currently, is the so-called working formulation of non-Hodgkin lymphoma, as suggested by the National Cancer Institute of the USA In this classification, the disease is divided into low-, intermediate- and high-grade lesions. Tumours containing small cleaved cells have a better prognosis. A follicular growth pattern has a better prognosis than a diffuse growth pattern.

Low-grade malignant lymphoma

- Small lymphocyte
- Follicular with predominantly small cleaved cells

Median survival – six years.

Intermediate-grade malignant lymphoma

- Follicular with predominantly large cells
- Diffuse growth pattern – small cleaved cells
- Diffuse growth pattern – mixed small and large cells

Median survival – three and a half years.

High-grade malignant lymphoma

- Large cell immunoblastic
- Lymphoblastic cells
- Small uncleaved cells

Median survival – 1,3 years.

Diverse malignant lymphoma

Mycosis fungoides and Sezary syndrome

Staging of Hodgkin disease and non-Hodgkin lymphoma

Stage I

Involvement of a single group of lymph nodes.

Stage II

Involvement of two or more groups of lymph nodes on the same side of the diaphragm.

Stage III

1. Involvement of lymph node groups on either side of the diaphragm, with abdominal involvement restricted to the upper abdomen.
2. Abdominal disease includes para-aortic, mesenteric and iliac lymph nodes.

Stage IV

Diffuse or disseminated involvement of one or more extralymphatic organs, with or without lymph node involvement. The symbol E denotes involvement of extralymphatic organs. A denotes the absence of fever, night sweats and weight loss and B denotes the presence of these systemic signs.

A thorough clinical examination must be performed, documenting all enlarged lymph nodes and organomegaly (hepatosplenomegaly) and observations of fever, mass loss, sweating and pruritis. The following special investigations are essential for forming a complete overview of the disease:

- Full blood count and erythrocyte sedimentation rate
- Liver functions
- Calcium
- Uric acid
- Serum-protein electrophoresis
- Chest X-rays
- Excreting urogram
- Sonar
- Lymphangiogram
- CT scan
- Bone marrow biopsy
- Biopsy of a lymph node

Staging laparotomy

The main objective of a staging laparotomy is to demonstrate undiagnosed abdominal disease. It is only of use if it will influence management. The importance of the staging laparotomy has recently been questioned, because clinical staging has now become more reliable with the growing availability of facilities for CT scanning and bipedal lymphangiography. Another reason is that management is now often modified to include chemotherapy as part of the treatment in any case.

Staging laparotomy still has the possible advantage that in a third of cases, staging may be altered by its practice and therapy changed accordingly, in that irradiation is adjusted and chemotherapy added to the treatment regimen.

Splenectomy also offers the advantage of limiting irradiation, thereby avoiding irradiation nephritis and pneumonitis. The morbidity of splenectomy is limited by the use of antibiotics and polyvalent pneumococcus vaccines. The mortality of laparotomy is 0,1%. Staging laparotomies ought only to be performed in Stage I, IIa and IIIa patients. Restaging laparotomy is indicated in highly selective cases where there is doubt as to whether occult disease still exists or where it is uncertain whether or not treatment can be terminated.

Staging laparotomy is not indicated in non-Hodgkin lymphomas, as 80% of cases are stage III and IV and the majority of the remaining 20% of cases are elderly patients. The usual treatment of choice is combination chemotherapy; and laparotomy would therefore not influence any management decisions.

Clinical presentation

In the majority of cases, the disease presents as enlarged lymph nodes, usually in the neck, in young, otherwise healthy individuals. Blood and bone marrow studies are usually normal and the diagnosis is confirmed by lymph node biopsy. In the more advanced stages of the disease, the patient presents with generalized enlargement of the lymph nodes and of one or more organs, eg hepatosplenomegaly. These patients sometimes present with mainly systemic complaints such as fever, loss of mass, weakness and anaemia.

Gastrointestinal tract involvement

Hodgkin disease does not usually present as a primary lesion in the gastrointestinal tract. In disseminated Hodgkin disease, there is a spread to the gastrointestinal tract. Non-Hodgkin lymphoma sometimes affects the gastrointestinal tract as a primary lesion. Of these primary lesions, 60% are found in the stomach, 22% in the small intestine, 15% in the colon and rectum and 3% in the appendix and pancreas. Lymphomas comprise 1-2% of all gastrointestinal tract tumours. Depending on which organ is involved, the patient may present with abdominal pain, fever and loss of weight. Haematemesis, abdominal distension and signs of obstruction and a palpable mass are also possible presentations. The tumour sometimes perforates and will present acute abdominal symptoms. In more diffuse gastrointestinal tract involvement, the patient may present with pain, loss of mass, diarrhoea and malabsorption syndrome.

Management of Hodgkin disease and non-Hodgkin lymphoma

Irradiation

- *Subtotal irradiation*
  Irradiation is directed only at affected lymph nodes. This is used mainly in stage I and II Hodgkin disease and sometimes in Stage I low-grade malignant lymphoma.
- *Total lymphoid irradiation*
  This is given in a mantle or inverted Y-field distribution. The irradiation thus covers all the major lymph nodes, major lymph node chains and the spleen. Total lymph node irradiation is used in Stage I and IIb Hodgkin disease. In Stage III Hodgkin and Stage II and III non-Hodgkin, it is used in combination with chemotherapy.

Chemotherapy

Various combinations of Vincristine, Adriamycin, Bleomycin, Cyclophosphamide and Prednisone are used, either with or without irradiation in advanced Hodgkin disease and non-Hodgkin lymphoma.

Surgery

In Hodgkin disease and non-Hodgkin lymphoma, the main role of surgery is to obtain tissue for the correct histological diagnosis and staging of the disease. Surgery plays a therapeutic role in lymphomas of the gastrointestinal tract.

Where possible, the primary lesion and the regional lymph nodes must be removed in toto, *always bearing in mind the risk related to the procedure and maintenance of reasonable function of the intestinal tract with primary repair of continuity. If the disease has penetrated through the serosa and/or if the lymph nodes are also affected, the patient must be treated with adjuvant combination chemotherapy. In some cases of inoperable gastric lymphoma, a combination of irradiation and chemotherapy may offer some palliation.*

Gastrointestinal lymphoma has a five year survival rate of approximately 35%. If total excision of a stage I lesion can be achieved, 75% of cases survive for five years. There is very seldom recurrence of the disease after five years.

Other primary tumours in the neck

Paraganglioma

The most common tumour is a carotid body tumour. The carotid body contains the largest collection of chemoreceptor tissue in the body and is situated in the bifurcation of the carotid artery.

There are other collections of chemoreceptor tissue on the jugular bulb, where a glomus jugulare tumour arises, and in the ganglion nodosum of the vagus nerve, the so-called intervagal tumour. Carotid body tumours are surrounced by a reddish-brown or greyish-red capsule, which is intimately interwoven with the adventitia of the carotid bifurcation.

Microscopically, these tumour nests or cell spheres comprise spindle-shaped, fairly large chief cells, surrounded by a vascular stroma of multiple capillary networks. As the tumour slowly enlarges, it has a tendency to encircle blood vessels and extend into the skull, exerting pressure on the cranial nerves.

The glomus jugular tumour can erode the petrous bone and cause seventh nerve palsy. It can present as a swelling in the external auditory canal. After a long course, up to a third of these tumours will show signs of malignancy with local infiltration and metastases.

Clinical presentation

The tumour presents as a potato-shaped, deep-lying, painless tumour, posterior to the angle of the mandible, partially covered by the sternocleidomastoid muscle. The tumour can move from side to side, but not up and down. It has a firm consistency, but is nevertheless slightly compressible, as it is very vascular. Pulsation of the external carotid, which is stretched over the tumour, is usually palpable and often a bruit is audible. If the tumour becomes large, it can be seen and palpated as an oropharyngeal mass. Sometimes it paralyses the recurrent laryngeal nerve, causing hoarseness. It can also paralyse the hypoglossal nerve and lead to multiple nerve palsies, including a glossopharyngeal nerve palsy with dysphagia. Although rare, functional tumours excreting catecholamines are sometimes found.

Differential diagnosis

The tumour must be differentiated from a branchial cyst, an aneurysm of the carotid artery, salivary gland tumours and primary or secondary lymph node tumours. It is usually necessary to perform carotid arteriography to confirm the diagnosis. This shows splaying of the carotid bifurcation by a tumour blush, or a tumour blush in the region of the jugular glomus near the base of the skull with a normal carotid bifurcation, indicating a glomus jugulare tumour.

Management

Although the tumour grows slowly, there is a danger of nerve palsy and malignant change. The tumour must be surgically removed while it is still small. It must be carefully separated from the adventitia of the carotid vessels on the plane of the so-called "white line", which forms the natural line of dissection. The blood supply usually comes straight from the bifurcation and finer branches from the external carotid artery. Bleeding must be carefully controlled. If the tumour is large, an intracarotid shunt (Javitt shunt) must be used to control bleeding. In some cases, it may be necessary to remove the carotid artery along with the tumour and to replace it with a venous transplant.

Surgery to carotid body tumours should be performed by experienced vascular surgeons. Because of the dangers involved in operating on these tumours, the diagnosis of carotid body tumours must always be considered and exploration or biopsy must not be undertaken by inexperienced medical pracitioners. If the tumour is irresectible, particularly in the elderly, irradiation will suffice. The tumour is radioresistant, but tumour growth is retarded. Jugular glomus tumours are often excised with the aid of an ear-, nose- and throat surgeon, as they often infiltrate the canal of the petrous bone and mastoid.

Inflammation of the lymph nodes

Nonspecific infection

This usually follows tonsillitis in children. If it presents in adults, a primary source of infection must be sought in the head and neck region or the oral cavity, especially the teeth. These nodes are enlarged, tender, warm and sometimes red. Treat with antibiotics. Sometimes an abscess will develop in the neck, and can be surgically drained.

Specific infections

Tuberculosis

The human tubercle bacillus enters through the tonsils and reaches the cervical lymph nodes. This disease has become far less common since tuberculosis in dairy cows has been controlled. The disease is still common among the black population.

Clinical presentation

The uppermost deep cervical nodes are affected. At the outset, the nodes are firm and clearly defined. As necrosis and caseation advance, the disease spreads beyond the capsule and the nodes clump together to form a mass. If the nodes liquefy completely, an abscess develops. At first the abscess may be painful, due to tension in the tissues. Later it breaks through the fascia to form the so-called "collar-stud" abscess. Because this is a chronic process, there is no hyperaemia and it is then called a cold abscess.

Management

Tuberculous lymphadenitis usually heals after antituberculous treatment. Currently, lymph node excision is very seldom necessary. Systemic treatment, comprising rifampicin, isoniazid and ethambutol or pirazinamide, is given.

Infective mononucleosis

This illness is common in children and young people. It is a benign, self-limiting lymphoproliferative disease which is caused by the Epstein-Barr virus. It is characterized by fever, sore throat, generalized lymphadenopathy and the presence of atypical lymphocytes in the peripheral blood. The spleen is often enlarged. Patients develop antibodies which agglutinate sheep red blood cells. This is known as the Paul Bunnel test. Anti-Epstein-Barr virus antibodies can also be demonstrated. Patients usually recover within two to four weeks.

Catscratch disease

This is probably caused by a virus. It is characterized by painful red lymph nodes. The glands sometimes liquefy and form an abscess. The patients are febrile. The disease resolves spontaneously within a few weeks. The histological appearance is typical of a granulomatous infection. The central necrotic focus is surrounded by mononuclear phagocytes, fibroblasts and giant cells.

Actinomycosis

Actinomyces are normally found in the mouth. The infection usually arises at the angle of the mandible. Induration is followed by breakdown, with sinuses which excrete watery pus with the characteristic sulphur granule appearance.

The treatment is longterm, high dosage penicillin.

Congenital conditions

During foetal development, branchial arches grow out into the branchial sinuses to close them. If this closure is not completed, a branchial fistula or branchial cyst is formed.

Branchial fistula

A small opening is visible just in front of the anterior border of the sternocleidomastoid muscle, at the level of the junction between the middle and lower thirds of the muscle. It is present at birth, but may only be noticed much later. At intervals, it excretes a shiny, sticky substance, and may become infected.

The treatment is excision of the tract. First the opening is excised and then the tract is followed along its course between the internal and external carotid arteries to where it opens into the supratonsillar fossa. The tract is too long to be dissected out through a single transverse incision, thus two transverse incisions are usually necessary.

Branchial cyst

The cyst arises from one of the branchial clefts, usually the second branchial cleft. The cyst is lined with squamous epithelium and has lymphoid tissue in its walls. It is filled with an opaque fluid containing cholesterol crystals. The cyst is situated deep to the upper third of the sternocleidomastoid muscle and usually presents as a cystic swelling at its anterior border.

The cyst may become infected because the lymphoid tissue communicates with the cervical lymph nodes and can then form an abscess. Such a cyst must be excised by means of a transverse incision. Avoid injury to the carotid artery and the internal jugular vein, which lie just deep to the cyst.

Cystic hygroma

This is a multilobular lymphoid congenital abnormality which arises from an embryonic remnant of the jugular lymph sac. It is usually found in the anterior or posterior triangle of the neck and can also extend into the axilla. It is compressible and transilluminable. It may develop secondary infection.

It must be removed, even if total excision is not possible. It is sometimes necessary to approach the neck and axilla via separate incisions. After excision, suction drainage must be applied, or lymphoid fluid may collect.

Pulsatile masses of the neck

Anterior cervical triangle

Aneurysm of the carotid artery

This usually arises from the common carotid or internal carotid artery. It is a very rare condition. In large series of aneurysms, only a few of these aneurysms have been reported, whereas thousands of other aneurysms are described.

A patient with a pulsatile mass in the neck is more likely to have a contorted, kinked, unfolded carotid artery (medical student's aneurysm). This is common in elderly, hypertensive, female patients. The mass sometimes disappears when the neck is rotated and the kinking is thus straightened out. Another diagnosis to be considered is a carotid body tumour. If there is any doubt, the diagnosis should be confirmed by means of an arteriogram.

Carotid artery aneurysms must be surgically corrected, because they can cause an embolism to the brain. It is usually necessary to use an internal bypass (shunt) during removal and replacement of the aneurysm.

Posterior triangle of the neck

A pulsatile mass in this region is usually a poststenotic dilatation of the subclavian artery after it has passed over a cervical rib. The hard underlying rib is palpable and can be seen on X-ray.

The aneurysm must be removed and replaced with a prosthesis, as it may cause embolism to the hand and can also rupture.

An aneurysm of the arch of the aorta, which may present in the neck, must also be considered.

THYROID

What does the patient complain of?

Complaints caused by thyroid enlargement

Patients present complaining that they or their families have noticed a swelling in the neck. They complain of discomfort when swallowing; not that they have trouble swallowing, but rather that it induces a heavy feeling and discomfort in the throat. They sometimes complain of difficulty with respiration. They often awake with a start, feeling dyspnoeic, just after having fallen asleep. They sometimes complain of pain, which can be acute and persistent, or vague and irritating.

Complaints secondary to disturbance of function

Hyperfunction

Patients complain of nervousness and an anxious sensation, tremor and palpitations. They may also have eye problems such as bulging eyes, eye discomfort or double vision.

Hypofunction

Patients complain of hair loss, weight gain, drowsiness and a sensation of coldness.

What must the clinician consider?

- Is the swelling in the neck a thyroid? A midline swelling, which moves on swallowing, is a thyroid mass.
- Is it diffusely enlarged?
- If it is diffusely enlarged without signs of hyperfunction, consider a colloid goitre, which is usually caused by iodine deficiency or thyroiditis.
- If it is a diffusely enlarged with hyperfunction, consider Graves/Basedow disease or thyroiditis.

Is it nodular?

- If multiple nodules are present without hyperfunction, consider multinodular hyperplasia.
- If multiple nodules are present with hyperfunction, consider secondary hyperthyroidism (Plummer disease).
- A single nodule without hyperfunction – consider an adenoma, a cyst, or a carcinoma.

- A single nodule with hyperfunction – consider an autonomically functioning adenoma.
- A painful, enlarged thyroid – consider thyroiditis, carcinoma (usually anaplastic) or haemorrhage into a colloid nodule.

What is found on examination?

The neck

A normal thyroid is not visible. Stand in front of a seated patient and observe the neck. Ask her to swallow; sometims a nodule which has been hidden behind the sternum becomes visible. If an enlarged gland is visible, note whether it is symmetrically or irregularly enlarged. Irregularity suggests nodularity. Palpate the neck. A normal thyroid is impalpable. Is it nodular? Is only a single nodule palpable? Allow the patient to swallow while palpating the neck. Sometimes a nodule on one of the inferior poles only becomes palpable on swallowing.

Palpate the cervical lymph nodes. Is there a bruit? A bruit can sometimes be discovered only on auscultation. Palpate the neck while standing behind the patient. Does the thyroid extend to behind the sternum? Percuss the sternum to confirm retrosternal extension. Is the trachea displaced away from the midline?

Systemic signs

Try to ascertain whether the thyroid has normal-, hyper- or hypofunction. In hyperfunction there is

- a raised metabolic rate
- increased sensitivity of the adrenergic receptors

Raised metabolic rate

The patient is losing weight despite a good appetite. She perspires excessively and prefers cold weather.

Increased sensitivity of B adrenergic receptors

She has a tachycardia and may even be fibrillating. She is nervous, her hands are sweating and she has a tremor. She has a staring gaze and prominent or bulging eyes.

Other signs

- Is her voice hoarse? This indicates involvement of the recurrent laryngeal nerve.
- Has she any bone pain, pretibial myxoedema or thickening of subcutaneous tissue?
- This is occasionally present in Graves disease and is an auto-immune reaction similar to retro-orbital thickening.

Hypofunction of the thyroid

Is the patient overmass, with the fat being mainly distributed over her back, neck and shoulders? Is there evidence of hair loss, particularly of the outer third of the eyebrows? Coarsening of the fingers and hands? Thickening of the eyelids? Slow speech? Does she always feel cold?

Which special investigations are necessary?

X-rays of the neck and thorax

- They can show calcification of the thyroid when haemorrhage into a multinodular goitre has taken place in the past.
- Displacement of the trachea is usually seen in multinodular goitre.
- Retrosternal extension of the gland can be demonstrated.
- Lung metastases in follicular or anaplastic carcinoma.
- Bone metastases in the ribs, claviculae or the humerus heads in follicular or anaplastic carcinoma.

Ultrasound

Single or multiple nodules, solid or cystic.

Thyroid functions

Direct and indirect measurement of thyroid hormone levels

- Direct radio-immunological assays
  Serum T_4 (tetra-iodothyronine)
  Serum T_3 (Tri-iodothyronine)
  TSH levels are raised when the thyroid is hypofunctional and lowered when the thyroid is hyperfunctional.
- Indirect measurements
  T_3 resin uptake test. In this test, unoccupied

receptors are counted. It is thus at its lowest when hormone levels are high.

- Thyroglobulin binding capacity
This test is unreliable, because false values are obtained in women who are either pregnant or on the "Pill", both of which cause a rise in the globulin. It is also unreliable when iodine has been ingested, e g in cough mixtures.
- Free thyroxine index
This is a good screening test.
FTI = T_4 / T_3 resin uptake x 100
This excludes the false positive readings obtained on thyroglobulin binding capacity tests. If it is high, hyperthyroidism can be confirmed by radio-immunological assays of the circulating hormone.
- Technesium (T^{99} – half life eight days)
- Iodine I^{131} and iodine I^{132} (half life – 2,5 hours)
The function of the gland and the pattern of uptake can be measured by means of radioactive technesium – or iodine tests. If there is any doubt about the thyroid functions, the thyrotropin-releasing factor (TRF) test can be carried out. TSH is measured 20, 40 and 60 minutes after an IV dose of 200 micrograms of TRF. In patients with normal function, TSH rises after 20 minutes and returns to normal within sixty minutes. There is no rise in cases with hyperthyroidism, because TSH is suppressed by high circulation T_4 levels.
- The Werner suppression test
I^{131} uptake is measured. The patient then takes 90 micrograms of T_3 daily for a week and the measurement is repeated. Patients with normal thyroid functions show suppression of I^{131} uptake in excess of 50%. In hyperthyroidism there is usually no suppression of I^{131} uptake.
- Needle aspiration cytology
A 0,7 mm (22 gauge) needle is inserted into the thyroid nodule. Suction is applied to the syringe, while the needle is plunged in and out a few times. The material thus obtained must be spread out on a glass slide and fixed with an alcohol spray or left to dry in the wind. This is a very reliable way of differentiating between a benign colloid goitre and hyperplastic nodules from a neoplasm. There has been no documentation of implantation of malignant cells in the tract. Needle biopsy and Trucut biopsy can make a histological diagnosis possible.

Auto-immune antibody measurements

- Hyperthyroidism
In this disease auto-antibodies against TSH receptors are found on the follicle membrane. Various immunoglobulins, the group of which is known as human thyroid-stimulating immunoglobulins (HTSI), are also found. LATS and LATSP are found less often.
- Auto-immune thyroditis
Antithyroglobulin and antimicrosomal antibodies are found in most cases of Hashimoto disease.

Classification of thyroid diseases

A. ABNORMALITIES OF EMBRYOLOGICAL DEVELOPMENT

- Thyroglossal cyst
- Lingual thyroid
- Lateral aberrant thyroid

B. FUNCTIONAL-PHYSIOLOGICAL ABNORMALITIES

- Diffuse colloid goitre
- Multinodular colloid goitre
- Inborn abnormalities of iodine metabolism

C. INFLAMMATORY CONDITIONS OF THE THYROID

- Acute purulent thyroiditis
- Subacute granulomatous thyroiditis (De Quervain disease)

D. AUTO-IMMUNE DISEASES

- Hashimoto thyroditis
- Primary hyperthyroidism (Basedow/Graves disease)
- Myxoedema

E. NEOPLASMS OF THE THYROID

(a) **Thyroid adenoma**

- Follicular adenoma
- Embryonic adenoma
- Colloid adenoma
- Foetal adenoma
- Hurthlé cell adenoma

(b) **Malignant tumours**

1. Well-differentiated tumours
   - Papillary carcinoma

- Follicular carcinoma
2. Poorly differentiated tumours
   - Anaplastic carcinoma
3. Medullary carcinoma of the parafollicular or C cells
4. Sarcomas
5. Metastases from other tumours

F. UNKNOWN AETIOLOGY

Reidl thyroiditis

A. ABNORMALITIES OF EMBRYOLOGICAL DEVELOPMENT

Embryologically, the thyroid develops from the floor of the mouth. It migrates downwards from the *foramen caecum* of the tongue to lie anterior to the body of the hyoid, then swings behind the body of the hyoid and comes to rest in the pretracheal space. A canal called the thyroglossal duct, is formed by this migration. This canal sometimes remains patent to form a sinus or a fistula. Cysts may arise in remnants of the canal. Sometimes the thyroid does not migrate and forms a lingual thyroid at the base of the tongue. The thyroid develops from a midline anlage from the pharyngeal floor in the region of the *foramen caecum*. While this main part of the thyroid is migrating to the neck, it receives two small lateral anlages from the ultimobranchial bodies, which develop from the fourth and fifth pharyngeal diverticula. This forms a very small contribution to the development of the thyroid, but probably explains the presence of the C-cells, which are of neuro-ectodermal origin. The so-called lateral aberrant thyroid, which is very rare, may also come from remnants of these lateral anlages.

Thyroglossal cysts

These are found in the midline, at any site from the chin to the isthmus of the thyroid. Most are found at the level of the hyoid bone. They may present in any age group, but are most common in young adults. The swelling is firm and painless. It is more mobile from side to side than upwards and downwards. When the patient puts his tongue out, the mass moves up and down. It also moves with swallowing, as it is attached to the hyoid bone. Sometimes thyroid tissue can be palpated at the base of the tongue. A small sinus may also be found in the neck. The cyst and the tract must be excised and because the tract is inseparably related to the hyoid, the middle third of this bone must also be removed. Care must be taken that the tract, which runs from the cyst in the direction of the thyroid, is also removed. This procedure is called the Sistrunk operation.

Lingual thyroid

This is a very rare condition, more common in women. In 70% of cases, the lingual thyroid is the only thyroid tissue the patient possesses. It is sometimes discovered by chance. It may enlarge and cause dysphagia, dyspnoea or a choking sensation.

In this condition hypofunction is more common than hyperfunction. A few cases of malignancy have been described. Radio-isotope studies with I^{131} confirm the diagnosis and can also show whether thyroid tissue is present at the normal site. If there is no urgent indication for surgery, the mass can be shrunken by exogenous hormone administration. If there is hyperfunction, it can be treated with radioactive iodine. If there is any danger of suffocation or suspicion of malignancy, the tissue must be excised. An intra-oral operation, pulling the tongue forwards and splitting the posterior tongue, is sometimes possible, failing which a lateral pharyngotomy must be performed to excise the mass *in toto*. Cases have been described where the thyroid tissue has been succesfully transplanted into muscle.

Lateral aberrant thyroid

A true lateral aberrant thyroid is extremely rare. Most cases are actually metastases of a papillary thyroid carcinoma in the lymph nodes. If so-called lateral aberrant thyroid tissue is found in the neck, no stone must be left unturned in excluding a primary papillary carcinoma in the thyroid tissue. Often the primary lesion is palpable; sometimes radioisotopes are necessary to confirm the diagnosis. If the diagnosis cannot be confirmed, surgical exploration of the thyroid, with a subtotal thyroidectomy and thorough examination of the excised tissue, must be carried out to find a small occult primary.

B. FUNCTIONAL-PHYSIOLOGICAL ABNORMALITIES

Diffuse colloid goitre

Iodine is essential for thyroid hormone synthesis. If there is an iodine deficiency and thyroxine levels fall, the pituitary is stimulated to excrete more TSH, which, in turn, causes thyroid hyperplasia. This results in increased thyroxine production, which suppresses TSH, causing involution and deposits of colloid. This cycle of hyperplasia and involution gives rise to diffuse colloid goitres. Sometimes the follicles rupture and heal by fibrosis. The hyperplasia can appear irregularly and give rise to a multinodular colloid goitre.

Causes of relative iodine deficiency include:

- *Iodine deficiency in the diet, for geographic reasons.*
- *Foodstuffs containing thiocarbamide, which retards the oxidation of iodine. These include cabbage, turnips and soya beans.*
- *Inborn enzyme abnormalities, which adversely affect deiodination of iodotyrosine, bonding of iodotyrosine and thyroxine release.*
- *Increased demand in puberty and pregnancy. Women are eight times more commonly affected than men.*

Multinodular goitre

Clinical presentation

The patient presents with a cervical swelling and complains of a heavy sensation when swallowing or a sensation of strangulation at certain head positions. This feeling often presents just as the patient is falling asleep and the neck muscles are relaxing. Kinking of the trachea takes place, with pressure being exerted by nodules and the patient will awake with a start, felling dyspnoeic. Haemorrhage into a nodule can cause respiratory distress. Sometimes the patient presents with hyperthyroidism due to hyperfunction, caused by multiple hyerplastic nodules which begin to function autonomically. This condition is found in older patients and is slow in onset. The diagnosis is sometimes not made, and patients present with tachycardia, arrhythmias and auricular fibrillation, with resultant cardiac failure in elderly patients with underlying heart disease. Thyroid functions must be tested in elderly patients with cardiac arrhythmias and weight loss. There are no eye symptoms. Some patients present with lethargy and the condition is then known as apathetic hyperthyroidism.

If a dominant nodule is palpable, or one nodule enlarges rapidly, malignancy must be considered.

Management

The majority of these patients are asymptomatic and need no treatment. They are discovered accidentally. The condition can be prevented in endemic areas by using iodised salt. If nodules have already developed, exogenic hormone can be tried, which may cause the nodules to regress or remain static.

Indications for surgery

- Pressure symptoms; difficulty with respiration or swallowing
- Cosmetic considerations
- Fear of malignancy

A subtotal thyroidectomy must be performed and tissue sent for histology. It is wise to put these patients onto permanent exogenous hormone supplementation, because nodules can sometimes recur or the patient may become hypothyroidic. Thyroxine and TSH levels can be measured to determine the correct dosage, but 0,2 mg thyroxine per day is usually adequate.

The management of nodular hyperthyroidism

The patient is prepared with bedrest, control of cardiac failure and a short course of lugol iodine. When the cardiac failure is under control, a beta blocker can be added. A subtotal thyroidectomy is then performed.

If the cardiac failure is uncontrollable, the patient must be treated with radioactive iodine. Here, higher doses are required than those for Graves disease, and the results are less predictable.

Inborn abnormalities of iodine metabolism

There are five different genetic enzyme abnormalities which can give rise to goitres with hypothyroidism in children.

- **Abnormal iodine absorption from the blood**

  This is a very rare genetic abnormality, where the thyroid is unable to concentrate iodine. It is treated with thyroxine replacement therapy.

- **Abornmal organic iodine binding**
  The thyroid absorbs iodine from the blood and concentrates it normally, but cannot convert the iodine so that it can bind with tyrosine. This defect is caused by a partial deficiency of thyroid peroxidase. Pendred syndrome (deafness and hypofunctioning goitre) is ascribed to this abnormality.

  It is treated with thyroxine replacement therapy.

- **Iodine-thyroxine binding abnormality**
  Binding of tyrosines to form thyroxines is abnormal.

- **Dehalogenase inadequacy**
  Mono-iodotyrosine and di-iodotyrosine are not broken down normally to free iodine for reuse. Mono- and di-iodotryosine build up in the blood and urine. This causes an iodine deficiency.

- **Abnormal iodoprotein synthesis**
  In this condition, abnormal iodo-albumin is formed, resulting in inadequate thyroxine production. Abnormal iodoproteins are also found in Hashimoto disease and thyroid carcinoma.

C. INFLAMMATORY CONDITIONS OF THE THYROID

Acute purulent thyroiditis

This is a rare condition, usually caused by pneumococci, staphylococci or *E. coli.* Often only one lobe is affected. The usual signs of acute inflammation – severe tenderness and redness – can be seen. Lymph nodes are enlarged and tender. The lobe can become purulent and fluctuation is then palpable.

Chronic infections such as tuberculosis, syphillis and actinomycosis, have been described.

In contrast to De Quervain thyroiditis, blood thyroxine levels are usually normal and radioactive iodine uptake is not impaired. Appropriate antibiotics must be given as soon as the diagnosis has been made, but it is often necessary to drain the purulent lobe. In chronic infections, a lobectomy is sometimes required.

Subacute thyroiditis

This condition is also known as pseudogranulomatous thyroiditis (De Quervain's disease). Its aetiology is, in all likelihood, viral. High titres of antibodies to mumps, coxsackie virus and influenza have been demonstrated in these patients. There has been no proof of any auto-immune aetiology. This disease is more common in women between twenty and fifty.

Clinical presentation

Patients usually present with a painful thyroid which is tender on palpation; and fever, weakness, fatigue and myalgia. The thyroid is moderately enlarged and one lobe is usually larger than the other and of a firm consistency. There is a variant which presents painlessly with signs of hyperfunction.

Confirming the diagnosis

Special investigations

T_4, T_3 and T_3 resin-binding tests are raised, while the radioactive iodine uptake is considerably lowered. The erythrocyte sedimentation rate is raised in the painful type, but is usually normal in the painless type.

Pathology

The thyroid is adherent to surrounding tissue, but can usually be detached, which differentiates it from Reidl struma. Histologically, there is widespread cell destruction with an early leucocyte infiltration which is followed by infiltration by large monocytes and lymphocytes. The follicles show hyperplasia and breakdown of the epithelial layer. Histiocytes cluster around colloid and form giant cells. When the inflammation resolves, a great deal of fibrosis remains. The histological picture eventually recovers, with only signs of fibrosis remaining.

Electron microscopy does not show viral inclusion bodies.

Natural course of the disease

In the early stages, signs of hyperthyroidism are evident, but later hypofunction occurs, with eventual recovery, which may take from two to six months. In rare cases, the patient may be left with myxoedema.

Differential diagnosis

This painful thyroiditis must be differentiated from purulent thyroiditis, which usually affects only one lobe; from Hashimoto disease, which does not cause as suppressed an I^{131} uptake; from anaplastic carcinoma, which infiltrates surrounding tissues and has associated lymph nodes; and from Graves disease which causes increased I^{131} uptake.

Management

Treatment is not always necessary, and salicylates are adequate for the fever and pain. If there are not rapid signs of improvement, steroids must be considered. Prednisone, in a dosage of 10 mg four times a day, usually has a dramatic effect. If hypothyroidism occurs, thyroxine replacement therapy must be given.

D. AUTO-IMMUNE DISEASES

Hashimoto thyroiditis

Hashimoto thyroiditis is one of a group of auto-immune thyroiditises. It varies from lymphocyte infiltration to a fibrous type, with very few lymphocytes found in the tissues. Hashimoto disease is probably related to Graves disease, but there are clearly recognizable differences.

A variety of auto-antibodies are found in the serum of patients with this disease. These auto-antibodies include antibodies against thyroglobulin, colloid, thyroid microsomes and antinuclear antibodies. Recently, specific autoreactive helper T-lymphocytes, sensitized to thyroid antigen, have also been identified. It would appear that specific helper T-lymphocytes are needed to stimulate specific B-lymphocytes to form thyroid auto-antibodies. The disease is more common in patients with HLA-DR5 antibodies. It would appear that the disease is rarer in areas with iodine deficiency and is found more often when iodine has been administered to the population. It is a known fact that the thyroid of a thyroiditis patient is far more sensitive to iodine, due to the Wolff-Chaikoff effect (inhibition of hormone synthesis caused by excess iodine in the gland).

Clinical presentation

The disease is usually found in women in their forties or fifties. Patients are often asymptomatic and the enlarged thyroid is noticed by themselves or their families. Sometimes the goitre develops more rapidly and is associated with pain. The thyroid is diffusely enlarged, firm and lobular. The patient usually has symptoms of hypofunction, such as fatigue and weakness. Sometimes hyperfunction is found early in the course of the disease. Thyroid-stimulating immunoglobulins may also be released, as in Graves disease. Depending on the underlying status of the thyroid tissue, the patient may by hyper- or euthyroid. The simultaneous presentation of Graves disease and Hashimoto thyroiditis is known as "Hashitoxicosis". Raised hormone levels may merely be the result of stored hormone release due to follicle damage, without any rise in TSH. Hashimoto disease usually results in ultimate hypofunction, due to auto-immune destruction of thyroid tissue.

Confirming the diagnosis

High titres of thyroid auto-antibodies are found. In lymphocytic thyroiditis in children and in atrophic thyroiditis, fewer antibodies are found. TSH levels are normal or raised.

Histology reveals degeneration of the acinar cells with reduction in the number of follicles and oxyphilic changes in the cytoplasm of the follicular cells. The gland is infiltrated by lymphocytes and plasma cells and germinal centres are a common finding. A fair amount of fibrosis is found.

Management

Patients must receive exogenous hormone treatment. Thyroxine, in dosages of 0,2 mg per day, will control hypofunction. The goitre does not usually enlarge on this dosage.

If the goitre is large, with associated pressure symptoms, or if the diagnosis is doubtful, a thy-

roidectomy is indicated. There is no increased incidence of thyroid carcinoma in these patients, but there is a slightly increased incidence of lymphoma.

Primary hyperthyroidism (Basedow/Graves disease)

Enlarged Thyroid + Hyper fx

This is defined as hyperthyroidism, with a diffusely hyperplastic gland, and is caused by stimulation by immunoglobulins. Although exophthalmos, ophthalmoplegia and pretibial myxoedema are found in this condition, one or all of these findings may be absent. Thyroid-stimulating immunoglobulins can be demonstrated in all cases. There are strong indications that the disease is caused by an inborn abnormality of immune regulation. Helper T-lymphocytes react with an antigen on the thyroid cell membrane, which starts a cell-mediated immune response in thyroid tissue. B-lymphocytes are then stimulated by the helper T-cells to bind thyroid-stimulating immunoglobulin onto the TSH receptors. This prevents TSH from binding onto its own receptors.

The exophthalmos found in Graves disease is also an auto-immune disease with a similar mechanism, but with different helper T-cells and immune-stimulating antibodies.

There is an associated genetic background, with HLA B8 and DW3 occurring in 60% of cases, as opposed to 20% in the general population. Sometimes other auto-immune diseases such as pernicious anaemia, diabetes, Addison disease, myasthenia gravis, rheumatoid arthritis and even chronic active hepatitis are found in these patients or their relatives.

Clinical presentation

The symptoms and signs of hyperthyroidism may develop slowly or suddenly, and may worsen rapidly. There is sometimes a history of a precipitating event, such as an accident or death in the family.

Symptoms include: anxiety, tremor, tachycardia, sweating and heat intolerance, a dry mouth and thirst, mass loss associated with an improved appetite, muscle weakness, dyspnoea, frequency and diarrhoea.

On examination, the patient is usually thin, restless, anxious and hyperactive, with a rapid pulse, sweating hands and a diffusely enlarged thyroid.

Eye signs

About 70% of patients with Basedow/Graves disease will have eye signs. The subtle signs are usually a staring gaze, with slight widening of the palpebral fissure and a mild proptosis. There is mild loss of convergence and lid retraction when the eyes are rotated downwards. The patients complain of pain and discomfort in the eyes, with lacrimation, headache, photophobia and blurred vision. Proptosis can become pronounced and later the exophthalmos can become so severe that the eyelids do not close properly and the patient develops corneal ulceration. Mild proptosis can be measured and is defined as eye protrusion of more than 20 mm.

Muscle weakness is a common finding. Loss of convergence is not very important. Weakening of the superior rectus muscle is more serious. Diplopia arises, and is very disabling for the patient. Patients with exophthalmos have an increased number of muscle fibres, with degeneration of these muscle fibres, infiltration by lymphocytes and macrophages and deposits of mucopolysaccharides, fat and oedema. These conditions are caused by an auto-immune process which is closely related to Basedow/Graves disease. The condition can present without associated Basedow/Graves disease.

The goitre

The thyroid is usually enlarged, but may be normal. The gland is diffusely enlarged, but may be asymmetrical. It is firm and may be lobular. The trachea is not displaced. A bruit is often audible.

The heart

There is a tachycardia; and fibrillation is found in 10% of cases, especially older patients. Sometimes there is an ejection systolic murmur. There is an increase in pulse pressure and skin capillaries are dilated. Cardiac failure is found in older patients.

Neuromuscular manifestations

Severe muscular weakness, which improves on treatment, may be a presenting symptom.

Pretibial myxoedema

Localized pretibial myxoedema is found in a small percentage of cases. This phenomenon can sometimes occur at other sites, such as the hands, fingers and neck. Histologically, the skin is oedematous, with deposits of mucopolysaccharides between the collagen fibres. It is associated with exophthalmos and Graves disease. These patients usually have high titres of thyroid-stimulating immunoglobulins. Control of the hyperthyroidism does not usually improve this condition. Systemic steroids and local steroid ointments are helpful. The condition sometimes resolves spontaneously.

Differential diagnosis

Basedow/Graves disease must be differentiated from:

Plummer syndrome

The thyroid is nodular and exophthalmos and pretibial myxoedema are absent. Thyroid-stimulating immunoglobulin cannot be demonstrated in this condition.

Graves disease can occur in patients who have previously had a multinodular goitre. It is then known as the Marine-Lenhardt syndrome.

Increased TSH secretion

This is caused by pituitary tumours or inappropriately raised TSH secretion without tumours. TSH levels are high and there is no associated exophthalmos.

Subacute thyroiditis

Radioacitve iodine uptake is not increased.

Increased thyroxine intake

Radioactive iodine uptake is not increased.

Jod-Basedow

Transient hyperthyroidism caused by iodine intake. Radioactive iodine uptake is not increased.

Tumours

Choriocarcinoma and hydatiform moles can cause hyperthyroidism, as many of these tumours secrete chorionic gonadotrophin, which binds to the TSH receptors and stimulates thyroid tissue. Follicular carcinoma of the thyroid and its metastases can hyperfunction and cause hyperthyroidism, but this is very rare.

Confirming the diagnosis of Basedow/Graves disease

- Raised circulating T_4 and T_3 serum levels. Sometimes only T_3 levels are raised, but this is rare.
- Low TSH levels.
- Increased I^{131} uptake with a diffuse uptake pattern. The presence of thyroid-stimulating immunoglobulins.

Macroscopic and microscopic appearance

A section through the lobes reveals a fleshy appearance without the normal glossy look, as there is much less colloid present than is found in normal thyroid tissue. Microscopically, diffuse hyperplasia with cylindrical epithelial cells is seen. The follicles are smaller, the thin colloid layer having a scalloped appearance. There are papillary outgrowths from the epithelium protruding into the follicles.

The natural course of Basedow/Graves disease

The disease can sometimes go into spontaneous remission. It can also remit permanently, or it can recur. Most cases will persist without treatment, and carry a relatively high mortality rate. Sometimes the thyroid can become so seriously damaged by antibodies that hypothyroidism arises. Patients who go into permanent remission usually lose their thyroid-stimulating immunoglobulins.

Management

There is no available treatment which can be directed at the cause of this disease. Initially symptoms must be controlled by drug therapy; and some patients go into remission even after medical treatment. If this does not occur, the thyroid must be partially destroyed, either surgically or by irradiation with radioactive iodine.

Drugs

Thionamides are the drugs used, namely thiourea or propyl-thiouracil, and neomercazole or the imidazole group.

Propyl-thiouracil (PTU) works in three ways. It inhibits the peroxidase enzymes which restrict oxidation of the iodine absorbed from the bloodstream. It also inhibits incorporation of iodine into iodotyrosine and iodotyramine; and it inhibits bonding of iodotyrosines. Lastly, it inhibits the conversion of L-thyroxine to L-tri-iodothyronine (T_3) in peripheral tissues.

The imidazole group acts on the peroxidase enzyme only, but despite the differences, it elicits a clinical reponse similar to PTU.

PTU is prescribed in dosages of 100 to 200 mg eight-hourly. As soon as the patient's symptoms are under control (usually after six weeks), the dosage is reduced to 50 mg per day.

Neomercazole or tapazole is given in dosages of 10–20 mg eight-hourly and then 5 mg daily. About 40% of patients with Basedow/Graves disease will go into spontaneous remission. Remission can be anticipated:

- *in patients with small goitres and relatively mild hyperthyroidism*
- *where TSI drops sharply during treatment.*

Remission is not usually achieved:

- *in patients with a large goitre and severe hyperthyroidism*
- *if the TSI does not drop during treatment*
- *in patients who carry the HLA DW3 gene.*

Potential complications of medical management

- *Enlargement of the goitre, usually when treatment causes hypothyroidism. This can be prevented by giving exogenous hormone in conjunction with neomercazole. It must not be given with PTU; the dosage of PTU should preferably be adjusted.*
- *Agranulocytosis. This occurs in less than 1% of cases. It happens so suddenly that this complication cannot be predicted by taking regular white cell counts. If the patient develops intraoral ulceration, fever, skin rash and pharyngitis, treatment must be stopped immediately and a white cell count performed. This agranulocytosis is usually reversible.*
- *Other complications include: dermatitis, joint pains, myalgia, jaundice, fever and lymphadenopathy.*

Surgical treatment

The patient must first be prepared until she appears to be euthyroid before the thyroidectomy is performed. Most surgeons use the thionamides to prepare their patients. There is controversy as to whether lugol iodine should be added for the last ten days preoperatively. Proponents of this therapy maintain that it makes the thyroid firmer and less vascular, thus facilitating surgery. Its opponents say that it makes the thyroid so firm or hard that it cannot easily be drawn together by continuous haemostatic sutures.

There are also differences of opinion as to the use of propanalol for beta blockade. Some surgeons use only Inderal for their preparation. They emphasize that the last preoperative dose should be given with the premedication and the next dose as soon as the patient comes round after the anaesthetic. Others use it in conjunction with the thionamides to achieve early control of symptoms.

The procedure of choice is a subtotal thyroidectomy. The amount of tissue to be left behind must be carefully calculated. If too little thyroid tissue is removed, hyperthyroidism will persist or recur; if too much is removed, the patient can be expected to become hypothyroid. This is often the case when thyroid antibodies have been demonstrated and the gland thus sustains further damage postoperatively, because of immune processes. A successful attempt to leave 8 g of tissue – 4 g either side – should lead to reoccurrence of hyperthyroidism in only 5% of patients and that of hypothyroidism in only 15%. Some surgeons weigh a piece of tissue to form an accurate idea of the size of 4 g of thyroid tissue. Usually a teaspoon will just cover 4 g of thyroid tissue.

Complications of thyroidectomy

The mortality is lower than 1%, because of good preoperative preparation.

Acute complications

Thyroid crisis

This life-threatening complication is fortunately rare, because of good preoperative preparation. It sometimes occurs unexpectedly in patients with undiagnosed hyperthyroidism, who undergo other operations. A crisis can also be precipitated by trauma or infection.

The clinical presentation is that of pronounced hyperthyroidism. This includes tachycardia, so rapid that it can cause cardiogenic shock; high fever, which may rise above 40°C; confusion and later apathy. Patients are nauseous, and they vomit and develop diarrhoea.

Sodium iodide must be given in a dosage of 0,5 g in a 1ℓ infusion over eight hours, after an intravenous dose of 500 mg Propylthioural. Propranalol must be given in doses of 1 mg IV per minute to a maximum of 5 mg, depending on the response. Corticosteroids can also be considered.

Acute postoperative respiratory distress

Despite suction drainage of the wound, a haematoma can develop in the neck. This causes respiratory depression through two mechanisms, namely:

- pressure on the trachea and
- restriction of venous drainage with acute oedema of the larynx and vocal cords.

  This crisis must be treated by opening the wound immediately in the ward, followed by immediate intubation. If intubation is not possible, two large needles must be pushed through the trachea to relieve the obstruction caused by oedema.
- Another rare cause of acute respiratory distress is injury to both recurrent laryngeal nerves. Injury to one side, which occurs in less than 5% of cases, does not cause respiratory distress. If both nerves are injured, which occurs in fewer than 0,5% of cases, acute obstruction can arise, necessitating tracheostomy as an emergency procedure.

Late complications

Hypoparathyroidism

With sophisticated investigations, hypoparathyroidism can be demonstrated in 10% of cases following thyroidectomy. However, before the diagnosis can be made, the calcium levels must be correlated to albumin levels. In the immediate postoperative period, there is an albumin leak which causes falsely high serum calcium levels. Only 1% of cases have severe hypoparathyroidism, which can lead to complications such as cataracts and metastatic calcifications. The condition must be treated with longterm vitamin D therapy.

Treatment with radioactive iodine (I^{131})

Radioactive iodine (I^{131}) has a half-life of eight days. The isotope is predominantly a beta-radiator and penetrates only 2 mm. Surrounding tissues are therefore not damaged. The irradiation destroys some cells and suppresses hormone synthesis. The clinical results of irradiation only become evident after a month. It is difficult to calculate the dosage accurately. Usually the mass of the gland is estimated and a dose of more or less 80 micro cu per gram of gland mass is given.

Complications of treatment with I^{131}

Hypothyroidism occurs in 20% of cases within a year of treatment. This percentage slowly climbs until most patients have hypofunction ten years later. This complication is, just as is found postoperatively, partially caused by auto-immune destruction of the cells. Other possible complications include:

Malignant change in the thyroid

Irradiation induces malignancy when given in low doses of 50 to 1 500 rads. The cells receive much stronger irradiation with I^{131}, between 5 000 and 10 000 rads. It is still feared that with patchy uptake, as in nodular hyperthyroidism, adjacent cells might not absorb I^{131} and could then receive lower doses of irradiation. In practice, no increased incidence of malignancy has ever been demonstrated in cases treated with I^{131}.

Increased incidence of mutation

The ovaries do not receive any more irradiation than from an ordinary abdominal X-ray. There is no increased incidence of mutation.

Abnormalities of leucocyte chromosomes

Fears of an increased incidence of leukaemia have never been confirmed.

Approach to the management of Basedow/Graves disease

Because some doubt still exists about the safety of I^{131}, it is used only in patients with Basedow/Graves disease who are older than forty. There are certain exceptions to this rule. Patients can be subdivided into:

- **A surgical group,** *where there are special indications for surgery.*
- **A medical group,** *where there is a special indication for medical management or a contraindication to surgery.*
- **An open group,** *the members of which have no special indications or contraindications for any particular form of management.*

Indications for medical management

- **Young patients** *with relatively mild hyperthyroidism and a slightly enlarged thyroid gland.*
- **During pregnancy:** *The drugs cross the placenta and can affect the foetal thyroid. Use the smallest doses needed to control the disease. The dose should be very carefully monitored, especially in the last trimester. At this time mild hyperthyroidism is more acceptable than hypothyroidism.*
- **Malignant exophthalmos:** *All three modalities of treatment – surgical, medical and I^{131} – can exacerbate exophthalmos. The clinician must attempt to achieve euthyroidism. Hyperthyroidism and hypothyroidism can both lead to exacerbation of exopthalmos.*
- **Recurrent hyperthyroidism:** *Medical management must be attempted, especially in cases where there is no palpable thyroid tissue. I^{131} is very effective against residual hyperthyroidism following surgery. The age limit is usually ignored in these cases.*

Indications for surgical intervention

- **Pressure symptoms:** *If pressure symptoms like stridor or a strangling sensation are already present, or if pressure can be predicted, eg in retrosternal or intrathoracic goitres, medical management must be avoided, as it may cause enlargement of the goitre.*
- **Fear of malignancy:** *If a malignant tumour cannot be excluded in patients with Basedow/Graves disease, surgery is preferable. Malignancy occurs concurrently in only 2% of Basedow/Graves disease cases.*
- **Failed medical management:** *Patients who are drug sensitive or drug resistant, must be operated on if they are too young to be given I^{131} therapy.*
- **Cosmetic reasons:** *A very large gland can in itself be an indication for surgery, as the gland usually enlarges on medical management.*
- **Socio-economic reasons:** *Surgery is indicated in patients who will probably not co-operate well with medical management requiring regular hospital visits.*

The "open" group

This group is the largest. They usually have no clear indications or contraindications for any form of treatment. Factors to be taken into account here are the patient's age, the facilities and skills available; and the patient's preference.

Younger patients between twenty and thirty-five, with severe hyperthyroidism, should preferably be treated surgically. These patients find that constant hospital visits interfere with their daily lives and are thus inclined to become non-compliant. Many patients are also inclined to develop hypothyroidism on medical management.

In the group aged between thirty-five and forty-five, good results can be expected with medical management if the TSI drops sharply during treatment and the patient does not carry the HLA DW3 gene.

Patients over forty should perhaps be treated with I^{131}.

In this "open" group, there is little choice between the three types of treatment and the patient's preferences should be taken into account.

Malignant exophthalmos

Malignant exophthalmos is difficult to treat. High doses of corticosteroids (120 mg Prednisone daily) are often necessary. Retrobulbar injections of corticosteroids can be given. If there is no improvement, irradiation of the retrobulbar tissue can be considered.

If medical treatment is not effective or cannot be used because of complications, surgery must be performed. A thyroidectomy can be performed with safety in the second trimester.

Myxoedema

Primary myxoedema

This condition can be defined as inadequate production or inadequate supply of thyroid hormone to the cells which require it to function. It is usually caused by inadequate production in the thyroid as a result of primary disease or abnormality of function (primary myxoedema), or as a result of inadequate stimulation by the pituitary due to abnormalities of the gland itself, or, rarely, of the hypothalamus (secondary myxoedema).

A third possibility is that the target cells do not respond to circulating thyroid hormone (Retetoff syndrome). This is a very rare familial syndrome.

Secondary myxoedema

In this condition, TSH levels are not raised. In primary pituitary inadequacy, T_4 will rise as TSH is given, but not if TRF is given.

Primary myxoedema is caused by agenesis or hypogenesis of the thyroid, auto-immune thyroiditis, destruction of thyroid tissue by irradiation, surgery or carcinoma, enzyme abnormalities, iodine deficiency and goitrogens.

The most important diagnostic finding is a raised TSH. The T_3 and T_4 may be low or low normal. Primary myxoedema can be excluded if TSH levels are not low. In Retetoff syndrome, TSH, T_4 and T_3 are raised.

All forms of myxoedema are treated with thyroid hormone replacement therapy.

Myxoedematous coma

This condition can be fatal if patients develop infection or undergo an operation. Large doses of thyroid hormone (500 micrograms of thyroxine) must be given IV. After this, 50 micrograms must be given orally on a daily basis. Corticosteroids must be considered and a glucose drip administered.

Sodium may be low due to inappropriate production of antidiuretic hormone. This must not be supplemented with hypertonic saline.

E. NEOPLASMS OF THE THYROID

Because the well-differentiated tumour usually presents as a single nodule in the thyroid, it is important to consider malignancy in such patients. It remains true that the vast majority of single thyroid nodules are benign (90%). If a single nodule is diagnosed in the thyroid, it is important to determine whether it is cystic and what its functional status is, using I^{131} radio-isotope studies. If the nodule is cystic, the chances are about 10% that it is malignant. If the nodule is cold on radio-isotope study, the malignant potential increases to 20%. If it is functional, in other words a warm nodule which absorbs all the I^{131}, the chances of malignancy are negligible.

The age and sex of the patient are important.

The following approach is useful in the assessment of a single thyroid nodule. A single nodule in a middle-aged woman is most likely a dominant nodule in a multinodular goitre, which is a common condition in women. 30% of women with a multinodular goitre are incorrectly diagnosed as a single nodule on clinical examination. Multinodular goitres are rare in children, young people and men. If a single nodule is palpated in a child, a young woman, or a man, a neoplasm must be strongly suspected.

If a nodule is cystic on ultrasound, the cyst can be aspirated and the fluid can be cytologically examined. Cysts are usually formed by degeneration in colloid nodules or sometimes in adenomas.

Thyroid adenoma

A distinction must be made between a well-differentiated carcinoma and an adenoma. Adenomas are usually follicular. If an adenoma has a papillary growth pattern, it is difficult to differentiate from papillary carcinoma. Infiltration of the capsule or blood vessels must be sought. The Hurthlé cell adenoma, with its oxyphilic cells, is also hard to differentiate from carcinoma. It is advisable to treat these two adenomas with lobectomy, as there is often doubt as to the final diagnosis.

Malignant tumours

Well-differentiated carcinoma

The high incidence of carcinomas reported on routine autopsies is probably not of clinical significance, because these tumours have never manifested clinically.

No association has been proven between nodular colloid goitres and carcinoma. Nodular colloid goitre usually arises under the stimulus of TSH. Although TSH plays a role in the growth of well-differentiated tumours of the thyroid, there is no proof that it can initiate carcinoma in humans. Only a small minority, not more than 5% of the thyroid carcinomas originate in nodular goitres.

Irradiation of the thyroid can cause carcinoma. It has been well documented that children who have been irradiated in the neck area develop carcinoma of the thyroid about fifteen years later. Only 7% of these children develop carcinoma, as the dosage of irradiation is a critical factor. The dose must be below 1 500 rads to initiate carcinoma. The dosage of irradiation with I^{131} in Basedow/Graves disease far exceeds this and thus destroys cells rather than causing cell division and mutation.

It is sometimes postulated that there is an increased incidence of carcinoma associated with Hashimoto disease. The more probable explanation is that focal thyroiditis is often induced in response to an underlying carcinoma in the thyroid gland – thus creating this impression. It is true that lymphoma is more common in patients with Hashimoto thyroiditis.

Papillary carcinoma

This is the most common type of malignant tumour (50%). It is four times more common in women than in men and usually occurs before the age of forty.

It usually presents as a single nodule in the thyroid and in 30% of cases a lymph node may be palpable in the neck.

It is a slow-growing tumour which remains restricted to the thyroid over a long period. It usually spreads to lymph nodes, but may metastasize to the lungs. The tumour is often multicentric but still carries a good prognosis. In young women who have a lesion smaller than 0,5 cm, restricted to one lobe, there is no shortening in life expectancy, even if there is a spread to lymph nodes, as long as the lymph nodes are removed along with the primary lesion. In patients over forty, the course is more malignant, with a tendency to local infiltration, especially into the trachea.

The histology shows papillary outgrowths covered by single layer cuboid or cylindrical epithelium. There is often a mixed picture of follicles, with or without papillary outgrowths and varying quantities of colloid material. Laminated calcified psammoma bodies are also found. If these bodies are noted on histological section, a tentative diagnosis of papillary carcinoma can be made.

Follicular carcinoma

About 20% of the well-differentiated tumours have a follicular growth pattern. It is a disease common to older women, usually over forty. Tumours spread via the bloodstream to the lungs and to bone. Usually this tumour presents as a single nodule in the thyroid. Occasionally, lung or bone metastases present first and the primary is discovered in the thyroid later. In exceptional cases, patients present with hyperthyroidism caused by widespread metastases.

The prognosis of follicular carcinoma is not as good as that of papillary carcinoma. 50% of patients survive ten years.

The histological appearance comprises micro- and macrofollicles and sometimes solid plates of tumour cells. The tumour often looks well encapsulated but infiltration of the capsule and blood vessels can usually be demonstrated.

Poorly differentiated carcinoma

About 15% of all thyroid carcinomas are anaplastic. These tumours grow rapidly, infiltrate local structures and spread to lymph nodes and via the bloodstream to the lungs, liver and bone. Most patients die within six months, and should a patient survive for longer than a year, the diagnosis must be questioned. The cells vary from small to large to spindle-shaped.

Medullary carcinoma

About 5% of thyroid carcinomas arise in the parafollicular or C-cells. These tumours form calcitonin and other hormones, such as ACTH, serotonin, prostaglandins and bradykinin.

Tumours occur sporadically, mostly in women over fifty, or in young patients as a familial tumour with autosomally dominant inheritance. In the familial syndrome, the tumour may occur alone, or as part of a multiple adenoma syndrome. It occurs in conjunction with phaeochromocytoma, sometimes bilaterally, and with parathyroid hyperplasia (Sipple syndrome or MEA. II.A). The MEA. II.B syndrome includes medullary carcinoma, Marfan-like appearance, oral mucusal neuromas and skeletal anomalies.

Medullary carcinoma is preceded by C-cell hyperplasia, with raised levels of calcitonin in the blood. It is sometimes necessary to do pentagastrin provocation tests to elicit these raised levels.

The tumour presents as a single nodule and metastases are found in the lymph nodes, lungs, liver and bone. The nodule is usually found at the junction of the upper third and lower two-thirds of the thyroid lobe. This is where the majority of the C-cells are located. If it is bilateral or multicentric, it is familial. Sometimes patients present with diarrhoea due to hormone excretion by the tumour and its metastases.

Histologically, the tumour consists of plates or polygonal or spindle-shaped cells. The presence of amyloid in the stroma is characteristic. The amyloid secreted by the tumour cells differs from normal amyloid in that it consists mainly of collections of precalcitonin.

The management of thyroid carcinoma

Well-differentiated carcinoma

In both papillary and follicular carcinomas, the primary must be removed by means of a lobectomy on the side of the nodule. In papillary carcinoma, the contralateral lobe must also be subtotally removed, because this tumour is multicentric and may be bilateral. The opposite lobe must be removed almost entirely, with preservation of only the posterior capsule to preserve the parathyroids and recurrent laryngeal nerve. This is done so that the rest of the lobe can be easily destroyed with I^{131}, to ensure that the metastases take up I^{131} without competition from residual normal thyroid tissue in cases of follicular carcinoma.

The use of radioactive iodine in well-differentiated carcinoma

Papillary carcinoma

Radioactive iodine treatment must be considered where the patient is older than forty, or where the disease is not limited to one lobe. This approach has a dual purpose. Any microscopic multicentric tumour cells and the remaining thyroid tissue may be destroyed by this irradiation and sometimes metastases do take up I^{131} if there is no competition from normal thyroid tissue in the neck.

Follicular carcinoma

The metastases of follicular carcinoma usually concentrate I^{131} well and can therefore be treated with this substance, provided all normal thyroid tissue which has remained after almost total thyroidectomy is destroyed with I^{131} beforehand. Response is usually good, but the less-differentiated cells remain behind and may proliferate again.

The management of lymph node metastasis

Lymph node metastasis is characteristic of papillary carcinoma. Lymph node metastases do not have much influence on prognosis in young people, provided the lymph nodes are removed, and removed again if other lymph nodes enlarge – so-called "berry picking". The prognosis is so good that a radical block dissection of the cervical lymph nodes is unnecessary.

Administration of exogenous hormone

Although TSH does not initiate tumours, well-differentiated tumours are relatively TSH-dependent. It is advisable to put these patients onto permanent TSH-suppressant doses of exogenous hormone, such as eltroxin.

Postoperative follow-up of well-differentiated carcinomas

Regular thyroglobulin levels must be taken. If normal or raised levels of thyroglobulin are measured, metastases must be sought.

The management of anaplastic carcinoma

The management of this disease is highly unsatisfactory. If the tumour is discovered while it is still restricted to the thyroid, a total thyroidectomy can be performed. In reality this is seldom possible, and the tumor can usually be treated only by means of irradiation from an external source. Sometimes the isthmus has to be split to prevent strangulation. Chemotherapy is of no use.

Management of medullary carcinoma

The management of the thyroid lesion is total thyroidectomy, ie total lobectomy ipsilateral to the lesion and removal of all the thyroid tissue of the contralateral lobe, with retention of the posterior capsule to preserve the parathyroids and recurrent laryngeal nerve.

The lymph nodes must be removed by means of a radical block dissection. In advanced cases, irradiation from an external source can be used. In sporadic cases, the prognosis is good where there is no lymph node metastasis (90% ten year survival rate).

If the lymph nodes are affected, the survival rate is less than 40%. Patients with familial type MEA. II.A have a relatively good prognosis, while those with MEA. II.B have a very poor prognosis. Calcitonin levels must be measured in family members of patients with medullary carcinoma. After provocation tests with alcohol, a calcium infusion or pentagastrin, a total thyroidectomy must be performed, even if only C-cell hyperplasia is present at this stage, otherwise the patients develop carcinoma in due course.

Other tumours

Lymphoma

There is an increased incidence in patients with Hashimoto disease. They respond well to irradiation if the lymphoma is restricted to the thyroid. About 20% of patients with disseminated lymphoma present with thyroid metastases.

Sarcoma

Anaplastic carcinoma is sometimes mistakenly diagnosed as sarcoma. Fibrosarcoma, haemangiosarcoma and even osteosarcoma have been described, but these conditions are all rare.

Metastases

Patients who die of other carcinomas sometimes have metastases to the thyroid. Very rarely, patients present with a metastasis in the thyroid which mimics a primary tumour. Tumours which metastasize to the thyroid include renal carcinoma, carcinoma of the lung, breast carcinoma and malignant melanoma.

F. UNKNOWN AETIOLOGY

Reidl thyroiditis

This is a very rare condition. Patients present with a very hard goitre and pressure symptoms such as dyspnoea, hoarseness and dysphagia. Signs of fixation and infiltration of surrounding tissues such as muscle, blood vessels and nerves are usually found, but the skin is loose. Because this condition is rare it is often clinically misdiagnosed as a carcinoma.

Patients are euthyroid and auto-antibodies are either absent, or present in very low titres. It is not an advanced stage of Hashimoto disease, although a few cases have been described who had both diseases concurrently.

In a few cases, mediastinal and retroperitoneal fibrosis, and sometimes even sclerosing cholangitis are found, which are indicative of systemic disease. Both lobes are affected, with infiltrating fibrosis, and a few inflammatory cells present. The fibrosis also extends beyond the gland to surrounding tissues. It is not usually possible to remove the gland surgically and it is advisable to remove just the isthmus to relieve dyspnoea.

THE ORAL CAVITY

What does the patient complain of?

- A swelling
  The swelling can be hard and solid
  It may be located on:
  - the lip
  - the tongue
  - the *diaphragma oris*
  - the palate

Related to teeth and gums

- A cyst
  Found on:

- the lip
- the *diaphragma oris*
- the gums, related to the teeth

- An ulcer
  Occurs on
  - the lip
  - the tongue
  - the *diaphragma oris*

It can be painful or painless

- A white patch on the mucosa (leukoplakia)
  This can occur at any site in the oral cavity, but is most often found on the tongue and lower lip
  - Usually painless
- A swelling (lymph node) in the neck can be painful or painless

What must the clinician consider?

An ulcer

The ulcer may arise as a fissure and ulcerate further. It may be either moderately or extremely painful.

- Common conditions

Trauma

Caused by a sharp tooth or ill-fitting dentures.

Aphthous ulcer

In younger people, on the tongue, very painful. Heals spontaneously.

Carcinoma

In older people. The ulcer has raised edges and a deep-lying mass is palpable. "Iceberg" effect.

- Rarer conditions

Chronic nonspecific ulcer

Painful ulcer on the tongue that does not heal spontaneously.

Tuberculous ulcer

Very painful, with undermined edges on the side of the tongue.

Syphilitic ulcer

Presents as a chancre or "snail track" ulcer.

Cysts

- Common conditions

Retention cysts

Of the mucus glands, especially on the lower lip.

Ranula

On the *diaphragma oris*, in the midline or slightly to one side.

- Rarer conditions
  Dermoid cyst on the *diaphragma oris*, in the midline
  Painful swelling on the floor of the mouth
  Ludwig's angina in the area of the *diaphragma oris*
  Peritonsillar abscess
  Retropharyngeal abscess

Swellings

Related to the gums

- Common conditions
  An epilus
  An alveolar abscess around the root of a tooth
  A dental cyst arises around the root of a tooth and can become infected
- Rarer conditions
  Dentigerous cyst arises around an unerupted tooth
  Inclusion cyst, usually of the upper jaw, at the junction of the premaxilla and the maxilla
  Adamantinoma: a painless swelling of the lower jaw
  Carcinoma of the maxillary antrum presents with loose upper teeth, or with a swelling in the maxilla or hard palate

Swellings elsewhere in the oral cavity

- Common conditions
  Carcinoma of the tongue and tonsil bed
  Mixed salivary gland tumours, especially on the palate
- Rarer conditions
  Benign tumours of the tongue
  Lingual thyroid, posteriorly at the *foramen caecum* of the tongue

Neck swellings (lymph nodes)

- Painful – consider inflammatory conditions of the oral cavity
- Painless – consider a malignant tumour in the oral cavity

Classification of diseases of the oral cavity

A. EMBRYOLOGICAL DEVELOPMENTAL ANOMALIES

1. Hare lip and cleft palate will not be dealt with in this text.
2. Lingual thyroid has already been discussed in the section dealing with thyroid diseases.
3. Anomalies of developmental fusion
   Dermoid cyst on the floor of the mouth
   Maxillary cyst at the junction of premaxilla and maxilla
   Dentigerous cyst, unerupted tooth

B. INFLAMMATORY CONDITIONS

Ulcers on the tongue

1. Aphthous ulcer, caused by viral or fungal infection.
2. Tuberculous ulcer – usually associated with advanced pulmonary tuberculosis
3. Syphilis – primary chancre or "snail track" ulcer

Intra-oral abscesses

1. Ludwig angina
2. Peritonsillar abscess
3. Retropharyngeal abscess

The teeth and gums

In conjunction with caries
1. Alveolar abscess
2. Tooth cysts
3. Granulomatous epulis

C. TUMOURS OF THE ORAL CAVITY

Benign tumours

1. Mixed salivary gland tumour of the palate
2. On the tongue (rare)
   Papilloma
   Angioma
   Lipoma
   Neurofibroma

The teeth and gums

1. Fibrous epulis – fibroma
2. Bony epulis – osteoclastoma

Premalignant conditions – leukoplakia

Malignant tumours

1. The lip – squamous carcinoma
2. The tongue – squamous carcinoma
3. The *diaphragma oris* – squamous carcinoma
4. The tonsil bed – squamous carcinoma 90%
   – lymphosarcoma 10%
5. Maxillary antrum – squamous carcinoma 95%
   – adenocarcinoma 5%
6. The jaws – adamantinoma

D. OTHER CONDITIONS

Ulceration

1. Traumatic ulceration – caused by a sharp tooth or ill-fitting dentures
2. Chronic non-specific ulcer – cause unknown

Cysts

Retention cysts

Ranula

Shortened frenulum of the tongue

A. Abnormalities of embryological development

Dermoid cyst

It arises from ectoderm which becomes embedded during development. It forms a painless cyst in the midline of the *diaphragma oris* in young people. It can occur superior or inferior to the myelohyoid muscle. If it is superior to the muscle, it can be surgically removed through the *diaphragma oris*. If it is inferior to the muscle, extra-oral surgery is necessary.

The maxillary cyst

This is a dermoid of the maxilla which forms at the junction of the premaxilla and maxilla between the incisors and the canines. The diagnosis is confirmed on X-ray. The treatment is excision.

Dentigerous cyst

This cyst develops around an unerupted tooth, usually related to the third molar of the lower or upper jaw. It is found in young people and is painful. There is a tooth missing in the area and X-rays show cyst formation around the unerupted tooth. The treatment is excision.

B. Inflammatory conditions

Ulcers on the tongue

Aphthous ulcer

This is a small, white, extremely painful ulcer found on the tongue, usually in young women. The ulcers heal spontaneously within ten to fourteen days. If an ulcer does not heal, histological confirmation of the diagnosis must be obtained.

Tuberculous ulcer

This is also very painful. It has undermined edges and may be multiple. These ulcers are rare and are found in association with pulmonary tuberculosis.

Syphilis

This is rare nowadays. All three stages can present in the mouth. Primary syphilis presents as a chancre on the lip or tongue. It starts as a flat, painless, pink blister, which breaks down and forms a painful ulcer. The patient's cervical lymph nodes enlarge. Later the ulcer heals spontaneously.

Secondary syphilis presents as a "snail track" ulcer covered with mucus. It is particularly common on the pillar of the tonsil bed.

Tertiary syphilis presents as a gumma on the tongue or palate. It is an indurated, painless, hard mass which is difficult to differentiate from carcinoma. The diagnosis is confirmed by blood tests.

Intra-oral abscesses

These have become rarer since free use of antibiotics for intra-oral infections has become practice.

Ludwig angina

This is a cellulitis or abscess caused by streptococci arising in the submental and sublingual spaces. Patients present with fever, pain, dysphagia and sometime dyspnoea. On clinical examination, a tender mass is found in the submental or sublingual areas. The tongue is displaced and its movements are restricted. This condition must be regarded as an emergency, because it can cause respiratory distress. The patient must be admitted to hospital and intravenous antibiotics and drainage via a cervical incision are essential. Preparations must be made for an emergency tracheostomy should this become necessary.

Peritonsillar abscess (Quinsy)

This is usually caused by streptococcus tonsillitis. The abscess develops between the tonsil capsule and the superior constrictor muscle. This displaces the tonsil medially and the uvula contralaterally. Patients present with fever, dysphagia and trismus, caused by spasm of the internal pterygoid muscle. The treatment includes antibiotics and drainage of the abscess via the anterior pillar of the tonsil bed.

Retropharyngeal abscess

This is found in young patients, especially children. It arises in the space between the superior constrictor muscle and the prevertebral fascia. Patients present with fever, stridor and dysphagia. On clinical examination, a soft, fluctuating, tender mass is palpable in the posterior pharynx in the midline.

Treatment includes antibiotics and drainage via the oropharyngeal mucosa, under general anaesthetic, with intratracheal intubation.

The teeth and gums

Alveolar abscess

These abscesses arise around carious dental roots. Patients present with a painful swelling of the jaw, often in the submandibular region. The diagnosis is confirmed on X-ray.

Treatment includes antibiotics and extraction of the affected tooth to facilitate drainage.

Dental cysts

These arise from the epithelial cells of the enamel organ around the roots of a carious tooth. If they become infected, an alveolar abscess forms. The diagnosis is confirmed on X-ray.

Treatment includes excision of the epithelial layer of the cyst. If it is infected, the dental caries must also be treated.

Granulomatous epulis

Granulomatous tissue heaps up around a carious tooth.

Treatment includes extraction of the tooth and curettage of the granulomatous tissue, with histological confirmation of the diagnosis.

C. Tumours of the oral cavity

Benign tumours

The palate

Mixed salivary gland tumours arise in the accessory salivary glands. As in the parotid, these tumours are not well encapsulated. They become malignant more frequently than those in the parotid. A slow-growing mass develops on the palates of elderly patients. The mucosa is usually intact and the tumour is mobile. The diagnosis and treatment include wide excision and histological examination.

A number of benign tumours are found on the tongue. These are all rare. They include papilloma, lipoma, angioma and neurofibroma.

Treatment includes excision and histological confirmation of the diagnosis.

A lingual thyroid must be borne in mind if a tumour is found on the posterior third of the tongue. Confirm the diagnosis with an I^{131} scan.

Fibromas arise on the gums. They must be excised and examined histologically, as they can undergo malignant transformation.

Osteoclastomas, or so-called gaint cell tumours, develop on the jaw. The gums overlying the tumour are oedematous. Excision is the treatment of choice and a bone transplant is sometimes necessary if the jaw has been weakened.

Malignant tumours

Adamantinoma

This is also known as an ameloblastoma and develops from the enamel organ of the jaw, usually in young people. The patient presents with a painless swelling of the jaw in the region of the molar teeth. On examination, an eggshell-like crackling effect is palpable. X-rays reveal locules and a honeycombed appearance. Histologically, the tumour is similar to a basal cell carcinoma.

Treatment includes excision, including a border of normal bone, otherwise the tumour recurs. Its malignant behaviour is similar to that of a basal cell carcinoma. It infiltrates locally but does not metastasize.

Carcinoma of the oral cavity

Before the various carcinomas can be discussed, attention must be given to premalignant conditions.

Leukoplakia

This is found most commonly in older men who smoke. It usually occurs on the tongue and lower lip, but can present anywhere in the *diaphragma oris*. It resembles spots of wet white paint on the mucosa. Later, it cracks and forms fissures and, still later, nodules.

Histologically, epithelial cell hyperplasia is seen (hyperkeratosis) and widening of the prickle cell layer (acanthosis). If atypia of cells, with loss of polarity and cell nuclei, begins to appear on the surface, malignant transformation has already commenced.

Treatment

If it covers a small area, or if there are any signs of malignancy (especially nodularity), the entire lesion must be removed if this is practically possible; or tissue must be removed for histology to exclude malignant transformation.

Larger areas without signs of malignancy can be followed up; and causes such as smoking, alcohol and other irritants must be eliminated. Serological tests for syphilis must be taken. Suspicious lesions must be biopsied to exclude malignant transformation.

Carcinoma of the lip

This is common in men over the age of sixty. There is often a history of smoking (especially pipe smoking) and sun exposure.

The ulcer, with its typical rolled edge, is found on the lower lip in 90% of cases. The rest are found on the upper lip or at the corners of the mouth. Carcinoma of the lower lip spreads to the submental lymph nodes, whereas carcinomas of the upper lip and corner of the mouth spread to the submandibular nodes. The diagnosis is confirmed by biopsy. The primary lesion must be excised as a wedge, along with a border of 0,5 cm of normal tissue. Irradiation achieves similar results. If the lymph nodes are palpable, a block dissection is necessary. Larger lesions and lesions of the corners of the mouth must be excised, and the defect repaired with plastic surgery procedures.

Carcinoma of the tongue

Carcinoma of the tongue is found mainly in men over fifty-five. There is often a history of smoking, dental caries and venereal disease.

Patients complain of pain, salivation, limitation of tongue movements and *foetor oris*. Examination will show an ulcer with rolled edges, a wartlike swelling, or a fissure. The ulcer is hard on palpation, with underlying induration. Hard, enlarged lymph nodes may be found on examination of the neck.

The primary lesion is most commonly found on the anterior two-thirds of the tongue, towards its edges. The lesion is sometimes situated on the posterior third of the tongue, where it is difficult to inspect. It is thus usually diagnosed by palpating the tongue.

The differential diagnosis of an ulcer of the tongue has already been mentioned. Any ulcer of the tongue which takes longer than fourteen days to heal, must be biopsied for purposes of histological diagnosis. Histology will confirm a squamous carcinoma and will indicate the degree of differentiation, which is of importance for prognosis and management.

Staging of carcinoma of the tongue

The TNM staging

T – tumour size
T1 – tumour smaller than 2 cm
T2 – tumour 2–4 cm
T3 – tumour larger than 4 cm
N – lymph nodes
NO – no palpable lymph nodes
N1 – homolateral mobile nodes smaller than 3 cm
N2 – single nodes 3–6 cm or multiple nodes larger than 6 cm
N3 – fixed or contralateral nodes
M – metastasis
MO – no distal metastasis
M1 – distal metastasis present

Carcinoma of the oral cavity spreads initially by local infiltration, later to homolateral lymph nodes and only then to other lymph nodes and to the bloodstream. The battle is often lost locally in this disease. It is thus very important that the lesion be diagnosed and optimally treated at an early stage.

Management of carcinoma of the tongue

Carcinoma of the anterior two-thirds of the tongue

Management of the primary lesion

Surgery and irradiation are adequate for T1 and T2 tumours, provided the lesions are well differentiated. Surgery is preferable, because it has rapid results, supplies useful information about the histology of the lesion and confirms that the primary lesion has been excised completely. The excision must be planned so that a 2 cm free border is included and function is not affected.

Radiotherapy is a good alternative, should the patient insist. If the lesion is poorly differentiated, irradiation is the preferred treatment, as surgery yields poor results in such cases. Irradiation does not give a very good result either.

Irradiation is preferable in larger lesions (T3), as an adequate incision (with 2 cm free borders) would impede function too much. The disadvantages of irradiation are:

1. *Duration – a course of irradiation takes four weeks*
2. *It damages adjacent tissues, giving rise to necrotic ulceration, dental caries, osteomyelitis and inhibition of salivary glands, causing a dry mouth.*

Salvage procedures

If surgical treatment fails, the residual lesion can be irradiated. If irradiation fails, radical surgery can be considered, if the patient is prepared to sacrifice function for possible healing.

The lymph nodes

If the primary lesion is T1 or T2 and well differentiated; and the lymph nodes are impalpable, then a policy of "wait and see" is adopted and lymph nodes are removed by radical dissection if and when they become palpable.

When the primary lesion is larger (T3), or the histology shows poor differentiation, the chances of lymph node spread are greater and elective resection or irradiation of lymph nodes must be considered. If the lymph nodes are palpable and the primary lesion has been cured, either by excision or irradiation, a radical block dissection must be performed. This applies to N1 and N2 lymph nodes. N3 nodes must be irradiated.

In T3 lesions, particularly those which have spread across the midline, bilateral lymph nodes may be affected. Bilateral block dissections are sometimes indicated.

Carcinoma of the posterior third of the tongue

This tumour is usually discovered at a late stage when it is already large and has often spread across the midline. Occasionally, patients present with a palpable lymph node and pain on swallowing. The lesion is discovered on palpating the tongue posteriorly.

Histologically, these tumours are often completely anaplastic. The primary lesion must usually be irradiated, because it is too large for excision. The lymph nodes are removed by block dissection. The prognosis is poor.

Carcinoma of the *diaphragma oris*

This presents as an ulcer on the anterior floor of the mouth near the frenulum. It is painless in the early stages, but it later becomes painful, especially if it becomes infected. It has a tendency to spread locally to the gums and jaw. It later spreads to the submandibular lymph nodes.

X-rays must be taken to exclude bone involvement.

Management involves wide excision of the ulcer, which usually means that the diaphragma oris *must be removed. The operation is completed by removing the lymph nodes* en bloc. *If the mandible is involved, a section of the jaw must be removed – the so-called commando operation. If the patient refuses surgery, the lesion can be irradiated, but this is a "second best" alternative as it is often followed by tissue- and bone necrosis. Despite biopsies, it can be difficult to differentiate between a residual ulcerating tumour and radionecrosis.*

Carcinoma of the tonsil bed

Carcinoma of the tonsil is found in patients over sixty. It presents with pain which radiates to the ear. The patient complains of dysphagia and foetor oris. *The tumour tends to infiltrate the pillars of the tonsil bed.*

The diagnosis must be confirmed by biopsy. The treatment usually involves irradiation of the primary lesion and block dissection of palpable lymph nodes. If the disease recurs after irradiation, radical surgery may be necessary.

Lymphosarcoma of the tonsil

This tumour is much rarer and is found in patients between forty and fifty. It is usually painless and ulceration and haemorrhage only occur late in its course. Radiotherapy is the treatment of choice.

Carcinoma of the maxillary antrum

This tumour arises in the antral mucosa in aged men. It usually becomes symptomatic only when it spreads out of the antrum into the maxilla, where it causes loosening of the teeth. It can also infiltrate the orbits, or break through the upper jaw to form an ulcer on the palate. The initial diagnosis is usually made on X-rays, which show obliteration of the antrum.

Biopsy confirms the diagnosis of squamous carcinoma. A small minority may have adenocarcinomas.

The treatment of choice is radiotherapy. If the tumour recurs, radical excision, maxillectomy and reconstruction may be performed.

The prognosis of oral carcinoma

If all cases of carcinoma of the tongue are considered, the five year survival rate is 30%. The more posterior the situation of the lesion, the poorer its prognosis. Prognosis is also strongly influenced by the size of the primary lesion and whether it has spread to lymph nodes.

Squamous carcinoma of the oral cavity has a fairly predictable behaviour pattern. The primary lesion tends to infiltrate locally. If the primary lesion is larger than 2 cm in diameter (T2–T3), the prognosis is much poorer. The fight against this disease is often lost because the primary lesion cannot be controlled.

If the primary lesion is smaller than 2 cm in diameter (T1), the lymph nodes are not involved (NO) and the tumour is well-differentiated, the prognosis is more than 90% five year survival with surgical excision and irradiation. If the primary lesion is larger than 2 cm and the lymph nodes are not involved (T2 NO), the prognosis deteriorates to 70% five year survival.

If lymph nodes are involved, the prognosis deteriorates drastically (T2 N1 prognosis 40% and T2 N3 prognosis 15%).

Because lymph node metastases are of such prognostic importance, there is debate as to whether impalpable lymph nodes should be removed electively and prophylactically. There have been objections to open lymph node biopsy, as it may contaminate the field. Aspiration cytology is a safe and useful method of making the diagnosis.

Because the size of the primary lesion can be used to predict the possibility of occult metastasis to the lymph nodes some surgeons suggest elective block dissection in poorly differentiated T2 lesions.

At present there is no clear evidence that elective, prophylactic block dissection influences the five year survival rate. Trials are currently being conducted to determine whether adjuvant chemotherapy plays a role in prognosis. Drugs which are useful in the treatment of squamous carcinoma of the oral cavity include CIS-platinum, bleomycin, adriamycin and methotrexate.

Regional administration of chemotherapy via intra-arterial catheters, which initially showed promise, is now only used palliatively in cases where surgery and irradiation are no longer possible.

Malignant melanoma

This can occur in the oral or nasal cavity. It is found more often in black patients and is a rare condition. The treatment of choice is wide excision of the primary lesion and block dissection of palpable lymph nodes.

D. Other conditions

Ulceration

Trauma

Sharp edges of carious teeth or ill-fitting dentures can cause ulceration of the mouth. It is important to view any oral ulceration as potentially malignant. Traumatic ulcers have a short course, are superficial and have no surrounding induration. A definite aetiological factor can be identified. The aetiological factor must be removed and if the ulcer does not heal within two weeks, a biopsy must be performed to exclude malignancy.

Chronic non-specific ulcer

These ulcers are usually found on the anterior two-thirds of the tongue. They are painful and do not heal. Tuberculosis and syphilis must be excluded, using appropriate special investigations. The diagnosis is confirmed and healing is accomplished by excision biopsy.

Cysts

Retention cysts

These cysts arise as a result of blockage of mucus-secreting glands anywhere in the oral cavity, but most commonly on the inner surface of the upper lip. The swelling is painless and semitransparent. The treatment is excision.

Ranula

This cyst is found in young peple on one side of the floor of the mouth between the tongue and the jaw. The cyst is smooth, semitransparent, transilluminable and painless.

It arises from blocked accessory salivary glands, the Blandin- and Nunes glands. It can extend from the floor of the mouth into the neck. The treatment is excision of the cyst or marsupialization into the oral cavity.

Shortened tongue frenulum

This is familial. Speech defects are often attributed to this condition but it is seldom the cause. The frenulum is short, wide and avascular. If it really prevents the child from putting his tongue out, the avascular part of the frenulum can be cut, but the underlying blood vessels must be avoided.

The oesophagus 2

Diagnosis

What does the patient complain of?

Dysphagia – difficulty in swallowing

Onset

- Sudden – consider obstruction by a foreign body.
- Rapid – carcinoma causes dysphagia that becomes worse within weeks.
- Slow – benign conditions like reflux oesophagitis with stenosis and achalasia take months or years to develop.

Site

- The patient can often indicate where the food sticks.
- Carcinoma can obstruct the oesophagus at any site.
- Pharyngeal diverticulum causes high dysphagia.
- Benign strictures are usually found at the lower end of the oesophagus.

Character

- If dysphagia for solids is exacerbated to dysphagia for liquids, suspect carcinoma if the progression is rapid, and a benign stenosis if the course is slow and the dysphagia is preceded by heartburn.
- If dysphagia for liquids is found from the onset, consider abnormalities of motility such as achalasia and diffuse oesophageal spasm.

Pain

Reflux of gastric juices into the oesophagus causes heartburn. It also causes a burning pain, felt retrosternally, associated with an unpleasant bitter taste in the mouth. The pain improves when antacids are taken. Indigestion followed by dysphagia usually suggests a hiatus hernia, with reflux oesophagitis.

Patients sometimes present with extremely severe retrosternal pain, which spreads to the arms and closely resembles ischaemic cardiac pain. Usually a good history will help the clinician to distinguish between the two. This severe oesophageal pain is caused by oesophageal spasm. Heartburn and dysphagia are often associated and the pain is not related to exercise. Reflux of gastric contents can be demonstrated.

Ischaemic pain is usually related to exercise, but sometimes the two types of pain are so similar that it is necessary to perform coronary vessel angiography.

Carcinoma is painless at first and later causes a vague, pressing, constant pain.

Achalasia is painless.

Regurgitation

This must be distinguished from vomiting. It is not associated with nausea and usually consists of undigested food, which appears in the throat without spasms. Sometimes this food is aspirated and patients present with coughing fits. Later, they develop severe pulmonary infection with restriction of lung function. If this sign presents, consider pharyngeal diverticulum and hiatus hernia. Often both conditions are found in the same patient.

What is found on examination

The oesophagus is situated almost totally intrathoracically. The pharyngeal-oesophageal junction is in the neck. A pharyngeal diverticulum is sometimes palpable in the posterior triangle of the neck just behind the sternocleidomastoid muscle.

Very rarely, a carcinoma of the oesophagus and stomach can be palpated high up in the epigastrium. Lymph node metastases sometimes present in the posterior triangle of the neck. Systemic signs such as loss of weight, anaemia and pulmonary disease must be sought.

Special investigations

Special investigations are essential for making a diagnosis, as the oesophagus is impalpable. These include chest X-rays, barium meal and endoscopy with biopsy. Normal X-rays do not suffice in a patient with dysphagia. Endoscopy and biopsy must always be performed.

Other special investigations such as pressure studies and pH measurements in the oesophagus are sometimes useful in diagnosing motility abnormalities. The application of specific special investigations will be explained when individual conditions are discussed.

Classification of oesophageal conditions

A. MOTILITY ABNORMALITIES

- Spasm of the cricopharyngeous muscle with pharyngeal diverticulum
- Oesophageal spasm and diverticula
- Hypertensive inferior oesophageal sphincter
- Achalasia
- Incompetent inferior oesophageal sphincter
- Schatzki ring
- Hypoperistalsis of the oesophagus

B. TRAUMA

- Swallowing foreign bodies
- Perforation and rupture of the oesophagus
- Bottletop explosion injuries
- Swallowing corrosive substances and irritant drugs

C. TUMOURS OF THE OESOPHAGUS

Benign tumours

- Leiomyoma
- Lipoma

Malignant tumours

- Squamous carcinoma
- Adenocarcinoma (arises in a Barrett's oesophagus)
- Adeno-acanthoma
- Leiomyosarcoma
- Carcinoid
- Melanoma

D. MISCELLANEOUS CONDITIONS

- Infections
- Webs
- External pressure on the oesophagus

MOTILITY ABNORMALITIES

Normal oesophageal motility

The oesophagus consists of a long muscular tube lined with squamous epithelium and is closed at its entrance and exit by sphincter mechanisms. The superior oesophageal sphincter (SOS), at the junction between the pharynx and the oesophagus, is formed mainly by the cricopharyngeal muscle. The inferior oesophageal sphincter (IOS) is not an anatomical structure, but an area of physiologically raised pressure, 2–4 cm in length. The resting pressure at both sphincters averages about 40 cm water. During swallowing, the sphincters contract after the bolus of food has passed through, preventing reflux into the pharynx at the SOS or into the oesophagus at the IOS.

Abnormalities of normal motility

Incoordination can arise on swallowing so that the SOS does not open on time. Swallowing then takes place against resistance. The IOS can be spastic, also known as a hypertensive IOS.

During swallowing, primary contractions drive the food bolus forward. Residual food is emptied from the oesophagus by secondary contractions. In elderly people, incoordinated small contractions take place, also known as tertiary contractions.

The IOS may contract weakly or not at all. This results in reflux of grastric contents from the stomach (zone of positive pressure) into the oesophagus (zone of negative pressure).

Pharyngeal diverticulum (Zenker diverticulum)

Aetiology

A pulsion diverticulum of mucus membrane pushes through the weak spot of Kilian in the lower part of the pharyngeal constrictor muscle. This is caused by incoordinated relaxation of the SOS, with functional obstruction. The reason for the spasm is not entirely clear. Often the patient also has a hiatus hernia with reflux oesophagitis and this may be the cause of the spasm.

Clinical presentation

This condition is found in older patients, more often in men. Patients complain of a typical dysphagia. The first few mouthfuls of food go down easily, but then the diverticulum fills and blocks the oesophagus, resulting in dysphagia which is felt high in the neck. Sometimes regurgitation takes place, with coughing fits, especially at night. Patients also develop pulmonary infections due to inhalation of food.

In about a third of cases, a mass can be palpated in the posterior triangle of the neck.

Special investigations

Do not begin with endoscopy, as the endoscope may perforate the diverticulum. Start with a barium meal, which will confirm the diagnosis. The diverticulum may just be a small bulge, or an obvious sac, several centimetres long. The spastic cricopharyngeal muscle is usually clearly visible as an indentation on the X-ray. Pressure studies show incoordinate peristalsis and sphincter relaxation.

Management

Infection, due to stasis, is often found in the diverticulum. Rinse out the diverticulum and give the patient fluids only for forty-eight hours. First treat the lung infection with physiotherapy and antibiotics.

The operation

The incision must be made at the level of the crycoid bone just anterior to the sternocleidomastoid muscle. The diverticulum is usually found most easily on the left-hand side and is dissected out up to its neck. It is helpful if the anaesthetist places a fairly thick tube into the oesophagus. Remove the diverticulum and close the mucous membrane. Do a myotomy of the cricopharyngeal muscle to relieve the spasm. If the diverticulum is just a small bulge, only the myotomy need be performed.

No fluids must be given by mouth for seven days. Do a gastrografin swallow at this stage – if no leak is demonstrated, the patient may begin to take fluids per os.

Oesophageal diverticula

These diverticula are found in the midoesophagus or at its lower end, lying in relation to the diaphragmatic hiatus.

Aetiology

Midoesophageal diverticula can either be pulsion diverticula, caused by raised oesophageal pressure, or traction diverticula, due to inflammation of hilar lymph nodes. The more distally situated, or epiphrenic diverticula, are pulsion diverticula, caused by raised intraoesophageal pressure. This raised pressure is caused by diffuse generalized oesophageal spasm, or a hypertensive IOS. In diffuse spasm, peristalsis is usually normal in the upper third of the oesophagus, but there is recurrent spastic contraction of the lower two-thirds.

Clinical presentation

Severe retrosternal pain is the most important symptom. Dysphagia and regurgitation are also found.

Special investigations

A barium meal confirms the diagnosis. Pressure studies can determine abnormal motility. Do not confuse an epiphrenic diverticulum with an epiphrenic ampulla, which is a normal finding. The oesophagus bulges out in the form of an ampulla just before the IOS relaxes. This must also be differentiated from a hiatus hernia.

Management

Often treatment is unnecessary. Anticholinergics sometimes relieve the pain. If symptoms are severe, diverticulectomy and myotomy of the oesophagus can be performed, in accordance with the area of spasm which has been demonstrated by manometry. If the IOS is hypertensive, a myotomy may be necessary to relieve symptoms.

Achalasia

This occurs in one in 100 000 of the population. It is found with equal frequency in men and women between thirty and sixty. It is rare in children.

Aetiology and pathophysiology

Degeneration and loss of ganglion cells in Auerbach's plexus are found in the dilated part of the oesophagus. The vagus nerve appears normal on light microscopy, but on electron microscopy, abnormalities of the Schwann cells can be seen. Degeneration of the myenteric plexus of the vagus nerve also takes place, probably secondary to changes in the vagus nucleus which shows a reduction in the number of nerve cells.

The true aetiology is unknown. Infection with Trypanosoma cruzi (Chaga disease), as seen in South America, causes degeneration of the Auerbach plexus, resulting in all the motor anomalics of achalasia.

Clinical presentation

Dysphagia, especially for fluids, is the most important sympton. Food can only leave the oesophagus by gravity. Patients develop various tricks to get their food down. They eat while standing or exhale strongly against a closed glottis. Regurgitation of food, especially at night, is an annoying symptom which can lead to chronic lung infections.

They break foul-smelling winds and halitosis can be a serious problem.

Pain is rare. Loss of mass is a late finding.

Special investigations

- A chest X-ray will show a widened mediastinum with a fluid level in the thorax and loss of the normal gastric bubble.
- A barium meal shows a widely dilated oesophagus, with a narrowed distal end, resembling a bird's beak.
- Manometry shows loss of peristalsis with a raised resting pressure of the IOS.
- The mecholyl test. If mecholyl is administered, a 20 cm rise in pressure occurs, lasting up to thirty minutes. It can be associated with severe pain. False negative results occur in longstanding achalasia and patients with diffuse oesophageal spasm.
- Endoscopy must always be performed to exclude carcinoma. Carcinoma is more common in achalasia, even where the condition is treated effectively.

Management

Management is aimed at relief of the high pressure zone at the IOS. This can be achieved by dilatation or surgery.

Hydrostatic stretching

A balloon with a diameter limited to 4,5 cm is used. The balloon is positioned at the level of the diaphragmatic hiatus, under X-ray guidance. It is then inflated to 200 mm Hg for one minute and to 300 mm Hg for a second minute. Dilatation has to be repeated often. Perforation occurs in 3% of cases and the mortality is 1%.

The Heller operation

A myotomy of the IOS is performed via a thoracic approach. The incision is 7 cm long and extends a few millimetres onto the stomach. It may not extend further than 1 cm onto the stomach, otherwise reflux becomes a serious problem. Some surgeons deliberately extend the myotomy to the stomach and then perform a Nissan fundoplication with the myotomy, to prevent reflux.

Perforation and fistula occur in 2% of cases and the mortality is 1%.

Prognosis

The Heller operation is successful in 90% of cases, while dilatation is successful in 60–70% of cases. Since there is no difference in mortality, the Heller myotomy is probably the treatment of choice. Reflux oesophagitis may present problems (10% of cases). Carcinoma must be borne in mind and follow-up endoscopy is essential.

Hiatus hernia and an incompetent IOS

Prevention of regurgitation of gastric contents into the oesophagus is dependent on the IOS mechanism. The most important component of this prevention is the zone of positive pressure at the lower end of the oesophagus (the sphincter). Other factors which play a role are the angle between the oesophagus and the stomach fundus (the angle of His), the mucous membrane rosette and the phreno-oesophageal ligament which fixes the IOS under the diaphragm. The IOS may have high, normal or no pressure on manometry. An IOS with good pressures can be competent even when displaced to the negative pressure zone of the thorax, thus preventing reflux.

A weak IOS will be competent in the abdominal cavity with its positive pressure, but incompetent in the negative pressure of the thorax. If the IOS is absent, the patient will reflux no matter where the cardia is situated.

A sliding hiatus hernia

A hernia consists of a defect (hiatus), a sac (peritoneal reflection) and contents of the sac (the stomach).

Definition of a sliding hiatus hernia

The content of the sac (stomach) forms part of the wall of the sac.

The IOS is displaced to the negative pressure area of the thorax.

Aetiology

Sliding hiatus hernias are common in people over fifty. Patients are usually severely obese. Sometimes the hernias are found in people of normal weight; and the reason for this is unknown.

Clinical presentation

The vast majority of patients with hiatus hernias are asymptomatic or have only mild symptoms. The most important symptom is heartburn. This is a burning, substernal pain. Sometimes the pain is very severe and is difficult to distinguish from angina, especially when diffuse spasm occurs in association with the hiatus hernia.

Regurgitation, especially at night when the patient is lying down, or during the day when they bend forward, is another important symptom. Dull pain in the region of the costal margin, disappearing suddenly when the patient stretches, is rare. Reflux oesophagitis can lead to inflammation, oedema and stenosis, with symptoms of dysphagia. Ulceration can occur, with chronic blood loss and anaemia.

On examination, severe obesity is a common finding.

Special investigations

- X-rays: A chest X-ray sometimes shows a second shadow behind the heart and a fluid level. A barium meal usually confirms the diagnosis. Gastric mucosa is visible above the hiatus and barium refluxes back into the oesophagus with ease. Stenosis and ulceration may be found; and reducibility of the hernia can be determined.

  A rolling hernia (rare) is sometimes seen. The fundus herniates through the diaphragm into the thorax but the cardia and IOS remain in the abdominal cavity and reflux cannot be demonstrated.
- Endoscopy: It is essential to determine the grade of oesophagitis and, if a stenosis is present, to determine the cause of the stenosis histologically. Carcinoma must be excluded.

Character of oesophagitis

Grade I: The mucosa is red and inflamed.
Grade II: There is mucosal ulceration.
Grade III: There is reversible inflammatory stenosis.
Grade IV: There is irreversible fibrotic stenosis.

Endoscopy is useful for excluding Barrett oesophagus (gastric mucosa in the oesophagus) and peptic ulceration in the stomach or duodenum.

- Pressure studies: The site and status of the IOS can be determined. Other conditions, such as achalasia, hypertensive IOS and scleroderma, can be differentiated.
- pH studies: Several tests have been described to demonstrate acid reflux in the oesophagus. They all include the positioning of a pH electrode in the oesophagus and measurement of reflux or acid into the oesophagus.

  The Bernstein test provokes pain when 0,1 N HCl is placed in the lower oesophagus.

Complications of sliding hiatus hernia

Stenosis is the most important complication, resulting from recurrent ulceration, inflammation and fibrosis. Inflammatory reflux is an early finding and can be reversed if reflux is prevented. Later, irreversible fibrotic stenosis occurs. Chronic haemorrhage, with iron deficiency anaemia, may present. A large bleed occurs very rarely.

Barrett oesophagus

This is an acquired condition, which evolves secondary to reflux oesophagitis, where the oesophageal mucosa is replaced by gastric mucosa. Often a stenosis is found higher than usual in the oesophagus. A deep ulcer may also be found at the junction between gastric and oesophageal mucosa.

Schatzki ring

This is an annular indentation of the oesophagus associated with a hiatus hernia. It can take one of two forms:

- Spastic muscle contraction due to irritation (temporary)
- Fibrotic ring due to recurrent inflammation (permanent)

Management of a sliding hiatus hernia

Conservative management

More than 90% of symptomatic patients can be treated successfully by conservative methods. Conservative methods must be aimed at:

1. *Reduction of intra-abdominal pressure by:*
   - *Weight loss. This is the most effective method.*
   - *Avoidance of corsets.*
2. *Use of gravity:*
   - *Avoid bending forward.*
   - *Sleep with the head of the bed propped up on bricks to prevent nocturnal reflux.*
   - *Do not lie down after meals.*
3. *Reduction of acid secretion in the stomach:*
   - *Avoid taking fluids with meals – eat "dry" meals.*
   - *Avoid acid-stimulating foods and irritants such as aspirin, alcohol and cigarettes.*
   - *Use antacids often, especially at bedtime.*

Surgical management

This is recommended only if symptoms persist in spite of adequate conservative treatment. Weight loss is the most important measure.

Surgery is also considered when complications such as stenosis and anaemia are already present. The operation of choice is a Nissan fundoplication. The gastric fundus is mobilized through an abdominal approach, pulled around the back and front of the lower oesophagus and sutured to form a valve. When pressure builds up in the stomach, it forces the lower end of the oesophagus closed and prevents reflux.

The Hill operation is similar. The lesser curvature of the stomach is pulled downwards to reduce the hernia and sutured to the dome of the diaphragm, over the aortic hiatus, to fix the stomach. The fundus is pulled anteriorly over the lower end of the oesophagus (a half-Nissan) and is also fixed.

In both operations, the crurae of the diaphragm are sutured.

If a stenosis is present, it is dilated. It may be necessary to repeat this a few times. If reflux is prevented, the stenosis will not re-form.

If the stenosis is fibrotic, it must be incised and the defect must be patched with gastric fundus, which is sutured onto it by means of a Nissan fundoplication. This is known as the Thal patching operation. It must be emphasized that the majority of stenoses can be dilated.

Patients are unable to vomit after a Nissan fundoplication and they sometimes complain of feeling bloated. A loose fundoplication, also called a "floppy" Nissan, allows for burbulence, but still controls reflux.

The rolling hernia

This is a herniation of the fundus through the diaphragm with the cardia in its normal position, thus reflux does not occur. Stasis can occur in the fundus in the hernia, with stasis ulceration and haemorrhage. Surgical repair is indicated. Rarely, a combination of sliding and rolling hiatus hernias is found. They are inclined to be irreducible and ought to be repaired surgically.

Sclerodermia

This is a collagen disease and a better name for it is systemic sclerosis, since, although skin involvement is usually the first manifestation of the disease and eventually occurs in 95% of cases, it is the involvement of the gastrointestinal tract, heart, lungs and kidneys which leads to serious complications. The disease occurs in women aged between thirty and fifty, who are affected three times more commonly than men.

The oesophagus is a common target organ. The smooth muscle of the distal two-thirds of the oesophagus atrophies, with loss of peristalsis and incompetence of the IOS. The patient complains of heartburn and dysphagia.

An early diagnosis can be made using pressure studies; later in the disease a barium meal will show a dilated oesophagus with stenosis and reflux. The disease follows a progressive course and must be treated symptomatically, as would the reflux of hiatus hernia. In selected cases, a Nissan fundoplication may be performed, following dilatation.

Other conditions

Diabetic and alcoholic neuropathy can cause hypoperistalsis. Other conditions include myasthenia gravis, myotonia dystrophica, polymyositis and dermatomyositis. These can all cause dysphagia.

Globus hystericus

This is a syndrome of dysphagia found in both young and older women. They complain of food sticking high in the throat. Psychological problems are often associated. Special investigations sometimes reveal spasm of the cricopharyngeal muscle.

B. TRAUMA

Swallowing foreign bodies

This is more common in children. Fish or chicken bones may be the cause in adults. If meat which has not been properly chewed sticks in the oesophagus, consider the presence of underlying disease.

Patients complain of dysphagia and salivation. If the foreign body sticks at the level of the cricopharyngeal muscle, it causes great discomfort. In adults, the foreign body often sticks in the distal end of the oesophagus.

The diagnosis is usually made on X-ray. The foreign body can be seen especially well on the lateral views. Look for free gas in the mediastinum which denotes perforation.

Management

Removal of the foreign body is not an urgent procedure unless it is sharp, or the patient experiences difficulty with respiration. If the foreign body lies in the distal oesophagus, sedate the patient and repeat X-rays a few hours later. Blunt objects and meat often pass through spontaneously.

Objects must be removed under general anaesthetic with a rigid oesophagoscope. In adults, this must be followed a few days later by a barium meal to exclude underlying pathology.

Perforations of the oesophagus

Common causes

- Rigid oesophagoscopy. This often occurs in older people when the neck is hyperextended. Osteophytes press on the oesophagus from behind when a foreign body is removed.
- Fibre-optic endoscopy. A rare cause, but it can happen when there is an unexpected pharyngeal diverticulum.
- Dilatation of strictures. Happens especially in malignant or long strictures.
- Foreign bodies.

Other causes

- Palliative intubation in carcinoma
- Vagotomy
- Sengstaken-Blakemore tube

Clinical presentation

There is usually a history of difficult endoscopy with slight bleeding after the procedure. Patients complain of pain, dysphagia and salivation. On examination, crepitus is palpable in the neck; and on X-ray air can be seen in the mediastinum or under the diaphragm. Patients have fever and leucocytosis.

Special investigations

- X-rays of the thorax and abdomen to show free air.
- Gastrografin to demonstrate leakage.

Determine the site and size of the perforation.

Management

Early diagnosis is important. Management depends on the time elapsed since perforation, the size of the perforation, the site of the perforation and whether there is underlying pathology.

Cervical perforation

Treat conservatively. Nil per os and antibiotics. Sometimes it may be necessary to drain an abscess.

Thoracic oesophageal perforation

If it is very small and extrapleural, without leakage on the gastrografin swallow, it can be treated conservatively. If it is larger and leaking intrapleurally, operate through a thoracic approach and suture the perforation, with drainage.

If there is an underlying carcinoma, resect it if possible, otherwise intubate. If the diagnosis is delayed for more than twelve hours, only an intercostal drain must be inserted and antibiotics administered. If the perforation is large, perform a cervical pharyngotomy and tie the oesophagus off temporarily.

Abdominal perforation

Always operate. Close the perforation and perform a Nissan fundoplication to patch the closure.

Spontaneous oesophageal rupture (Boerhaave syndrome)

This is a full thickness rupture of the oesophagogastric junction, usually after a rapid rise in intra-abdominal pressure, as caused by vomiting, labour or pressure on stooling. There is usually an underlying sphincter muscle incoordination caused by alcohol.

Clinical presentation

It is most often found in men over fifty. Severe pain, shock and slight haematemesis follow vomiting after severe alcohol abuse. Dysphagia, dyspnoea and cyanosis are found. A left-sided pneumothorax and cervical crepitus are present.

Special investigations

X-rays reveal haemopneumothorax and mediastinal emphysema. Gastrografin swallow demonstrates rupture.

Management

A thoracotomy must be performed immediately, with suturing of the tear and patching by means of a Nissan fundoplication, followed by underwater drainage. If the diagnosis is delayed, perform a cervical oesophagotomy, close the lower end of the oesophagus and insert an intercostal drain.

Give appropriate antibiotics and intravenous alimentation for a few weeks. Delayed diagnosis leads to increased mortality.

Bottletop explosion injuries of the pharynx

Children put dry ice into Coke bottles and close the top so tightly that it cannot be loosened. They then attempt to unscrew the top, with their teeth. An explosion takes place in the mouth, causing the following injuries:

- Laceration of the soft palate, tonsil bed and posterior pharynx due to the bottletop missile.
- Laryngeal, tracheal and oesophageal laceration with mediastinal emphysema or even pneumothorax as a result of the blast injury.

Management

Explore the neck and suture the pharyngeal lacerations. Tracheostomy may be necessary in laryngeal injuries. Endoscopy must be performed to exclude tracheal and oesophageal lacerations. Remember that a pneumothorax is possible and an intrathoracic underwater drain may be necessary.

Swallowing corrosive substances

Strong alkalis or acids are swallowed by accident or during suicide attempts. The strong alkali is usually caustic soda (NaOH) and the acids can be battery acid (H_2SO_4) or swimming pool acid (HCl). Alkalis cause liquidifying necrosis, while acids cause coagulation necrosis. Shock is usually absent. If pain and shock are present, consider a perforation. Burns on the lips or mouth do not necessarily mean that the oesophagus and stomach have also been burnt.

Management

Nothing should be given per os. It is not advisable to insert tubes for lavage. The treatment is as follows:

- *Establish an IV line and give analgesics.*
- *Although there is no definitive proof that they prevent strictures, steroids are given by most clinicians, namely hydrocortisone 200mg IV six-hourly. If the patient is able to swallow later, give prednisolone 1 mg/kg for three weeks.*
- *Give broad spectrum antibiotics and antifungal agents.*
- *Physiotherapy to minimize pulmonary complications.*
- *Do a careful oesophagoscopy to assess the extent of the lesion. If the lesion is small, stop the steroids.*
- *After ten days, a barium meal can be done to assess the oesophageal and gastric lesion fully. Alkalis usually cause oesophageal strictures and acids cause gastric strictures. Sometimes both the oesophagus and the stomach are affected. Single, short oesophageal strictures respond well to dilatation, which should be repeated often. If the strictures are too long or too extensive, bypass procedures may be considered. The colon is usually used for this purpose.*

There is an increased incidence of carcinoma in damaged oesophagus and this must be borne in mind during the follow-up period.

The gastric strictures can take on an hourglass appearance, or they can cause gastric outlet obstruction. A gastrogastrostomy can be performed for the hourglass strictures and a distal gastrectomy must be performed when there is gastric outlet obstruction.

Drugs and the oesophagus

Cases of pain and dysphagia have been described, due to ulceration of the oesophageal mucosa. Drugs which can cause this include aspirin, Cetiprin, tetracycline, 5-fluouracil and potassium chloride (Slow K). Drugs which are taken when the patient is lying down can remain in the oesophagus for a long time. Pills and powders must be swallowed with copious amounts of fluid.

C. TUMOURS OF THE OESOPHAGUS

Benign tumours

Leiomyomas and lipomas are rare tumours of the oesophagus that may sometimes cause dysphagia. They bulge into the lumen in barium meal, but the mucosa is intact on endoscopy.

Sometimes fibrovascular polyps, covered by normal squamous epithelium, develop, especially in the proximal third of the oesophagus. Duplication cysts of the oesophagus have also been described.

Malignant tumours

Carcinoma of the oesophagus has assumed epidemic proportions among black patients. The incidence is 100 or more per 100 000 of the population. In the Transkei, it forms 41% of tumours in men and 36% of tumours in women.

In training hospitals, it is the third most common reason for admission, following trauma and sepsis, and is the most important cause of hospital death. There is a fivefold increase per decade in the incidence of the disease.

Among whites, the disease occurs in 3,5 per 100 000 of the population.

Aetiology

The disease is more common in South Africa, China and Iran. It is more common in men, with an average age of sixty. Environmental factors which may play a role include mineral-deficient soil with high heavy metal content. Nutritional factors are also of importance, such as diets which are composed mainly of grain products and are deficient in proteins and vitamins, especially riboflavin, thiamine, nicotinic acid and vitamins A and C.

Carcinoma of the oesophagus is a disease of poverty and malnutrition. Alcohol and tobacco have been considered as causative agents, but these would not apply in Iran. Contamination of grain products with fungi and the development of nitrosamines have also been singled out, but there is not definite proof.

Viruses, such as human papilloma virus and herpes virus, may be involved. The rapid increase in the incidence of the disease in urban blacks suggest a possible contagious causative agent.

Premalignant conditions associated with the disease in whites include irradiation, corrosive substances, chronic iron deficiency (Plummer-Vinson syndrome), achalasia, scleroderma and Barrett oesophagus.

Pathology

Site of occurrence

- 20% are found in the proximal third
- 50% occur in the middle third
- 30% are found in the distal third

In whites, it is often postulated that most tumours are found in the distal third, but this includes adenocarcinomas, which originate in the stomach.

Macroscopic types

- Infiltrating. An infiltrating, stenosing lesion with ulceration is the most common type.
- Fungating lesion. The tumour presents as an irregular filling defect on a barium meal.
- An ulcer. An ulcer is found with typical raised, rolled edges. It also infiltrates the wall, with stenosis.

Microscopic picture

- Squamous carcinoma (95%). Tumours range from well-differentiated with central keratinization and pearl formation, to poorly differentiated with pleomorphism and many mitotic figures.
- Adenocarcinoma. At the distal end, it is usually gastric carcinoma which affects the oesophagus. Adenocarcinoma may arise in Barrett's oesophagus, submucosal glands and islands of gastric mucosa. Rare variants include adeno-cystic and muco-epidermoid tumours.
- Adeno-acanthoma. Rare mixed squamous and adenoid tumours.
- Poorly differentiated. Consist of strings of small dark cells which resemble oat cell tumour of the lung.
- Miscellaneous: Leiomyosarcoma. Carcinoid. Melanoma.

Spread

- **Intra-oesophageal spread**: Tumours are inclined to spread adjacent to submucosal lymphatic vessels. They most commonly spread proximal to the wound, to as far as 10 cm. Distal spread does not usually extend as far.
- **Extra-oesophageal spread**: Tumours spread to the adjacent trachea and bronchi. Ten per cent of cases already have fistula on admission. Spread also occurs to fascia, thyroid, carotid sheath and vertebrae.
- **Lymphatic spread**: More than 50% of patients already have lymph node involvement on admission. Spread takes place to the para-oesophageal, peri-oesophageal and lateral oesophageal lymph nodes. Postoperative survival is directly linked to lymph node involvement.
- **Blood spread**: It spreads to the lungs, liver, bone and brain at a later stage.

In black patients, about 10% of cases are limited to the oesophagus at the time of diagnosis. If the resected specimen is examined later, spread beyond the oesophagus has already taken place in most cases.

Clinical presentation

Patients usually present with swallowing problems. This means that the disease is already advanced. The early symptoms and signs of pain, regurgitation of food and saliva can be elicited on thorough enquiry . The presentation of the more advanced disease is more typical, with pain, dysphagia and loss of weight. Later, pulmonary infections follow, with hoarseness and sometimes haemoptysis and haematemesis.

On clinical examination, physical signs, other than emaciation, are seldom found.

Special investigations

- **Chest X-rays:** A soft tissue mass, with an obscured trachea, may be seen. There are signs of pulmonary infection and later, metastases.
- **Barium meal:** Irregular narrowing and a rat's tail appearance are typical signs. The proximal oesophagus is slightly dilated and there may be shoulder formation.

The fungating mass appears as a series of filling defects, often with ulceration on its surface. An isolated malignant ulcer is a rare finding. The early sign of a slightly irregular mucosa, as described by the Japanese, is rare in black patients.

A barium meal is the best method of assessing the status of the disease and feasibility of surgery. If the long axis of the oesophagus is preserved on both AP and lateral views, the tumour is probably resectible. If the axis is disturbed, it usually means that infiltration has taken place outside the oesophagus, causing distortion. Other signs of advanced disease include tracheo-oesophageal fistula, a mediastinal sinus and a tumour longer than 10 cm.

- **Oesophagoscopy:** This must always be performed to make a histological diagnosis, to determine the level of the tumour and to assess the fixity of the tumour.
- **Bronchoscopy:** This must also always be done. Oedema and contact bleeding indicate tracheal infiltration. Distortion and obvious infiltration indicate advanced disease. Flattening of the carina indicates lymph node metastases.
- **Computer tomography and ultrasound:** Computer tomography is useful to demonstrate spread outside the oesophagus into the mediastinum. It is also useful in showing infiltration of gastric and coeliac lymph nodes. Liver metastases are also diagnosed by this test.

In black patients who are emaciated and have no remaining fatty tissue, CT is not very helpful. Ultrasound can contribute.

- **Lymph node biopsy:** Biopsy of the supraclavicular or palpable cervical lymph nodes can be useful in diagnosing spread of the disease.
- **Mediastinoscopy and laparotomy:** This is not undertaken very often these days, as noninvasive investigations, particularly CT, provide similar information.
- **Other investigations:** Fluid and electrolyte balance, renal functions and nutritional status of the patient must be determined to assess how much preoperative preparation is necessary or whether the patient is more suited to palliative intubation.

In a patient with dysphagia and an oesophageal stricture, carcinoma must always be considered and must be differentiated from:

- reflux oesophagitis with stenosis
- achalasia
- corrosive substances
- webs

Management of oesophageal carcinoma

The aims of management are to:

- *restore the ability to swallow*
- *heal the disease*

Restore the ability to swallow

The best way to restore the swallowing ability is undoubtedly to resect an early lesion totally and restore continuity. Unfortunately, such early lesions are extremely rare.

A second possible method is to heal the disease by radical irradiation.

The third possible way of effecting healing is multimodality management – surgery, irradiation and chemotherapy. There is no real documented proof that the addition of irradiation and chemotherapy improves healing.

Heal the disease

Three factors play a role in deciding what form of treatment is to be used:

- *The general condition of the patient.*
- *The site of the tumour.*
- *The pattern of spread of the tumour.*

Factors which influence management

The general condition of the patient

Before resection and restoration of continuity can be considered, the patient must either be fit or be made fit for surgery. The nutritional status must be improved, with hyperalimentation if necessary. Intensive physiotherapy and antibiotics may be necessary to improve the lung functions. The general condition of the patient will greatly influence the decision whether to perform a bypass or only palliative intubation.

The site of the tumour

If it is situated in the cervical part of the oesophagus, a curative operation will mean that the larynx must also be removed. Cervical carcinoma is usually treated by irradiation. In midthoracic and distal oesophageal lesions, surgical removal must be considered.

Spread

If there are no signs of spread to be found beyond the oesophagus and the patient is fit for surgery, the lesion must be resected and continuity restored. If there are already signs of spread and the patient is fit for surgery, a surgical bypass must be peformed. If there are signs of spread and the patient is not fit for a bypass, intubation must be performed.

There are differing opinions as to which method offers the best palliation; intubation or bypass. If very advanced metastases are present, intubation is preferable, regardless of the general condition of the patient, because survival is less than six months.

Principles of surgical procedures

A prominent characteristic of carcinoma of the oesophagus is the fact that it spreads extensively proximally in the submucosa. At least 10 cm of macroscopically normal oesophagus must be removed proximal to the lesion, to ensure that no incision is made through microscopic spread of the carcinoma.

Carcinoma of the distal end of the oesophagus

Squamous carcinoma

Since it is a carcinoma of the oesophagus, the oesophagus must be cut through at the level of the arch of the aorta. This means that two incisions are necessary for exposure. First, a laparotomy is peformed, and the upper two-thirds of the stomach are dissected for resection. Then a right-sided thoracotomy is performed to cut through the oesophagus at the level of the aortic arch. Two-thirds of the stomach and its lymphatic drainage, plus the oesophagus, are resected up to the aortic arch, and the distal one-third of the stomach, after mobilization, is pulled up into the thorax to be joined to the oesophagus.

Carcinoma of the thoracic oesophagus

This operation involves a triple-incision approach:

- *Laparotomy to mobilize the stomach.*
- *A right-sided thoracotomy to mobilize the thoracic oesophagus.*
- *A right-sided cervical approach to prepare the cervical oesophagus for anastomosis to the stomach, which has been pulled up.*

Opinions differ as to whether pyloroplasty should be performed, as gastric stasis sometimes occurs. Although this causes problems in only a minority of cases, it is probably still advisable to prevent it.

Transhiatal oesophagectomy

Only a laparotomy and cervical approach are used in this operation and the oesophagus is mobilized transhiatally by means of blunt finger dissection in the thoracic cavity. Surprisingly few problems occur with postoperative haemorrhage.

Surgical bypass procedures

The bypass of choice is to suture the entire stomach to the cervical oesophagus. The stomach is pulled upwards through a retrosternal tunnel. The distal and proximal oesophagus are closed, except in cases where an oesophagotracheal fistula is already present. In these cases, the distal oesophagus is drained by suturing it to a Roux small intestine loop, thus resolving infection of the respiratory tract.

Intubation

If the patient is not fit for bypass, or if there is extensive metastasis, intubation is performed.

Pulsion intubation

Indications

Lesions of the upper and middle third: The tube of choice is the Proctor-Livingstone tube, which is inserted from above with a rigid oesophagoscope, following dilatation of the lesion.

Traction intubation

Indications

Lesions of the distal third: *A laparotomy and an oesophagoscopy are performed simultaneously. A guide is passed from above through the lesion into the oesophagus and a tube is pulled through into the stomach. The Celestin tube is most commonly used. The tube is fixed in the stomach.*

Other treatment alternatives

Radiotherapy

This does not improve the lot of patients who have tubes in situ. *Patients are usually able to swallow reasonably well as long as a semi-solid and liquid diet is followed. The tube can migrate to the stomach. Often patients develop pressure necrosis, with fistula formation. Survival averages six months. Radiotherapy can be useful in patients with advanced local lesions which are inoperable, but it does not improve survival in patients with metastases.*

Chemotherapy

Several drugs have been shown to be effective against these tumours. Bleomycin, adriamycin, cisplatinum, methotrexate, 5-fluouracil, vindecine and vincristine have all been tried.

Bleomycin elicited a response in over 20% of cases, with slightly prolonged life expectancy. Multidrug response is better, but the risk of toxicity is increased.

The nutrition of patients on radiotheraphy and chemotherapy must be attended to and improved.

Laser treatment

Laser resection may be useful in the rarer fungating lesions.

Prognosis

Less than 10% of black patients present with lesions which have not spread at all. Less than 50% of patients are fit, or can be made fit, for resection or bypass surgery. The operation mortality of curative operations is about 10%. The mortality of bypass operations (sicker patients, more advanced lesions) is about 12%.

The mortality for intubation procedures (even sicker patients, or even more advanced disease) is 15% for pulsion tubes and 21% for traction tubes.

The five year survival rate of black patients who have undergone curative resection, is less than 10%. In white patients, the prognosis is somewhat better. Figures as high as 35% have been reported in the literature.

Gastrostomy

This form of palliation must be used only in exceptional cases, where nothing else is possible. This does not solve the main problem, dysphagia, and patients usually die of the complications of aspiration.

D: MISCELLANEOUS CONDITIONS

Infections

Moniliasis

This is common in immunosuppressed patients or in patients who have been treated with longterm oral antibiotics.

Clinical presentation

Patients complain of painful dysphagia. A barium meal shows ulceration and a cobblestone appearance. Oesophagoscopy demonstrates white lesions and candida organisms can be seen on curettage.

Management

Terminate immunosuppression and antibiotics if possible. Give oral nystatin, suspended in water, hourly. If no response is noted, give amphoteracin lozenges.

Herpes viruses

These cause ulceration of the mucus membranes in immunosuppressed patients.

Management

Terminate immunosuppression, if possible. Administer acyclovir.

Sideropaenic dysphagia (Patterson-Kelly syndrome, Plummer-Vinson syndrome

Aetiology

Changes take place in the oesophageal mucosa, and lead to web formation. These changes are often associated with iron-deficiency anaemia, but this is not always the case.

Pathology

Mucosal atrophy, basal cell hyperplasia and hyperchromatism of cell nuclei, with fibrosis and lymphocytic infiltration, take place. A web usually forms at the upper oesophageal sphincter.

Clinical presentation

Patients complain of dysphagia and choking. Examination reveals atrophy of the tongue, koilonychia and anaemia.

Special investigations

A barium meal demonstrates the web which arises from the anterior wall of the upper oesophagus. Oesophagoscopy must be performed to exclude carcinoma. Usually the membrane is perforated by the instrument.

Management

Treat the underlying anaemia. Dilate the web. Follow up annually with oesophagoscopy and exclude carcinoma with biopsy or brush cytology.

External pressure on the oesophagus

Conditions which can cause dysphagia due to external pressure include:

- Enlarged nodular thyroid, vascular anomalies (dysphagia lusoria), aneurysm of the great vessels.
- Tumours of the bronchus.
- Tumours of the lymph nodes in the bronchial mediastinum.
- Osteophytes of the vertebral column.

Stomach and duodenum 3

What does the patient complain of?

Pain

The patient often presents with no symptoms other than pain. The exploration of the nature of this symptom is therefore of cardinal importance.

Site

The patient will usually indicate the upper abdominal area. On further enquiry, it is often possible to localize the pain to the epigastrium. The patient can also sometimes say whether the pain is deep or superficial. The most important point is to determine whether it really is an upper abdominal pain, which narrows the diagnosis down to stomach, duodenum, biliary tract and pancreas.

Onset of the pain

Was it sudden or gradual? A sudden, very severe pain in the epigastrium, which becomes worse and is still present, usually suggests a perforated peptic ulcer. Differentiate this from pain which begins gradually and develops over a long period. Pain caused by inflammation or malignant conditions has a gradual onset and becomes worse over a shorter or longer period.

Intensity of the pain

A perforated peptic ulcer causes extremely severe pain. A good way of judging the severity of the pain is by determining whether it wakes the patient and keeps him awake, whether it prevents him from going to work and whether it impels him to consult a doctor or go to a hospital. A pain which forces a patient to see his doctor, or, even more importantly, makes him come to a hospital, is a pain which indicates organic disease.

The nature of the pain

Gastrointestinal pain has two main causes, namely inflammation of the tissue, which causes a persistent, burning pain; or stabbing pain and partial or complete obstruction of a hollow organ, which causes intermittent cramping pain, that does not disappear entirely (colic). Peptic ulcer causes a vague, burning, epigastric pain, which is described as indigestion, or a more severe, persistent, nagging pain. Carcinoma can be painless or it can cause a nagging, persistent, dull pain.

Further progression of the pain

A pain which begins, becomes worse and is still present when the patient consults his doctor, has an underlying organic cause.

Functional pain has usually disappeared by the time the patient consults his doctor.

Factors which influence the pain

- What exacerbates the pain? Eating aggravates the pain – consider a gastric ulcer. Movement aggravates it – consider a perforated peptic ulcer.

- What alleviates the pain? Eating alleviates the pain – consider a duodenal ulcer. Food buffers the acid which irritates the ulcer.

Antacids alleviate the pain – both gastric and duodenal ulcer pain are relieved by antacids.

The pain of carcinoma does not improve. Vomiting relieves the pain – consider a gastric ulcer.

Radiation of pain

Radiation of pain means that the original pain is still present but has extended to an adjacent area. This usually means that inflammation has spread. The pain from a penetrating gastric or duodenal ulcer radiates to the back.

Vomiting

How often does the patient vomit? What is the nature and volume? Does it happen shortly after meals?

If the patient vomits after meals, especially to relieve pain and discomfort, consider a gastric ulcer. If the patient vomits old food every second or third day, consider gastric outlet obstruction. This is caused by peptic ulceration or by carcinoma.

If the patient vomits bile, consider bile reflux. This can occur spontaneously in patients who have a gastric ulcer, or it can be a complication of previous gastric surgery.

Haematemesis

Has the patient vomited blood? Large amounts of blood, preceded by nausea, suggest a peptic ulcer, gastric mucosal erosions, or oesophageal varices.

Small amounts of red blood can suggest a milder haemorrhage due to the same conditions. Also consider carcinoma. Visible haematemesis due to carcinoma is rare.

Coffee ground vomiting

This is old blood, of relatively small proportions, which has been in the stomach for quite some time and has already formed acid haematin.

Change in appetite

Has there been a decrease in appetite? Is this due to a loss of appetite or a fear of eating because it causes pain? Have certain food preferences or dislikes developed?

If there is a fear of eating because it causes discomfort or even pain, consider a gastric ulcer. If food alleviates the pain and there is thus a tendency to eat more often, consider a duodenal ulcer. If there is total loss of appetite, consider gastric carcinoma. If there is a particular distate for meat, consider gastric carcinoma.

Indigestion and flatulence

Indigestion is a term which is used loosely by patients to describe a variety of symptoms such as pain, discomfort after meals, heartburn and regurgitation.

Flatulence is discomfort in the upper abdomen and a tendency to break wind. The entire symptom complex, which centres the clinician's attention on conditions of the stomach, duodenum, biliary tract and pancreas, is nonspecific. Such patients must be investigated further.

Melaena

The patient complains of having passed black, tarry stools. Only 50 ml of blood from the stomach or duodenum is necessary to produce a melaena stool. This is ascribed to production of acid haematin by the action of gastric acid on haemoglobin and the production of sulphides by the action of hydrogen sulphide on the iron in the haem molecule.

If a large bleed has taken place, more than 1 000 ml, the patient can continue to pass melaena stools for up to five days afterwards and, in the absence of other signs, this does not necessarily indicate continued bleeding.

Other causes of black stools, such as certain types of food and preparations containing iron, must be borne in mind. Melaena stools imply haemorrhage from the oesophagus, stomach or duodenum. If a large, rapid bleed takes place, the patient can pass blood clots which have not yet undergone changes.

What does the clinician find on examination

There is relatively little to find on clinical examination. Tenderness on deep palpation of the epigastrium is often the only positive sign and is nonspecific. A vague mass is sometimes palpable. This indicates a gastric carcinoma.

A distended stomach may be visible and peristalsis is also sometimes visible. Succussion may be elicited. This indicates gastric outlet obstruction, usually due to a peptic ulcer. In carcinoma, the stomach is not usually overly distended.

Enlarged supraclavicular nodes (Virchow-Troisier nodes) are indicative of gastric carcinoma.

Special investigations

- **Fibre-optic endoscopy:** Patients with symptoms suggestive of gastric or duodenal pathology must be examined endoscopically. Multiple biopsies must be taken of any lesion encountered.
- **Barium meal:** This must be performed where endoscopy is not available. A barium meal is also useful in providing information about gastric function.
- **Acid secretion in the stomach:** Basic and stimulated acid secretion are useful in diagnosing Zollinger-Ellison syndrome and gastric carcinoma (achlorhydria).
- **Gastrin measurements:** Useful in the diagnosis of Z-E syndrome.
- **Gastric emptying studies:** Studies using radioisotope methods are especially useful in postgastrectomy syndrome.

Classification of gastric and duodenal disease

It is convenient to classify these diseases according to their importance and incidence, as encountered in surgical practice.

A. Benign ulcers of the stomach and duodenum

- Peptic ulcer
- Gastric ulcer
- Duodenal ulcer
- Stomal ulcer
- Zollinger-Ellison syndrome
- Stress ulcer

B. Tumours

Benign tumours

- Hyperplastic polyps
- Adenoma
- Leiomyoma

Malignant tumours

- Carcinoma
- Lymphoma
- Leiomyosarcoma
- Carcinoid

C. Miscellaneous

- Giant mucosal folds of the stomach
- Bezoars
- Gastric volvulus
- Gastric and duodenal diverticula

BENIGN ULCERS

Peptic ulcer

There has been a definite decrease in the incidence of peptic ulcer in the western world. The incidence is now 50% of what it was thirty years ago. This decrease is largely attributable to a decrease in the incidence of duodenal ulcer.

Peptic ulcer is found in a 3 : 1 ratio in men as compared to women. The ratio in duodenal ulcer (DU) is 4 : 1, while in gastric ulcer (GU) it is 2 : 1. In Pretoria, the incidence of peptic ulcer in men as opposed to women is only 1,3 : 1. The ration between DU and GU is 2 :1 for men and 1 : 1,2 for women.

Gastric ulcer

Aetiology

A gastric ulcer is probably the result of normal acid and pepsin attacking the mucosa, the normal defence mechanisms of which have been damaged. Acid levels are usually normal or subnormal in patients with gastric ulcers.

Theories to explain the change in resistance of the gastric mucosa

Reflux gastritis (Du Plessis)

If the duodenal contents, comprising a mixture of bile and pancreatic juices, reflux into the stomach through the pylorus and remain there for some time, chronic gastritis developes. The extent of the chronic gastritis varies. Ulcers always arise at the boundary between the gastritis and the normal acid-producing mucosa. The higher the area of gastritis extends up the lesser curvature of the stomach, the less acid the stomach secretes. If the patient presents with gastric acid secretion which is lower than normal, it can be predicted that the ulcer is situated high up on the lesser curvature.

It is not known why the pylorus is incompetent in certain patients, but there are indications that in these patients, it does not react normally to stimuli such as secretin and cholecystokinin.

The gastric stasis theory (Dragstedt)

Chronic irritation of the gastric mucosa, due to stasis of gastric contents, causes gastritis, which lowers the resistance of the gastric mucosa. Patients with delayed gastric emptying due to duodenal ulcers do develop secondary gastric ulcers. In an ordinary gastric ulcer, no clear reason can usually be found for delayed gastric emptying.

Damage to the mucosa by drugs and other irritants

This is caused by damage to the lipoprotein layer of the epithelial cells; by influencing the cell turnover due to suppression of bicarbonate secretion; and by stimulation of acid secretion. Drugs which play a role include aspirin and indomethacin. Smoking may also play a part.

Clinical presentation

This condition is common in middle-aged men and women. The patient complains of epigastric pain which comes on after meals. The pain is relieved by antacids. There is often a history of similar episodes which lasted for a few weeks and then disappeared for a few months. On examination, the patient is usually found to be thin, with deep tenderness on palpation of the epigastrium.

Special investigations

Barium meal

This will show an ulcer, usually situated on the lesser curvature of the stomach. The ulcer may also lie prepylorically or in the pyloric canal. Sometimes the ulcer is found very high up on the lesser curvature. A gastric ulcer must be differentiated from a malignant gastric ulcer. The following are useful characteristics to note on barium meal:

- **Size:** The larger the ulcer, the more likely it is to be a carcinoma. Large benign gastric ulcers are also found on the lesser curvature.
- **Site:** Although most carcinomas are found on the lesser curvature, as are benign ulcers, an ulcer situated away from the lesser curvature, eg on the greater curvature, is more likely to be malignant.
- **Ulcer crater:** The ulcer crater of a benign ulcer extends beyond the lesser curvature, because a benign ulcer tends to penetrate through the normal gastric wall. A malignant ulcer arises in an underlying tumour. The crater does not therefore extend beyond the silhouette of the lesser curvature, but does have raised edges.
- **The mucosa around a benign ulcer:** The mucosal folds run into an ulcer crater. Inflammation tucks the folds into the crater. The folds around a carcinoma do not run into the crater, because the mucosa around the crater is infiltrated by tumour.

Endoscopy

Fibre-optic endoscopy is essential to show the nature of the ulcer and to take multiple biopsies to exclude carcinoma.

Measurement of gastric acid

A carcinoma must be strongly suspected when achlorhydria is present.

Duodenal ulcer

Aetiology

It has been generally accepted that DU is a disease of acid hypersecretion. The details are not watertight, but the following findings have been described:

- As a group, patients with DU secrete more acid than normal patients. This applies to both the basal and stimulated acid secretion. This is ascribed to an increased parietal cell mass. Following pentagastrin stimulation about 50% of patients secrete more acid than the upper limit of normal patients.

- It has also been found that patients with DU have a lower gastric juice pH for longer periods of time than normal patients.
- It can thus be broadly postulated that, as a group, patients with DU secrete more acid, but that most DU patients secrete acid at levels which fall within two standard deviations of the average acid secretion of normal patients.

Campylobacter pylori

There has recently been a lot of interest in the role that this bacterium plays in the aetiology of duodenal ulcer. The bacterium can be demonstrated in the gastric mucosa of certain patients. It has been suggested that the presence of this bacterium plays a role in the high recurrence rate, following healing on H_2 receptor antagonists, found in some patients with DU.

Clinical presentation

This ulcer is more common in younger patients and is found more often in men than in women. The presenting complaint is epigastric pain which begins two to three hours after meals. The pain can wake the patient at night. The pain is relieved by eating and antacids. Patients are often overweight, because eating relieves the pain.

The symptoms tend to persist for a month or two and then disappear completely for a few months.

Special investigations

- **Barium meal:** This reveals an ulcer crater in the duodenal cap (first part of the duodenum). Sometimes the cap is deformed due to spasm secondary to the inflammation.
- **Endoscopy:** This confirms the diagnosis but is not essential as malignancy is not a problem in these cases.
- **Acid measurements:** These are not of any practical importance.

Management of peptic ulcer

The management of DU and GU will be discussed together, in order to compare and contrast the two.

Peptic ulcer must be treated conservatively, provided certain conditions are met. If a gastric ulcer is diagnosed, endoscopy must be performed and the benign nature of the ulcer must be confirmed histologically. If there are no complications and the patient has never before been properly and intensively treated by conservative methods, medical treatment must be commenced. Remember that 40% of peptic ulcers heal spontaneously after six weeks of placebo administration. They also tend to heal and then recur in a cyclical manner.

General principles

In the past, much emphasis was placed on dietary advice. Frequent intake of soft, bland foods throughout the day was often recommended. The buffering action of this food on the gastric acid was supposed to contribute to healing. There is no proof that this approach helps in healing ulcers. These days, three normal meals per day are recommended.

Smoking and alcohol are forbidden.

There is no doubt that bedrest heals ulcers, but this advice is not readily accepted by patients nowadays.

Acid supression

Parietal cells, which secrete acid, have H_2 (histaminic), gastrin, M_2 (muscarinic) and probably prostaglandin receptors on their surfaces. These receptors all play a role in acid secretion. There are two basic approaches to reducing acid in the stomach and duodenum. The acid can be neutralized by antacids, or acid secretion can be inhibited by receptor antagonists.

Antacids

Fifteen ml of liquid antacid neutralizes four hours of basal and one hour of maximal gastric acid secretion. Thirty ml of liquid antacid per day provides a 1007 m.eq neutralizing capacity and can heal just as many ulcers as the H_2 receptor antagonists can. Antacids are inconvenient for the patient (large bottles to carry around) and cause constipation.

Antacids containing magnesium hydroxide (Merasyn) prevent constipation. Antacids which contain aluminium hydroxide (Mucaine, Aludrox) tend to cause constipation. There is definitely still a place for antacids in the treatment of patients with mild symptoms and unproven peptic ulceration.

Receptor antagonists

Stimulation of H_2, gastrin and M_2 receptors activates the second messenger systems, which stimulate the H^+, K^+, ATP-ase proton pump to secrete acid. Antogonists to each of these receptors already exist and also a coupling antagonist to the H^+, K^+, ATP-ase proton pump.

H_2 receptor antagonists

- Cimetidine *(Tagemet). Dosage: 400 mg twice daily. This drug heals 80% of DU's and 70% of GU's after six weeks of treatment. Side effects which have been described include gynaecomastia and hyperprolactinaemia, raised liver enzymes and inhibition of the cytochrome P450 system, which has lead to interactions with Diazepam and Warfarin. Confusion and even toxic psychosis have been described in elderly people. Rash and diarrhoea are possible. These side effects are only found at high dosages and the drug can be regarded as very safe.*
- Rinitidine *(Zantac). Dosage: 150 mg twice daily. It heals 80% of DU's and 70% of GU's within six weeks. Side effects are rarer. Rinitidine also binds the cytochrome P450 system, but to a lesser degree. Headache and diarrhoea have been described. Both these drugs are convenient and easy to use.*

  Other H_2 receptor antagonists such as Famatodine and Nizatidine are now available in South Africa.
- M_2 receptor antagonists. *Pirenzepine tablets. Dosage: 50 mg twice daily. They block the muscarinic cholinergic receptors, inhibit acid production and heal ulcers.*

  The side effects – dry mouth and blurred vision – make the drug unacceptable.
- Gastric receptors. *There are no antagonists available to these.*
- Prostaglandin receptors. *These receptors have not yet been irrefutably proven, but there is every indication that they do exist. The synthetic prostaglandins (Misoprostol) heal ulcers just as effectively as the H_2 receptor antagonists. They work in two ways. They inhibit acid secretion and play a role in protecting the cells.*
- Proton pump antagonists. *Omeprozole. Dosage: 20 mg in the morning (single dose). The drug turns off the total H^+, K^+, ATP-ase proton pump, inhibiting acid production almost entirely. Eighty percent of DU's are healed within two weeks.*

Mucosal protectants

The disadvantage of this group of drugs is that they must be taken on an empty stomach, which may be inconvenient for the patient.

- Sucralphate *(Ulsanic). Dosage: 1 g half-an-hour before meals and in the evenings. The drug heals 80% of DU's and GU's within six weeks. It works by coating the ulcer and also neutralizes acid. Side effects such as nausea and constipation do occur.*
- Colloidal bismuth *(BCP, De Nol, Ulcerone). Dosage: 5 ml four times daily, half-an-hour before meals and in the evenings. It heals 80% of peptic ulcers within six weeks. The drug has an unpleasant ammonia-like smell and causes black discolouration of the tongue and stools. There are also doubts about long-term treatment because of the possible dangers of bismuth absorption.*
- Carbenoxolone *(Biogastrone). This drug probably works via a prostaglandin mechanism. It stimulates mucus secretion and has cytoprotective properties. It heals peptic ulcers, especially GU's, just as effectively as the H_2 receptor antagonists, but is not really used because of severe side effects. It has a mineralocorticoid effect, causing water retention and encouraging potassium loss, thus causing hypokalaemia.*

The natural course of a duodenal ulcer when treated

The diagnosis is usually confirmed by endoscopy. The patient is put onto a course of Tagemet or Zantac. Symptoms usually disappear within a few days, but the course must be completed (six weeks). The ulcer heals in 80% of cases. If the patient falls into the 20% group which does not heal, full treatment must be continued for three months. Some patients heal after more prolonged treatment.

If the ulcer still does not heal, there are two alternatives. Further medical treatment with sucralfate or colloidal bismuth can be attempted, or an operation can be performed in this select group. Surgery is preferable.

If the patient falls into the group who have healed on H_2 receptor antagonists, the treatment must be terminated after six weeks and the patient must be followed up. Twenty per cent of these patients will have no further trouble from their ulcers. The ulcer will recur within a year in the majority of patients and within three years in another group. The natural tendency of peptic ulcers is to recur cyclically after having healed on treatment. Endoscopy must be peformed first to confirm that the symptoms are due to a recurrent ulcer, before the patient is treated again with an H_2 receptor antagonist, until the ulcer has healed.

Patients with early recurrence are placed on long-term maitenance doses. Cimetedine, 400 mg, is given in the evenings. Even on a maintenance dose, 40% of the ulcers recur within the following year. There are two alternatives nowadays. Patients can be placed on full dosages or the treatment can be changed to sucralfate or colloidal bismuth. There are indications that the recurrence rate is greater in patients who test positive for *Helicobacter pylori* on gastric mucosal biopsies. There is a lower recurrence rate in these patients if they are treated with colloidal bismuth (De Nol).

The second alternative is surgery.

In patients who remain healed for years, each recurrent ulcer can be regarded as a new ulcer and can be treated with a full course of H_2 receptor antagonists until healed. The treatment can then be withdrawn in the expectation that the ulcer will remain healed again for years.

In practice, surgery is only performed on patients who do not heal, or who do not remain healed on maintenance doses of H_2 receptor antagonists. About 40% of patients with DU will undergo surgery within two years.

Operations which can be performed for peptic ulcers

The aim is to reduce acid secretion and, when necessary, to remove damaged mucosa, including the peptic ulcer itself. Acid secretion takes place in the body of the stomach under the stimulus of the vagus nerve and gastrin, which is secreted in the antrum of the stomach.

Gastrectomy

This operation involves the partial removal of the distal stomach, which includes the pylorus and antrum (gastrin secretion) and a part of the parietal cell mass (acid secretion).

After part of the stomach has been removed, continuity must be restored. This can be achieved by suturing the open duodenal stump to the stomach so that food passes directly from the remainder of the stomach into the duodenum (Bilroth I anastomosis).

The Bilroth I gastrectomy is the operation of choice for a gastric ulcer. It is an extremely successful operation, because it reduces acid secretion (removal of the gastrin-producing antrum and part of the parietal cell mass). It removes the gastritis segment of the gastric mucosa and the ulcer and it improves gastric emptying (pylorus also removed). It retains normal physiology to a certain extent, in that food mixes normally with the duodenal contents.

If a gastrectomy has to be done higher up to remove the ulcer, or if the open duodenal stump is not suitable for anastomosis, the stump can be closed and a loop of jejunum sutured to the remaining gastric stump (Bilroth II anastomosis).

The B II gastrectomy is very seldom performed for a peptic ulcer, because it is less physiological and postgastrectomy syndromes occur more often. It is the operation of choice for gastric carcinoma. It is only considered for peptic ulcer if the anatomical problems already discussed make it necessary.

Vagotomy

Severance of the vagus nerve supply to the stomach reduces acid secretion and the motor function of gastric emptying. If the vagus is totally severed (truncal vagotomy), a drainage procedure, pyloroplasty or gastro-enterostomy, must be done concomitantly to prevent the annoying problem of gastric stasis.

If one severs the vagal supply only to that part of the stomach which secretes acid and preserves the nerve supply to the distal antrum – pylorus area (Latarjet's nerve), it is not necessary to do a drainage procedure because the stomach can still be emptied adequately by the action of the pyloroantral pump mechanism.

- **Truncal vagotomy and drainage**

The left (anterior) and right (posterior) vagus nerves are severed on the abdominal oesophagus. Usually a Heineke-Mikulicz pyloroplasty is done concomitantly. The pylorus is cut lengthwise and sutured transversely. A posterior gastro-enterostomy can be used as an alternative drainage procedure. The gastro-enterostomy is done to the distal antrum near the pylorus to effect good drainage of the antrum.

- **Truncal vagotomy and antrectomy**

The two trunks of the vagus are severed. An antrectomy is then performed, and if the duodenal stump is suitable, a B I anastomosis is done. If the stump is not suitable for anastomosis, it must be closed and the operation completed by means of a B II anastomosis.

- **Highly selective vagotomy**

The anterior and posterior vagus nerves are dissected out on the oesophagus, with care being taken not to damage them. Latarjet's nerves are spared anteriorly and posteriorly where they descend in the gastric omentum to end as crow's foot branches supplying the pyloroantral pump.

The small branches between Latarjet's nerve and the lesser curvature of the stomach, which supply the parietal cell mass, which secretes acid, must all be carefully identified and severed. Because the nerve supply to the pyloroantral pump remains intact, a drainage procedure is not necessary.

Choice between the three operations

Technically, a truncal vagotomy and pyloroplasty is the easiest operation.

The mortality is lower than 1%, but the recurrence rate is 10%. Truncal vagotomy and antrectomy has a mortality of about 2%, but the recurrence rate is lower than 2%. Postgastrectomy syndrome follows more commonly than after truncal vagotomy and pyloroplasty.

A highly selective vagotomy is a difficult and time-consuming operation. The mortality is less than 0,5%. Postgastrectomy syndrome virtually never occurs, but the ulcer recurrence rate is more than 10%.

Our standard operation for DU is a truncal vagotomy and pyloroplasty. We prefer truncal vagotomy and antrectomy for pyloric canal ulcers. Highly selective vagotomy is preferable in young women and thin patients.

Other operations

- *The Madlener-Kelly gastrectomy. The ulcer is so close to the cardia that a high B II gastrectomy is not possible. A B II gastrectomy is peformed distal to the ulcer. The ulcer usually heals spontaneously following this procedure.*
- *The Pauchet manoeuvre. The ulcer is situated high up on the lesser curvature. In order to remove it, the entire lesser curvature must be removed up to the cardia and a new lesser curvature is created by rotating the stomach.*

Complications of peptic ulcer

Upper gastrointestinal tract haemorrhage

Peptic ulcer is the most common cause of this acute emergency. More than half of these patients will bleed because of a DU or GU.

The second most common cause (20%) is gastric erosion.

Oesophageal varices cause about 10% of cases.

The remainder of haemorrhages are caused by Mallory-Weiss tears of the mucosa at the cardia, tumours (leiomyoma or carcinoma) and, in a small percentage, the cause is never found. Because the treatment of each of these conditions differs, it is important to make a definitive diagnosis.

Clinical presentation

History

The patient may provide a history of a previously confirmed diagnosis of a peptic ulcer. There may also be a history of chronic alcohol abuse (portal hypertension with varices) or analgesic abuse (gastric mucosal erosions).

Consider Mallory-Weiss tears if the patient vomited gastric contents first, and then blood.

Clinical findings

It is important to determine whether the patient has bled to shock. Shock usually indicates a large bleed, such as would be found in bleeding varices or bleeding chronic peptic ulcer. Signs such as jaundice, visible collateral vessels on the abdominal wall, ascites and hepatosplenomegaly, confirm portal hypertension and the possibility that the patient has bleeding varices.

Special investigations

- **Endoscopy.** Currently, the diagnosis is usually made by fibre-optic endoscopy. The resuscitated patient's stomach is emptied by means of a nasogastric tube and lavaged well until clear fluid is drawn off. Take care that aspiration of gastric content does not occur, as this can cause mortality. Insert the endoscope and examine the lower end of the oesophagus to exclude varices. Mallory-Weiss tears of the the mucosa of the gastro-oesophageal junction can also be seen. Examine the stomach for an ulcer, erosions or a tumour. Examine the pylorus and duodenum for an ulcer. If an ulcer is found, it must be carefully examined for an underlying blood vessel or a clot embedded in the crater.
- **Barium studies.** If endoscopy is not available, a barium swallow and -meal must be performed. Varices form long tortuous filling defects, but bleeding cannot be confirmed. A peptic ulcer can be seen in the stomach or duodenum, but once again bleeding cannot be demonstrated. An ulcerated tumour can be seen. Erosions are not usually visible on barium studies.

Management

The management of bleeding oesophageal varices will be discussed in the next chapter. Haemorrhages of the upper gastrointestinal tract are treated conservatively unless there is a special indication for surgery.

Conservative management

A nasogastric tube is essential for emptying the stomach and to eliminate any danger of aspiration. It is also useful to ascertain whether the patient is still bleeding.

An intravenous infusion must be established. If the patient is not in shock, put up an electrolyte/dextrose solution to provide maintenance fluids and to keep the vein open in case it should be needed urgently. Meanwhile, send a sample to the blood transfusion services for cross-matching.

If the patient is in shock, resuscitate with a balanced electrolyte solution until blood is available. Blood must be given soon enough to restore the systolic blood pressure to 100 mm Hg or more.

In elderly patients, it is advisable to insert a central venous pressure catheter to ensure that the heart is not overloaded by fluid. Pulse, blood pressure, central venous pressure and urine output are the parameters used for ongoing monitoring of the patient's general condition.

Suppression of the gastric acid secretion

Administer cimetidine in doses of 20 mg/kg body weight per hour. The infusion must not exceed 150 mg/hour. Also give mucaine 30 ml per os. About 80% of haemorrhages will resolve on conservative treatment. Twenty per cent of cases will require surgery.

Indications for surgery

Relative indications

- **Clinical indications**

  Patients over the age of 50, who have bled to shock and therefore need a blood transfusion. Their blood vessels are atherosclerotic and do not constrict very effectively.

Gastroscopic indications

A deep, chronic ulcer.

Absolute indications

Clinical indications

- *Persistent bleeding despite conservative treatment.*
- *Bleeding that resumes, following cessation after conservative treatment.*

Gastroscopic indications

A chronic, deep ulcer which is still bleeding. A deep, chronic ulcer with a thrombus which cannot be easily rinsed off. A visible blood vessel in the base of the ulcer.

Absolute and urgent indications

A massive haemorrhage. The stomach cannot be rinsed clean for diagnostic endoscopy. The patient bleeds so rapidly that resuscitation is difficult.

What type of surgery

The diagnosis is known

- **A bleeding gastric ulcer:** *Do a B I gastrectomy*
- **A bleeding duodenal ulcer:** *Do a truncal vagotomy. Cut through the pylorus to open the duodenal cap. Undersew the duodenal ulcer with nonabsorbable suturing material (silk or prolene). Do a pyloroplasty by suturing the incision transversely. A small percentage of patients rebleed after undersewing. If there is any doubt as to whether the undersewing will be successful, an antrectomy must be performed in conjunction with the vagotomy, with excision of the bleeding DU. Restore continuity by means of a B II reconstruction.*
- **Bleeding erosive gastritis:** *The majority of these cases stop bleeding spontaneously after conservative treatment. If bleeding continues and large volumes of blood are required to resuscitate the patient, surgery may be essential, especially in patients over fifty.*

A truncal vagotomy and antrectomy are indicated. Undersew bleeding points in the gastric mucosa and monitor under direct vision. If the bleeding stops, complete the procedure with a B I or B II reconstruction. If the bleeding persists and is not controlled by either reconstruction, do a total gastrectomy with reconstruction by means of a Roux loop of jejunum brought up to the oesophagus. Such radical surgery is seldom necessary, but it must be done if indicated.

- **Mallory-Weiss tears:** *Most resolve on conservative treatment. If bleeding continues, the bleeding point must be undersewn.*

The diagnosis is unknown

Usually the patient is bleeding copiously and endoscopy is not possible. Endoscopy is unavailable and barium studies cannot confirm the diagnosis.

At laparotomy, inspect the stomach and duodenum. Sometimes the ulcer can be seen or felt. If the cause of bleeding is not apparent, open the pylorus and first inspect the lumen of the duodenum. If nothing can be found, lengthen the incision and inspect and palpate the gastric mucosa. If an ulcer is found, follow the procedures already described.

If bleeding erosive gastritis is found, follow the protocol already described.

Prognosis

If the aforementioned principles are observed in the treatment of bleeding peptic ulcer, the mortality will be lower than 5% and the operative mortality only 10%.

Perforated peptic ulcer

Both gastric and duodenal ulcers can perforate, but DU's perforate about twice as frequently as GU's.

Clinical presentation

History

There may be a preceding history of peptic ulcer, or it may happen without any previous symptoms. The onset of the pain is sudden, it is very severe and affects the whole abdomen.

Clinical findings

The patient lies very still and is afraid to breathe. The abdomen is diffusely tender, with boardlike rigidity. This muscular rigidity is caused by a chemical peritonitis. Later, patients lose a lot of fluid into the third space (intraperitoneally and into the intestinal lumen if ileus develops) and may show signs of hypovolaemic shock.

Special investigations

Standing and supine X-rays of the chest and abdomen must be taken. The domes of the diaphragm are best seen on chest X-ray. In most cases, air under one or both diaphragmatic domes confirms the diagnosis.

Differential diagnosis

Acute pancreatitis must be differentiated from perforated peptic ulcer. The pain associated with pancreatitis has a slower onset. A history of severe alcohol intake during a weekend is common. The pain starts on Sunday afternoon and slowly becomes worse until it becomes extremely severe at the time of admission, on Monday afternoon. There is also often a history of previous similar episodes.

The patient moves restlessly in the bed and crouches on all fours to relieve the pain. The abdomen is very tender, with a doughy rigidity, as opposed to the boardlike rigidity found in perforation. The patient loses a lot of fluid into the third space and may have hypovolaemic shock. Pancreatic calcifications may be visible on abdominal X-rays. There is no air under the diaphragm, and serum and/or urine amylase levels are elevated.

Management

All patients require certain urgent procedures preoperatively.

- **Nasogastric tube:** *Because the stomach or duodenum are perforated, acidic gastric contents leak into the peritoneal cavity and cause a chemical peritonitis. Insert a nasogastric tube immediately and apply continuous suction to drain the gastric contents.*
- **Intravenous infusion:** *Because a chemical peritonitis occurs, the patient loses a great deal of fluid into the third space, the peritoneal cavity, leading to hypovolaemic shock. These patients need large volumes IV fluids to replace the losses.*
- **Central venous pressure catheter:** *With the large volume of fluid that may be required, older patients are especially at risk for fluid overload, causing cardiac failure. The CVP must be monitored constantly to prevent this.*
- **Antibiotics:** *Patients must be put onto a broad spectrum antibiotic to prevent any secondary infection which may arise in the peritoneal cavity.*

The operation

Surgery is performed as soon as the patient has been adequately resuscitated. There are two possible approaches. The perforation can merely be closed, or the final ulcer operation can be performed during the emergency surgery.

- **Simple closure:** *Sutures are placed through the ulcer to close the perforation and a patch of omentum is sutured over the closed perforation.*
- **The final operation:** *If the perforation is duodenal, the ulcer can usually be excised and the opening lengthened through the pylorus to convert it into a pyloroplasty. A truncal vagotomy is also peformed.*

If the duodenum is not suitable for pyloroplasty, the perforation can be closed as has already been described, a gastrojejunostomy created for drainage and a truncal vagotomy performed to complete the operation.

If the perforation is in the stomach, a B I gastrectomy is performed.

Indications for the final ulcer operation

If the perforation is merely closed and the patient is treated conservatively, 50% of cases can be expected to present with recurrent ulcer within a year and 40% will require further surgery within the next three years. The chronic ulcers usually cause later problems. The following protocol is now generally applied:

The final operation is performed if:

1. *It is a chronic ulcer, ie a history of peptic ulcer which has been present for longer than six months, or if it becomes obvious during surgery that this is a chronic ulcer with pronounced fibrosis.*
2. *The patient is fit enough for the longer procedure.*
3. *There has not been too much delay, with widespread contamination of the abdominal cavity.*
4. *The surgeon is capable of performing the more extensive operation.*

If the abovementioned preconditions are not met, the perforation must simply be closed.

If this protocol is followed, about 50% of perforations will merely be closed. If closure alone is performed, the patient must receive a complete course of H_2 receptor antagonists and healing of the ulcer must be confirmed.

Reperforation occurs in 10% of patients.

Conservative management

Patients who are totally unfit for surgery can be treated conservatively. This consists of: nasogastric suction, fluid replacement, antibiotics and the drainage of intraperitoneal abscesses under local anaesthetic, should they arise.

Prognosis

The mortality of perforated peptic ulcer is 7%. Death is more common in patients over sixty. Applying the protocol (to select cases) for final operation does not raise the mortality rate. Three times more people die annually from haemorrhages then from perforations. Haemorrhages occur three times more commonly than perforation.

Gastric outlet obstruction

The stricture is usually distal to the pylorus in the duodenum, where the peptic ulcer was situated. Carcinoma of the distal antrum can also cause gastric outlet obstruction. Duodenal stricture is caused by swelling and oedema of a large chronic DU or by a fibrotic stenosis which has arisen after repeated ulcer recurrences and has healed by fibrosis over a long period of time.

Clinical presentation

History

There is a long history of chronic peptic ulceration. The patient has begun to vomit recently; at first daily, but later large amounts of old, undigested foul-smelling food. The patient breaks foul-smelling winds.

If it is an acute ulcer with oedema, epigastric pain will also be present.

Clinical findings: Patients are often emaciated and dehydrated. A dilated stomach, sometimes with visible peristalsis, can be seen. A succussion splash can be elicited.

Special investigations

A barium meal is very useful. It will show a large distended stomach filled with food residue and pyloroduodenal stenosis.

Endoscopy

This is often unsuccessful due to food residue. The stomach must be rinsed clean for a few days before endoscopy, which is useful for excluding malignancy or, in the case of an active ulcer for determining whether a stenosis is fibrotic or inflammatory.

Differential diagnosis

Gastric carcinoma

If the obstruction is caused by carcinoma, the stomach is less distended than it might otherwise be. The deformity is in the stomach rather than in the duodenum and a malignant ulcer can be seen. Endoscopy is then necessary to confirm the diagnosis histologically.

Management

Electrolyte and fluid imbalance must be corrected. Malnutrition and anaemia must be treated. The stomach must be rinsed very thoroughly. If the obstruction is being caused by an active ulcer with oedema, the patient must be treated conservatively with acid suppression. A number of patients will recover on conservative treatment. If this does not happen, or if the stenosis is fibrotic, surgery must be performed, after the patient has been carefully prepared.

Operation of choice

If an active ulcer is present, a truncal vagotomy and gastrojejunostomy (for drainage), must be performed. If a fibrotic structure is present, the ulcer has usually already healed. It is still safer in these cases to do a truncal vagotomy and gastrojejunostomy.

Malignant transformation in an ulcer

Rarely, gastric ulcers do undergo malignant transformation, but this is not a common problem. A benign gastric ulcer and an early carcinoma are difficult to differentiate from each other on barium meal or on macroscopic endoscopic appearance. It is essential to differentiate these two conditions from each other, because gastric carcinoma has a good prognosis (50% five year survival) if it is operated on before lymph nodes are affected. All gastric ulcers must be examined endoscopically and multiple biopsies must be taken for histology. Brush cytology is also useful in making the diagnosis. Remember that a carcinomatous ulcer can shrink misleadingly on treatment with Tagemet and may almost heal. Never take healing to mean that a lesion is benign.

The postoperative management of patients who have undergone gastric surgery

The nasogastric tube

After gastric surgery it is essential to keep the stomach empty until function has resumed and the stomach can empty normally. This usually takes between forty-eight and seventy-two hours.

If the patient has passed flatus and bowel sounds are audible, the nasogastric tube must be removed. If there is any doubt, a test for gastric emptying must be peformed. With the nasogastric tube in situ, 100 ml of water is given every half-hour for one and a half hours. Wait half-an-hour and apply suction to empty the stomach. If less than 200 ml of fluid is recovered, the nasogastric tube can be removed. Begin with oral fluids three hours later.

Intravenous fluid

Patients need basic maintenance fluid and electrolytes as well as replacement of abnormal losses. Remember that after surgery, the patient's normal metabolic response to trauma is activated. At a neuro-endocrine level, the ADH secretion is stimulated, causing the kidneys to retain fluids and sodium and to lose potassium.

The normal losses per 24 hours are:

Urine – 2 000 ml water 80 mmol Na^+
60 mmol K^+
Insensible sweating 800 ml
Respiration 200 ml
Total fluid required for maintenance:
= 3 000 ml/24 hours

This can be administered as follows:
Maintenance fluid (Maintelyte) 3 000 ml. This provides 105 mmol Na, 75 mmol potassium, 7,5 mmol Mg, 195 mmol Cl — and 5 040 kj energy.

The fluid requirements can also be administered as follows:
500 ml 0,9% Na Cl + 1,5 g KCl and the other 2 500 ml as 5% dextrose with 1,5 g KCl added to 2 further bottles.

Abnormal losses

These are calculated by keeping a careful record of the volumes of fluid suctioned from the stomach. If the patient sweats excessively, this must also be replaced. It can be assumed that if the patient is feverish, he will lose an additional 200 ml/per day per °C that the temperature is raised. Sweat contains 30–70 mmol Na^+ and about 10 mmol potassium per litre.

Because gastric juices contain 50 mmol Na^+, 10 mmol K^+, 80 mmol Cl^- and 40 mmol HCO_3 per litre, and duodenal fluid contains 140 mmol Na^+, 10 mmol K^+, 100 mmol Cl^- and 60 mmol HCO_3, abnormal losses must be replaced with Plasmalyte B or Ringer lactate.

Daily fluid losses and replacement must be carefully charted and a balance must be calculated so that fluid and electrolyte replacement is kept up to date.

Laboratory electrolyte measurements can also give a good indication whether the balance is being maintained. As soon as the patient has regained normal gastric function, the infusion must be removed and fluids must be given orally.

Peritoneal drainage tubes

A corrugated drain is left at the site where the stomach or duodenum has been sutured or at the site where the duodenal stump was closed. Breakdown of the suture line does not usually take place before the fifth day. The drain is shortened on the sixth day and removed on the seventh day if all is well.

Urinary catheter

The urinary catheter must be inserted in the theatre under sterile conditions and removed within forty-eight hours if the patient is stable.

Postoperative complications

Certain complications can be expected after any major abdominal operation, but there are also complications specific to certain gastric operations.

Post-operative fever

- A mild fever, which arises in the first twenty-four hours and resolves spontaneously within seventy-two hours, is the normal metabolic response to trauma.
- A relatively high fever, present on the first day, usually suggests pulmonary atelectasis. There is patchy collapse of the alveoli in the lungs due to secretions and inadequate respiration after the operation.

Active lung physiotherapy usually resolves this problem. If thick secretions block the bronchi, a bronchoscopy must be done to remove the secretions.

- Fever on the fifth or sixth day. Consider wound sepsis, especially if the wound is painful and throbbing. The wound is red and tender on inspection. Remove the cutaneous sutures, do a sensitivity test and put the patient onto broad spectrum antibiotics.

- A single peak of fever on the fifth or sixth day. Consider deep venous thrombosis. Examine the legs. The early signs are oedema posterior to the medial malleolus and calf tenderness. The diagnosis must be confirmed by means of radionuclide venography or contrast venography. Treat with heparin. Give a loading dose of 100 units per kilogram, followed by a twenty-four hour dose based on the following formula: Body mass (kg) x 1 000/2.
  The activated thromboplastin time must be maintained between 50 and 80 seconds. On the fifth day, Warfarin therapy must be commenced.
- Other causes of fever to be borne in mind after the fourth day are lung infections and urinary tract infections, especially if the patient has had a catheter *in situ* for a few days.

Wound dehiscence

This often occurs in patients with bad lungs who cough a lot postoperatively. Poor nutrition, especially hypoalbuminaemia, plays a role. Underlying wound sepsis is sometimes a contributory factor.

On the sixth or seventh day, the patient complains of discomfort in the wound. A watery yellow discharge is found on clinical examination. Intestine is sometimes visible between the cutaneous sutures. The patient must be taken to theatre and the wound must be resutured with interrupted nylon or prolene sutures which penetrate the full thickness of the abdominal wall. There is mortality related to this complication. A wound which has been secondarily sutured usually heals well.

Subphrenic abscess

If the patient develops fever with no obvious cause, a subphrenic abscess must be suspected. There is a swinging pyrexia, pain on compression of the lower thorax and an air/fluid level visible between the liver and diaphragm on standing X-rays. Ultrasound usually confirms the diagnosis. The abscess must be drained and the patient must be given broad spectrum antibiotics.

Prolonged ileus

Although postoperative ileus usually resolves within seventy-two hours, it can sometimes persist, particularly if oral feeding is commenced too soon. It may be caused by an electrolyte imbalance or intraperitoneal sepsis.

Sometimes ileus is perpetuated by fibrinous adhesions. Treatment includes adequate gastric suction and restoration of the fluid and electrolyte balance. If sepsis is present, it must be drained. If the fibrinous adhesion obstruction does not resolve, it must be loosened operatively.

Specific complications

Breakdown of the duodenal stump of a B II gastrectomy

This complication is probably due to a partial obstruction at the gastrojejunostomy, which raises the pressure in the duodenal loop. Stump leakage usually occurs on the fifth or sixth day. The patient feels ill, develops a fever and bile begins to leak past the corrugated drain. The duodenal fistula must be treated conservatively.

The principles are:

- *Maintain fluid and electrolyte balance. Feed the patient parenterally.*
- *Protect the skin against the erosive effects of the activated pancreatic fluids by sticking a "stomahesive" ring around the opening and attaching a colostomy bag.*
- *If the partial obstruction resolves, the fistula will close spontaneously. It is rarely necessary to operate. Do not attempt to suture the fistula. Place a catheter into the fistula to create a so-called "controlled fistula" and ensure that there is no distal obstruction.*

Leakage at the anastomosis of a B I gastrectomy

The fistula which arises must be treated conservatively.

Delayed gastric emptying

Large quantities of gastric juices are drained, despite the patient having good bowel sounds and the ileus having resolved completely.

Oedema of the stoma is sometimes the cause and abnormal motility sometimes plays a role. Very rarely, a mechanical cause, such as kinking or an adhesion, is responsible. A gastrografin meal will demonstrate that the stoma is open.

Management

Continue gastric suction, correct hypoalbuminaemia and electrolyte imbalances and be patient. Metaclopromide can sometimes stimulate gastric emptying. It is seldom necessary to remake the stoma.

Postgastrectomy syndrome

Metabolic abnormalities

Loss of mass

This is common when part of the stomach has been removed and it is repaired unphysiologically, for example when the duodenum does not receive the food bolus from the stomach.

Loss of mass is very common after BII gastrectomy. It may be due to loss of appetite. Sometimes it is the result of a type of blind loop syndrome, with overgrowth of bacteria in the afferent loop causing malabsorption and steatorrhoea.

Anaemia

Iron deficiency anaemia is very common. Three reasons have been postulated:

- Malabsorption of iron. Iron absorption is acid dependent and occurs mainly in the distal duodenum and proximal jejunum. Anaemia is especially common following a BII gastrectomy. Female patients ought to take supplementary iron after a gastrectomy.
- Chronic blood loss. This is mainly due to bile reflux gastritis.
- Anaemia due to a B12 deficiency. This is rare, but is found after a subtotal gastrectomy. Loss of intrinsic factor causes the anaemia. The patient must receive Vitamin B12 parenterally for the rest of his life.

Calcium malabsorption

This occurs commonly in women after a BII gastrectomy and this operation should not be performed in postmenopausal women, as they develop osteoporosis.

Dumping syndrome

This occurs ten minutes after meals. The patient experiences epigastric discomfort, begins to sweat, has palpitations, feels faint and must often lie down.

There is an increase in bowel sounds, sometimes with colic and then sudden diarrhoea. This clinical picture lasts for thirty to sixty minutes.

It is caused by rapid dumping of hyperosmolar food from the stomach into the duodenum, where it draws fluid from the circulation into the intestinal lumen. Intestinal distention causes the discomfort. The fluid shift is probably responsible for the rest of the picture. The syndrome tends to improve with time and must be treated conservatively.

Small dry meals must be taken and hot, sweet meals must be avoided completely. Fluids must not be taken with meals. This syndrome seldom requires surgery. However, if conservative management does fail, the operative options available are the following:

- Convert a BII gastrectomy into a BI gastrectomy.
- An interposition loop of jejunum can be placed between the gastric stump and the duodenum.

It must be emphasized that surgery should be avoided for as long as possible, because results have been shown to be poor in cases where conservative methods have failed.

Reactive hypoglycaemia

The rapid absorption of carbohydrates from the jejunum causes hyperglycaemia, stimulating insulin, which results in reactive hypoglycaemia. This syndrome occurs one and a half to two hours after meals. It occurs in 5 to 10% of postgastrectomy patients, but is usually mild and transient.

Patients must adhere to a low carbohydrate diet avoid exercise after meals. An attack can be treated with oral glucose.

Diarrhoea

This is common following a truncal vagotomy and drainage. About 30% of patients experience an increase in stools after this procedure.

Most patients welcome the change in bowel pattern. The diarrhoea is a problem in less than 5% of cases, but even in these cases the problem can be successfully treated by dietary means and the use of codeine phosphate and lomotil. In resistant cases, cholestyramine can be tried. In rare cases the diarrhoea can be urgent, with incontinence, and can disrupt the patient's lifestyle.

The cause of this diarrhoea is not completely clear. It does not occur after highly selective vagotomy and is probably caused by gastric incontinence, with dumping of hyperosmolar food into the jejunum and withdrawal of fluid from circulation. This causes hyperperistalsis and diarrhoea. It must thus be related to dumping.

The patient must be treated conservatively. In severe cases, surgery can be considered. Several options are possible, namely:

- *Restoration of pyloric continence after pyloroplasty: The plasty must be opened and sutured again in the opposite direction to repair Torgeson's muscle.*
- *Closure of the gastro-enterostomy: At this late stage drainage is no longer necessary and the stoma can thus be repaired.*
- *Reversed ileal loop: This is only considered when the above operations have not worked. A loop of intestine (8 cm long) must be inverted (antiperistaltically) 100 cm distal to the duodenojejunal junction. It is sometimes successful.*

Vomiting bile

This occurs after all the types of ulcer operation, but is more common after a BII gastrectomy.

Clinical presentation

History

It begins within weeks of the operation. The patient feels uncomfortable after meals and experiences epigastric pain and nausea. After having suddenly vomited bright yellow bile, the patient feels much better.

Endoscopy

The stomach contains bile and the mucosa looks red and oedematous. There may be erosions, especially round the stoma.

Differential diagnosis

Vomiting of bile must be differentiated from chronic obstruction of the afferent loop. There is sometimes a partial obstruction of the afferent loop, which can be caused by oedema and stomal swelling or a mechanical cause, such as adhesions or kinking of the loop. The patient has severe pain, which is sometimes colicky. He vomits large amounts of bile and this affords relief.

Barium studies can show a large, distended loop. Bile can also reflux through an incompetent inferior oesophageal sphincter and cause alkaline oesophagitis. Patients then complain of indigestion and regurgitate small amounts of bile. The diagnosis can usually be confirmed endoscopically. A hiatus hernia with bile reflux oesophagitis is the most common finding.

Management

Bile vomiting improves with time and must always be treated conservatively. It is helpful to bind the bile and to neutralize the acid. Hydrotalcite (Altacite) is useful in this regard. Metoclopromide (Maxolon) must be given half an hour before meals. Chlolestyramine, which binds bile salts, is sometimes helpful.

If the patient has not improved after a year at least, surgery can be considered. Various operations have been tried in the past. If a BII gastrectomy was done originally, it can be converted into a BI gasterectomy, with interposition of a jejunal loop. If a gastroenterostomy was done for drainage, it can be closed.

Because these operations were often unsuccessful, most surgeons nowadays prefer to do a Roux-and-Y bypass. The afferent loop is sutured to the jejunum at least 50 cm below the gastric stomal end. Bile can therefore not enter the stomach at all. The loop must be long enough to prevent reflux of bile back against peristalsis.

In all cases, a truncal vagotomy must be performed in conjunction with the Roux loop, otherwise these patients develop stomal ulcers.

Although this operation is very successful in preventing bile vomiting, there is a tendency towards stomal stenosis postoperatively. The reason for this is not always clear, but inflammation with fibrosis, secondary to erosive gastritis and relative ischaemia of the loop, may be the cause.

Stomal ulcer

After all peptic ulcer surgery, there is a possibility of a residual ulcer. Bearing in mind the dictum "no acid, no ulcer", the implication is that recurrence is directly related to the effectiveness of the operation in reducing acid secretion. Truncal vagotomy and antrectomy, which influences both the neural and gastrin stimulation of gastric acid secretion, has the lowest recurrence rate (less than 2%). In a Billroth II gastrectomy, where the antrum (gastric secretion) and part of the parietal cell mass are removed, the recurrence rate is lower than 4%.

A truncal vagotomy and pyloroplasty, which only influences the neural stimulation of gastric acid secretion, has a recurrence rate of 10%. A highly selective vagotomy, which also influences the neural stimulation of gastric acid secretion, has an ulcer recurrence rate exceeding 10%.

These recurrent ulcers are mostly due to incomplete vagotomies. It is more difficult to do a highly selective vagotomy effectively, than a truncal vagotomy. When a Hollander test (insulin stimulation of acid secretion) is performed on patients who have undergone truncal vagotomies, to determine adequacy of the surgery, the following is found:

- Recurrent ulcer following total truncal vagotomy, 3%.
- If the Hollander test is positive early on, 20%.
- If there is a delayed positive Hollander test, 10%.

Other cases of stomal ulceration must be considered, namely:

Ulcer caused by sutures which do not disolve

Silk sutures are no longer used for gastric anastomoses. In the past they caused ulceration along the suture line. The black silk sutures could be seen endoscopically in the ulcer.

Antral remnant

The antral mucosa contains G cells which secrete gastrin. The presence of acid inhibits gastrin secretion. If part of the antrum is not removed during a BII gastrectomy and the stump is closed, this means that the residual G cells of the antrum which will secrete gastrin continuously, because the inhibiting acid cannot reach this area. This is sometimes the cause of a stomal ulcer.

The diagnosis is made on finding high levels of gastrin, which are inhibited by secretin. A "warm" area can be seen on a technesium scan where the antral mucosa takes up the isotope. It may also be useful to examine the surgical specimen to determine whether or not the incision through the duodenum was free of antral mucosa.

The Zollinger-Ellison syndrome

This sometimes causes ulcer recurrence. The diagnosis is confirmed by finding very high gastrin levels, which are elevated even more by secretin. The Z-E syndrome will be discussed later.

Reflux gastritis

A stomal ulcer which is situated proximal to the gastric stoma is usually caused by damage to the mucous membrane round the stoma through reflux of duodenal contents, bile and pancreatic juices into the stomach. Endoscopy shows bile in the stomach, with inflammation and erosion around the stoma and an ulcer just proximal to the stoma. Often the gastritis is the underlying predisposing factor and analgesics containing aspirin taken by the patient are the final precipitators.

Clinical presentation

The patients develop the same pain they had before surgery. The pain is associated with flatulence, nausea and vomiting. Cholemesis is often a presenting complaint. These stomal ulcers also have a greater tendency to develop complications. Patients may bleed or perforate. They sometimes have symptoms and signs of gastric outlet obstruction which can also perforate right into the adjacent colon. This happens commonly when a retrocolic anastomosis has been done in a BII gastrectomy. The bacteria colonize the stomach and jejunum through the fistula and this leads to vomiting, diarrhoea and malabsorption, causing loss of weight.

Special investigations

- **Barium studies** are useful in diagnosing gastric outlet obstruction and in determining the exact nature of the previous surgery, if this is unknown. A barium enema is more reliable than a barium meal in demonstrating a gastrocolic fistula. A barium meal is not reliable for diagnosis of a stomal ulcer, as the deformity caused by the previous surgery makes the diagnosis difficult.
- **Fibre-optic endoscopy** is very helpful in diagnosing stomal ulceration. It is important to determine the exact location of the ulcer. An ulcer distal to the stoma implies continued acid secretion. An ulcer proximal to the stoma implies bile reflux gastritis and irritating drugs.
- **Serum gastrin levels** must be measured. If levels are raised, a **secretin suppression test** must be carried out. Secretin, 1 unit/kg, is injected rapidly IV. A 100% rise in the gastrin level indicates Z-E syndrome, a drop suggests residual antral tissue.
- **The Hollander test.** Basal gastric acid secretion is measured every 15 minutes, for one hour. Twenty units of insulin are then given IV and gastric juice is collected every fifteen minutes for two hours. Blood is taken after forty-five and ninety minutes to ensure that hypoglycaemia is present (blood glucose of less than 1,7 mmol/litre).

  The test is positive if:
  - a rise in acid of 20 mmol/litre is shown in any fifteen-minute specimen as compared to the highest fifteen-minute basal acid secretion;
  - a basal acid secretion of more than 2 mmol per hour is measured;
  - there is a rise of more than 2 mmol per hour after insulin compared to basal acid secretion. If this occurs during the first hour, it is described as an early response; and if it occurs during the seconed hour, it is described as a late response.

Management

Patients with stomal ulcers must be treated conservatively with H_2 receptor antangonists for long periods. Most of them will heal. About 40% will require further surgery, which will depend on the underlying cause. Most ulcers will be due to inadequate ulcer surgery.

Incomplete vagotomy

If it is known that a main branch of the vagus was not found at surgery, it may be advisable to complete the vagotomy. This is not usually the case and an antrectomy or B II gastrectomy should be performed. Attempts to look for remaining vagus nerve branches or to do a vagotomy through the thorax, are usually unsuccessful.

If a gastrocolic fistula is present, the patient must be prepared (including colonic intestinal preparation) and then operated on. If the patient is very ill, a defunctioning colostomy can be considered as a preparatory procedure.

The Zollinger-Ellison syndrome

This is very rare, but is sometimes the cause of recurrent, resistant ulcers and especially recurrent complications such as haemorrhage and perforation. The syndrome can be divided into two main types:

- **Sporadic nonfamilial gastrinoma.** This represents 70% of cases. In 70% of these cases, the gastrinoma is found in the pancreatic islets, 15% of the tumuours are found in the duodenum and the rest in other places such as the liver, the stomach and the lymph nodes. Sometimes no tumour can be located, only a gastrinoma in a lymph node. More than half these cases are either multicentric or have already spread to lymph nodes and the liver.
- **Multiple endocrine adenopathy type I (MEA I).** This is a familial disease. Adenomas or hyperplasia are found in the parathyroids, the pituitary gland and the adrenal glands. There are usually multiple gastrinomas in the pancreatic islets.

Clinical presentation

The excess gastrin stimulates excessive acid secretion by the stomach. Patients complain of epigastric pain and sometimes diarrhoea. Occasionally, diarrhoea is the only presenting symptom.

The ulcers may be situated in unusual places, such as the distal duodenum and jejunum. They do not respond well to conservative treatment and tend to bleed and perforate. Sometimes the ulcer is less aggressive initially and can become worse over a period of years.

About 20% of cases are diagnosed because a peptic ulcer does not respond well to adequate treatment. In the familial type, signs of endocrine adenopathy can be found. The most common sign is hypercalcaemia due to hyperparathyroidism.

Special investigations

- Plasma gastrin levels are raised. If levels are very high, there is no doubt as to the diagnosis. In cases where the diagnosis is doubtful, stimulation tests must be performed. Hypergastrinaemia is found in cases of hyperchlorhydria. Examples of such causes include previous vagotomy, pernicious anaemia, atrophic gastritis and gastric carcinoma.

  The Z-E syndrome can be diagnosed only where hypergastrinaemia and hyperchlorhydria are present.

  Conditions which must be differentiated from Z-E syndrome include:
- **Antral G cell hyperplasia of the gastric antrum:** The secretin stimulation test does not cause a significant rise in gastrin. A protein meal does cause gastrin to rise.
- **Residual antral tissue after a B II gastrectomy:** Secretin stimulation and a protein meal does not raise gastrin levels.
- **Z-E syndrome:** Secretin stimulation raises the gastrin level by at least 200 pmol/litre. A protein meal causes no rise in the gastrin. Liver metastases must be sought using ultrasound and computer tomography.

Management

Although it must be realized that most patients have either multiple multifocal lesions or existing metastasis, there will be a small group in whom removal of the gastrinoma is appropriate. After having excluded the groups with the MEA I syndrome and metastasis, an attempt must be made to locate the gastrinoma, with a view to excision.

Endoscopy can sometimes reveal a tumour in the duodenum. Ultrasound and computer tomography may demonstrate the primary tumour in the liver or pancreas. Arteriography is sometimes useful, but unfortunately gastrinomas are not very well vascularized tumours. Placing catheters percutaneously and transhepatically into the portal venous system and taking blood for gastrin levels can be useful in pinpointing the location of the tumour. Lastly, exploratory surgery must be performed to try and locate the tumour.

An area which must be closely examined at surgery is the triangle of Stabile, bounded by the cystic duct/bile duct junction, the junction of the second and third parts of the duodenum and the neck of the pancreas. If a tumour or lymph node is found, they must be removed without removing the pancreas.

Unfortunately, the majority of cases are not suitable for removal of the gastrinoma because of metastasis, or because the tumour cannot be found. In the past, a total gastrectomy would have been performed in these cases. Currently, conservative treatment is used. Three groups of drugs are available, namely:

- **The H_2 receptor antagonists:** *High doses of Tagemet or Zantac (two to three times the normal doses) may be necessary to control acid secretion.*
- **The ATP-ase inhibitor Omeprazole** *must be given if the H_2 receptor antagonists fail.*
- **Somatostin:** *This drug supresses gastrin secretion very effectively and several cases treated with this drug have shown significant declines in gastrin levels. If the disease cannot be controlled with any of these drugs, a total gastrectomy must be performed.*

Streptozotosin and 5-fluoro-uracil can sometimes bring about remission.

Stress ulcer

These ulcers start as superficial erosions which deteriorate and start bleeding. They sometimes penetrate the wall of the stomach or intestine and can perforate.

Damage to the protective mechanism of the mucosa permits increased rediffusion of hydrogen ions. The lowered mucosal resistance can be caused by a variety of factors, such as ischaemia due to shock, reflux and the use of drugs such as aspirin. Disseminated intravascular coagulation can also play a part. Changes in the mucosa have been described:

- **Curling ulcer:** This is found after severe burns, usually involving more than 50% of the body surface. It is more commonly found in the duodenum but does occur in the stomach.

- **Cushing's ulcer:** This is found after intracranial trauma or surgery to the oesophagus, stomach or duodenum. Acid secretion is increased, probably due to raised intracranial pressure. These ulcers are often inclined to penetrate and to perforate.
- **Gastric erosions:** These follow trauma, sepsis, operations and myocardial infarctions. The gastric mucosa shows a haemorrhagic gastritis and multiple erosions. These erosions tend to bleed.

Clinical presentation

These complications must always be borne in mind, especially in patients being nursed in intensive care wards. Patients develop epigastric pain and begin to bleed. Often the patient is on a respirator and the bleeding occurs totally unexpectedly. The diagnosis is made on endoscopy.

Management

It is very important to anticipate this complication in patients in intensive care units who are subjected to severe stress. Preventative measures must be taken by treating the patients hourly with 15 ml of antacid administered through the nasogastric tube. If there are already signs of bleeding, IV cimetidine should be given in doses of 5 mg per hour for 48 hours, together with antacids, followed by oral cimetidine. There are indications that stress ulceration is rarer in patients who receive hyperalimentation during their stay in the intensive care unit.

If the bleeding does not stop, surgery must be performed. A truncal vagotomy and undersewing of the bleeders must be done initially and the mucosa must be inspected intraoperatively to see whether the bleeding is under control. If bleeding cannot be controlled, a total gastrectomy must be performed, because this condition carries a high mortality rate.

- **Dieulafoy erosions:** This is a rare condition where severe bleeding occurs in the gastric mucosa, usually in the fundus. There is repeated massive bleeding. The barium meal is normal. The bleeding point can be identified on endoscopy. This condition is ascribed to rupture of a small aneurysm in the blood vessels of the gastric wall.

B. TUMOURS

Benign tumours

Hyperplastic polyps

These are usually multiple, found by chance and are probably hamartomas.

Adenomas

These adenomas are found in the antrum or on the lesser curvature. They have a villous or tubulovillous growth pattern and are premalignant. If the adenoma is larger than 2 cm in diameter, there is a 30% chance that it is malignant.

Clinical presentation

They are often asymptomatic. Sometimes pain and bleeding are presenting symptoms.

Management

They can be removed endoscopically if they are pedunculated. Multiple polyps are usually hyperplastic polyps and must merely be followed up. If the adenoma is larger than 2 cm, it must be operated on, especially if it cannot be removed endoscopically.

Leiomyoma

This is just as common as adenoma, occurs in the smooth muscle of the gastric wall and projects into the lumen.

Clinical presentation

Small tumours are usually asymptomatic. Larger tumours undergo typical central ulceration and the patient presents with discomfort, loss of appetite and pain. The ulcer also tends to bleed.

Special investigations

A typical smooth, polypoid tumour with central ulceration can be seen on barium meal. The diagnosis can be confirmed endoscopically. Biopsy is not useful, because usually only mucosa is snipped by the biopsy forceps.

Management

All symptomatic tumours which are larger than 2 cm must be excised, with a 2 cm free border. It is difficult to differentiate a leiomyoma from a leiomyosarcoma. The malignant tumour is larger and has more mitotic figures on histological examination. Ultimately, the two are differentiated by signs that the tumour is infiltrating locally or metastasizing.

Malignant tumours

Carcinoma of the stomach

The incidence of gastric carcinoma is on the wane in the western world. It is very common in Japan. In South Africa it is particularly common in coloured men. Gastric carcinoma is almost twice as common in men as in women.

Aetiology

- **Genetic factors:** There is a familial incidence. Blood group A is more common in patients with gastric carcinoma.
- **Diet:** It would appear that certain communities ingest carcinogens in their diet. A probable link with polished rice has been described in Japan. Smoking of fish or meat, as is done in Scandanavia and Germany, may play a rôle. Nitrosamine, a known carcinogen, is also commonly found in smoked foods.
- **Pernicious anaemia:** The atrophic gastritis and metaplasia found in these patients is probably responsible for the increased incidence of carcinoma.

Gastric ulcer

There is not much documentation to support a link between gastric ulceration and carcinoma. It is more important to differentiate between gastric ulceration and gastric carcinoma.

Previous gastric surgery

Certain researchers have postulated that gastric carcinoma is found more commonly in the gastric stumps of patients who have undergone gastrectomies. It has also been found that such patients have, for example, an increased incidence of lung carcinoma. Many of these patients smoke and there may also be other predisposing social factors. On the other hand, it is possible that the gastritis which caused the ulcer could also have prepared the ground in which the gastric carcinoma would later arise.

Pathology

Five microscopic types are found:

- **Superficial carcinoma (6%).** Although this is found in any population, it has mainly been described in Japan. Researchers there have divided it into three types:

Type I: Polypoid carcinoma. This takes the form of a polyp which is difficult to differentiate from a benign polyp.

Type II: Superficial carcinoma. This is divided into three further subgroups, namely:

- Raised type.
- Flat type. Only a mucosal colour change is visible.
- Diffuse type. This is a diffuse mucosal lesion with erythema and bleeding.

Type III: Ulcerative type. A small ulcer, which cannot be distinguished from a benign ulcer, is found. Superficial carcinomas are limited to the mucosa and submucosa.

In Japan, superficial carcinomas represent 33% of cases, while in the west, they form only 6%. About 5% spread to the lymph nodes.

- **A fungating mass (36%).** A large cauliflowerlike mass which ulcerates and infiltrates the surrounding mucosa.
- **An ulcer (25%):** It is sometimes difficult to distinguish a malignant ulcer from a benign ulcer, but they usually do have typical malignant characteristics. The edges are raised, the crater is necrotic and irregular and there are often signs of lateral infiltration.
- **Diffuse infiltrating tumours (linitis plastica, leatherbottle stomach) (26%).** A large part of the stomach is thickened and infiltrated. The mucosal folds are obliterated and superficial ulceration is sometimes present.
- **Polypoid tumours (7%):** An actinomorphic large polyp which is difficult to distinguish from an adenoma. It is possible that some arise from benign adenomas.

Carcinomas can thus be divided into:

- A fungating growth pattern which tends to form a mass
- an infiltrating growth pattern.

Microscopic appearance

These tumours are adenocarcinomas. Two cell types are found, metaplastic intestinal and gastric cells which secrete mucus. Both cell types may be present. Mucus builds up in the cell and displaces the cytoplasm to form so-called signet ring cells. These cells are particularly common in the infiltrating type of carcinoma. Mucus can also be secreted from the cell to fill the glandular lumens. The cell may also be poorly differentiated without any signs of mucus secretion.

Staging of gastric carcinoma

The TNM staging

T_1 Limited to the mucosa
T_2 Infiltrates the wall but does not involve the serosa
T_3 Infiltrates through the serosa
T_4 Diffuse infiltration of the gastric wall.
N_0 No lymph nodes involved
N_1 Perigastric nodes involved
N_2 Distal nodes involved
M_0 No metastasis
M_1 Metastasis

Clinical presentation

History

Loss of appetite, especially for meat, must arouse the clinician's suspicion. Epigastric pain and dyspepsia, especially when found in patients older than forty, must be further investigated by means of endoscopy. Remember that pain caused by carcinoma also improves on antacid treatment. Dysphagia may also present if the carcinoma is situated near the cardia. Nausea and vomiting indicate possible gastric outlet obstruction.

Examination

A palpable mass is found in less than 30% of cases. There may be signs of weight loss. If the tumour is already advanced, signs such as left-sided supraclavicular lymph nodes (Virchow-Troisier's sign), a palpable liver, ascites, jaundice and a palpable rectal mass may be evident.

Special investigations

The diagnosis is usually made on barium meal or endoscopy.

Barium meal

A double contrast barium meal must be done. Polypoid and fungating tumours show as large filling defects. These masses are irregular and may have irregular ulceration on their surfaces. The surrounding stomach is oedematous and there is loss of mucosal folds, a sign of lateral infiltration. An infiltrating tumour (leatherbottle stomach) presents as a narrowed oedematous, rigid stomach with loss of mucosal folds. Ulceration may also be evident. Carcinomatous ulceration is sometimes difficult to differentiate from benign ulceration. A malignant ulcer is an ulcer which is situated on the surface of an infiltrating lesion. It is inside the lumen and has visible raised edges, in contrast to a benign ulcer which penetrates outside the lumen. The mucosal folds round the ulcer are absent, indicating infiltration. Mucosal folds run into the crater of a benign ulcer.

The site – lesser curvature or greater curvature – and the size of the ulcer are not reliable indications.

Endoscopy

This investigation has become extremely important. Not only can it reveal the macroscopic appearance of the ulcer but it also allows for histological or cytological confirmation of the diagnosis. Multiple biopsies, preferably more than six, must be taken. If cytology is done along with biopsy, the diagnosis is even more reliable. A brush is drawn across the ulcer and cytology is performed on the cells which are washed from the brush.

Achlorhydria

If the patient has an ulcer and achlorhydria, carcinoma must be strongly suspected.

Management

The management is surgery. Patients must first be prepared for surgery. They are often anaemic and have low albumin levels. The type of operation depends on the site and stage of the tumour.

A curative operation must be performed, and if this is not possible, a palliative operation is the alternative. If the tumour is macroscopically confined to the stomach, a curative procedure is carried out. Most tumours are found in the distal third of the stomach. Perform a subtotal gastrectomy, leaving a small piece of stomach in the region of the cardia to facilitate anastomosis. Include the hepatogastric and greater omentum. The reconstruction is a B II anastomosis with a stoma running the full width of the stomach.

If the tumour is situated in the middle third, or corpus, a total gastrectomy is preferable. It is sometimes also necessary to perform a splenectomy. Anastomose the jejunum to the oesophagus by means of a Roux loop. The Roux loop must be at least 50 cm long to prevent bile reflux. If the tumour is situated at the cardia, resect the proximal two thirds of the stomach, the omentum and the spleen via a thoraco-abdominal incision. Anastomose the distal third of the stomach to the oesophagus.

Palliation

It is always better to resect the stomach if possible. This provides better palliation than a bypass, because the lesion causing blood and protein loss, is removed. If the tumour is so widespread that it cannot be removed, do a gastroenterostomy to relieve obstruction. If the irremovable tumour is situated at the cardia, insert a Celestin tube.

Adjuvant management

The palliative contribution of radiotherapy and chemotherapy is very limited. Combinations which include 5-fluoro-uracil are being tried.

Prognosis

The five year survival of all cases is lower than 10%. If a curative operation is performed, the survival rate is 25%. If the lymph nodes are negative in the surgical specimen, the survival rate is 40%. A small minority of patients will have negative lymph nodes.

In Japan, where early superficial carcinoma is discovered in screening tests, the five year survival rate is 90%.

Lymphoma of the stomach

This forms 5% of all malignant gastric tumours. Gastric lymphomas form 50% of all gastrointestinal lymphomas. These tumours occur in the corpus of the stomach, presenting as ulcerating, polypoid or infiltrating lesions. Histologically, they are lymphosarcomas, usually of the diffuse histiocytic type. Clinically, they present exactly like gastric carcinoma. They resemble carcinoma on barium meal. Endoscopically, they are also very similar to carcinoma and the diagnosis is made on histology and cytology.

Gastrectomy, followed by radiotherapy and chemotherapy, yields the best results. The five year survival rate is 50%. If the tumour is not removable, good palliation can be achieved with radiotherapy and chemotherapy.

Leiomyosarcoma

This represents less than 1% of malignant gastric tumours. It presents like leiomyoma with a tumour bulging into the lumen and often ulcerating on its surface. The treatment is gastrectomy and the five-year survival rate is 50%.

Carcinoid of the stomach

Tumours of neuro-endocrine origin, with argentaffin-positive cells, are sometimes found in the stomach. They can secrete a variety of hormones, including histamine and 5-hydroxytryptamine.

C. MISCELLANEOUS CONDITIONS

Giant mucosal folds of the stomach

Primary giant folds

There are two main types:

- **Giant folds with protein loss and normal acid secretion (Ménétrier's disease):** Patients present clinically with hypo-albuminaemia. The disease is usually found in adults. When it occurs in young people, it tends to resolve spontaneously.

- **Giant folds with increased acid secretion and normal albumin (Schindler disease):** These patients develop duodenal ulcers with complications. The condition must be distinguished from the Z-E syndrome, where high gastrin levels are found. The treatment of primary giant folds is a radical B II gastrectomy. In Schindler disease, a vagotomy must also be performed.

Secondary giant folds

Hypertrophic mucosal folds are also found in the Z-E syndrome, lymphoma, carcinoma and tuberculosis of the stomach.

Bezoars

Two types, phytobezoars (plant material) and trichobezoars (human hair) have been described. Bezoars made up of plant material are usually found in patients who have undergone previous gastric surgery. Trichobezoars are most commonly found in young women who are mentally disturbed. Patients present with pain, nausea and vomiting. Sometimes ulcers arise in the stomach, with haemorrhage. Barium meal confirms the diagnosis.

Phytobezoars can usually be broken down and removed endoscopically. Trichobezoars often necessitate a gastrostomy.

Fungal infections of the stomach

This condition is known as mucormycosis. The fungi can be found in the stomach without any lesions being present on the walls. Sometimes the fungi infiltrate the gastric walls, especially in weak, malnourished patients with gastric ulceration. The fungi are found in the lumens of the blood vessels. The blood vessels clot, causing necrosis of the gastric mucosa. The only treatment is radical resection and administration of amphoteracin B. The prognosis is poor, but fortunately the condition is rare.

Gastric volvulus

A large para-oesophageal hiatus or an eventration of the diaphragm is usually associated with this condition. The stomach either twists organo-axially, i e around its long axis, or mesenterio-axially, i e around its transverse axis. An acute presentation of closed-loop gastric obstruction, or one of chronic presentation of discomfort, flatulence and borborygmi, are both possible.

Barium meal usually demonstrates the volvulus and the associated hiatus hernia.

The treatment is surgery, with repair of the hernia and gastropexation.

Gastric and duodenal diverticula

Gastric diverticula are very rare. They are most commonly found in the prepyloric region and must be differentiated from an ulcer. On barium meal, normal mucosal folds are usually found in the diverticulum. The diagnosis can be confirmed endoscopically. Surgery is not necessary.

Duodenal diverticula

These diverticula, which are found in about 2% of barium meals, have now become significant because they can impede canalization of the sphincter of Oddi during ERCP. The diverticulum is related to the papilla of Vater and the bile duct often opens into its walls, or even into its depths. Patients with diverticula have a higher incidence of gallstones.

The most important point to remember is not to ascribe the patient's symptoms to the duodenal diverticulum. There is usually another cause. The removal of a diverticulum is a very difficult and dangerous operation.

Diverticula can sometimes cause complications such as haemorrhage, perforation and pancreatitis. These serious complications justify surgery, but this should be tackled only by a very experienced surgeon.

MORBID OBESITY – SURGICAL TREATMENT

A patient has morbid obesity when his mass is twice the ideal mass for his height and he has maintained this weight for five years, despite attempts by the patient, his family and his doctor to reduce his mass to a more acceptable level.

Life insurance company statistics show that the mortality of men between fifteen and thirty-nine with a mass greater than 115 kg is three times that of the normal population. This can be ascribed to an increased incidence of degenerative diseases of the blood vessels supplying the cardiac muscle and brain, and diseases of the gastrointestinal canal, particularly fatty infiltration of the liver and even cirrhosis. Obese patients have an increased incidence of hypertension, diabetes, thrombosis, arthritis (especially of the knees) and disc prolapse of the vertebrae.

Obesity is not only a health hazard, but is also a social, psychological and economic problem. It affects interpersonal relationships and hinders a person's ability to find and retain suitable employment.

Morbid obesity arises when caloric intake consistently exceeds energy consumption. The ideal treatment would thus be to reduce food intake and to increase energy consumption by means of exercise. Unfortunately, morbidly obese people have compulsive eating habits and take no physical exercise at all. There are various theories to explain the habit of overeating in the morbidly obese. It has been postulated that such people have an abnormal satiation centre and that decreased physical activity causes increased insulin sensitivity in the muscle fibres, which in turn stimulates increased insulin secretion. This suppresses the blood sugar level, which then stimulates appetite. It has been postulated that they sleep more and take less exercise than others.

Morbid obesity is familial. It is unclear whether this can be ascribed to genetic factors or whether it is merely the result of psychological and emotional factors present in the family situation. The morbidly obese very seldom succeed in maintaining a diet and exercise programme. Findings show that 90% of patients in mass loss clubs regain their original mass within a year. Only 25% of patients lose 10 kg and only 5% 20 kg on medical treatment. Because morbid obesity is a life-threatening condition and because medical treatment usually fails, surgery is an option which must be considered.

The Payne and De Wind operation

The jejunum is transected within 35 cm of the ligament of Treitz and sutured end-to-side to the ileum, 10 cm from the ileocaecal valve. Ninety percent of the gastrointestinal tract is thus bypassed. Because food can reflux into the ileum, the loss of mass is inadequate in many cases.

The Scott operation

In this operation, 30 cm of jejunum is sutured end-to-end to 10 cm of distal ileum. This long excluded ileojejunal section (90%) is closed proximally and the distal open end is sutured to the colon for drainage of the blind loop. This operation is more effective in inducing mass loss.

Complications

The mortality of this operation is 5%. Complications such as wound infection, thrombosis, pulmonory embolus, coronary thrombosis and peritonitis are common after this operation in these very obese patients.

Diarrhoea

This always follows the operation. In the initial phase twenty stools a day are not uncommon. Later this improves, but the patients usually still pass more than five stools daily. They often develop perianal complications such as haemorrhoids, fissures-in-ano and inflammation. Sometimes the diarrhoea is so severe that the intestinal anatomy must be repaired.

Fluid and electrolyte losses

There are large losses of potassium, calcium and magnesium in the multiple stools. Patients develop weakness, muscle cramps and anorexia.

Hepatic complications

The majority of morbidly obese patients have fatty infiltration of the liver. This usually improves postoperatively, but about 5% develop hepatic failure. Patients present with anorexia, nausea and vomiting, oedema and ultimately, jaundice and coma. Luckily the condition is reversible when amino acids are administered intravenously. If the patient does not improve rapidly, the intestinal anatomy must be repaired. Hepatic failure is probably caused by a variety of factors. Protein malabsorption, endotoxins from bacteria colonizing the blind loop and toxic bile acids such as lithocolic acid, which accumulate due to malabsorption of bile salts in the shortened small intestine, probably all play a rôle.

Other complications include arthritis, oxalate renal calculi and alopecia. Pseudo-obstruction, due to gaseous distention of the blind loop, also occurs. In about 10%, intestinal anatomy will have to be repaired becausc of irreversible diarrhoca, excessive weight loss or hepatic failure. Because of these serious complications after intestinal short circuits, they are no longer performed for morbid obesity.

Gastric reduction procedures (the Mason operation)

This procedure has undergone several alterations over the years. It is based on the following principles: The stomach is surgically altered to create a small reservoir so that the patient can ingest only 50 ml of food per meal. If more food is ingested, abdominal discomfort is experienced. There is a small opening between the reservoir and the rest of the stomach, allowing for slow emptying. The most popular operation is the Mason vertical staple gastroplasty. The advantage of the operation is that the patient's food intake is limited. The wellknown complications of malabsorption seen after intestinal bypass, do not occur.

Complications

The mortality of 2%, wound sepsis, thrombosis and pulmonary embolus can occur. Peritonitis, with subphrenic abscess formation, is a complication of leakage at the staples. Stasis gastric ulcer in the gastric reservoir has also been described. Loss of mass is not always satisfactory, as patients may cheat by ingesting liquid foods, especially chocolate and soft drinks. Other causes of failure are that the opening between the reservoir and the main part of the stomach stretches open and that staples come undone.

Facts to be emhasized

- Only morbid obesity is an indication for surgery.
- Cosmetic reasons must not be taken into consideration.
- It is a very difficult operation, with a risk of mortality and many complications.
- To reduce the incidence of complications, the operation should be performed by skilled surgeons only.
- It is essential that the patient be followed up adequately.

The liver, bile ducts, pancreas and spleen 4

The liver, bile ducts and pancreas are discussed as a unit, due to their anatomical and functional interdependence and the similarity in the symptom complexes caused by their diseases.

What does the patient complain of?

Pain

The pain is experienced in the upper abdomen. Severe, colicky pain, arising in the right hypochondrium and spreading to the back and right shoulder is suggestive of gallstone colic.

Vague pain or discomfort in the right hypochondrium, especially after fatty meals, suggests chronic cholecystitis (stones in the gall-bladder). Pain arising in the epigastrium, spreading to the back and relieved by movement, especially by bending forward, suggests pancreatic pain.

Dull, throbbing pain in the right hypochondrium, suggests hepatic conditions which cause tension in the hepatic capsule, such as hepatitis, abscess or tumour.

Jaundice: introductory remarks

This is a yellow discolouration of the tissues, caused by abnormal accumulation of bile pigments, especially bilirubin, in the tissue fluids. The discolouration is especially noticeable in tissues containing a lot of collagen. Jaundice is best observed in the sclerae, skin, palate and eardrums.

Jaundice is observable when the serum bilirubin exceeds 40–50 micromol/litre. Jaundice is one of the key signs of diseases of the liver-bile tract-pancreas complex.

Cholestatic jaundice

This is a condition in which the flow of bile to the duodenum is impeded. Cholestasis can be caused by obstruction of the

- extraphepatic bile duct or
- intrahepatic bile stasis.

Accumulation of bile in the bile canaliculi can be histologically confirmed.

Overproduction of bilirubin or congenital abnormalities of bilirubin metabolism

It is essential to distinguish cholestatic jaundice caused by extrahepatic obstruction from other forms of jaundice, because surgical correction is often possible.

In order to view the significance of jaundice in the right perspective, various other factors must also be taken into consideration, namely:

The age and sex of the patient

Children and young people with jaundice

- Congenital abnormalities of bilirubin metabolism
- Viral and other infections

Middle-aged men

- Alcoholic cirrhosis

Middle-aged women

- Gallstones
- Intrahepatic cholestasis

Older patients

- Malignant tumours of the pancreas, bile tract and liver

More than one family member affected

- Congenital abnormalities of bilirubin metabolism
- Viral infections

Pain, fever and jaundice

- Pain, fever and jaundice suggest an infective cause
- In viral hepatitis, fever and malaise usually precede the pain and the pain improves when jaundice develops
- In bacterial cholangitis there is pain, rigor and jaundice, which become progressively worse
- Pain and jaundice without fever indicate a mechanical biliary tract obstruction, usually caused by gallstones
- Pain is less prominent in jaundice caused by malignancy

Pruritis and the colour of the jaundice

- A dark green jaundice associated with pruritis suggests extrahepatic cholestasis
- An orange-yellow jaundice associated with pruritis suggests intrahepatic cholestasis
- A light yellow jaundice without pruritis suggests haemolytic jaundice

Systemic symptoms and signs

- Jaundice associated with loss of weight, fatigue and dyspnoea suggests a malignant cause.

What else does the clinician want to know from the history?

1. Was there exposure to
   - Drugs
   - Alcohol
   - Injections
   - Blood transfusion or other blood components
   - Anaesthesia
   - Surgery to the bile ducts
   - Industrial toxins
2. Has the colour of the urine darkened? Excess bile pigments in the urine, indicating obstructive jaundice, cause a yellow discolouration in the foam on shaking the urine.
3. Have the stools become pale? Greyish-white stools suggest obstructive jaundice. The loss of colour is caused by a loss of bile pigment and excess fat. If the obstruction involves both the bile ducts and the pancreas (carcinoma of the head of the pancreas), the fat content is so high that the stool usually floats in the toilet bowl.
4. Were black, tarry stools noted? This suggests an upper gastro intestinal tract bleed; and when this is associated with jaundice, portal hypertension with bleeding varices must be considered.

What is found on clinical examination?

A palpable gall-bladder

Courvoisier's law is a very useful clinical sign. If the gall-bladder is palpable in a jaundiced patient, carcinoma of the head of the pancreas is highly likely. Gallstones cause fibrosis of the gall-bladder wall due to recurrent attacks of chronic cholecystitis and do not therefore dilate easily when a gallstone causes obstruction of the gall-bladder.

There are exceptions to the rule. If the gall-bladder has not been severely damaged by chronic cholecystitis, it can dilate when obstructed by a stone. This can then give a false positive sign. Carcinoma of the gall-bladder can also cause a palpable gall-bladder and jaundice.

Sometimes the gall-bladder is tucked so far behind the liver that a dilated gall-bladder is not palpable. This is a false negative sign. Sonar will show an enlarged dilated gall-bladder and an extrahepatic bile duct.

Hepatosplenomegaly

This suggests liver disease, probably with portal hypertension. If a mass is palpable, malignancy must be considered.

Large dilated veins, especially periumbilically (caput medusae), are a sign of hepatic disease with portal hypertension.

Ascites may indicate cirrhosis or malignancy.

Other signs include – spider nevi on the thorax, neck, face and upper arms and palmar erythema. This phenomenon is probably due to hormonal imbalance, but the mechanism is not fully understood.

Patients may also have clubbed fingers. Palpable, hard lymph nodes in the supraclavicular region or nodules per rectum suggest malignancy. A bruit is sometimes audible at the umbilicus and disappears when hard pressure is applied on the umbilicus. There is usually a large collateral vein between the umbilical vein and the left portal vein. This is known as the Cruveilhier-Baumgarten syndrome.

Special investigations

Biochemistry

A. Liver function tests

Three functions are usually tested, namely:

- Excretory function:
  Bilirubin: Total bilirubin and the conjugated fraction are measured. A raised conjugated water-soluble fraction indicates obstructive jaundice.
- Metabolic function:
  Albumin, fibrinogen and prothrombin are synthesized in the liver. Globulin is synthesized inside and outside the liver in the reticulo-endothelial system.

  A fall in albumin levels and a rise in globulin, or a disturbance in the albumin/globulin ration indicate hepatocytic disease. There is a simultaneous drop in fibrinogen and prothrombin.
- Enzymes:

(a) *Transaminases:* Aspartate aminotransferase (AST) and alanine aminotransferase (ALT) are found in the cytoplasm and mitochondria respectively. A rise in serum levels of these enzymes indicates hepatocyte damage.

(b) *Gamma-glutamyl transpeptidase (Gamma GT):* This enzyme is found in the hepatocytes and the epithelium of the bile canaliculi in the liver. It is usually raised when there is hepatocyte damage with cholestasis. Most patients with alcoholic hepatitis have high levels.

(c) *Alkaline phosphatase:* This enzyme is synthesized in the liver, small intestine and bone. The various phosphatases can be distinguished from each other by measuring their iso-enzymes. Bile duct obstruction increases synthesis of alkaline phosphatase by the intrahepatic bile duct cells. A rise in alkaline phosphatase usually precedes the rise in bilirubin. When the obstruction is relieved, it takes longer than bilirubin to fall. Although raised alkaline phosphatase associated with raised conjugated bilirubin strongly indicates extrahepatic bile duct obstruction, it must be remembered that an intrahepatic lesion such as a metastasis can cause alkaline phosphatase to rise without raised bilirubin levels.

(d) *Lactic acid dehydrogenase (LDH):* This enzyme has five iso-enzymes. Iso-enzyme LDH5 is usually raised in liver disease. The enzyme is very nonspecific.

B. Viral markers

Hepatitis A and B surface antigen and antibodies must be measured in conjunction with immunoglobulins.

C. Auto-immuno antibodies

Measurement of antinuclear, anti-smooth muscle and antimitochondrial auto-antibodies is useful in the diagnosis of auto-immune liver disease.

D. Other useful tests

These include

- Alpha fetoprotein: This is an alpha globulin which is usually raised in patients with hepatoma. It can be raised in patients with viral hepatitis or chronic active hepatitis. It is sometimes raised in cases with gastric or pancreatic carcinoma.
- Alpha-1-antitrypsin: This is raised in patients with cholestasis due to liver disease.

Congenital alpha-1-antitrypsin deficiency causes severe liver damage due to cirrhosis.

- Bile salts: These are synthesized in the liver and secreted in the bile, whereafter they are reabsorbed in the distal small intestine (enterohepatic circulation of bile salts). A rise in bile salts is a very sensitive indicator of cholestasis.
- Serum amylase: A tenfold increase is pathognomonic of pancreatitis. A raised serum or urine amylase associated with a typical clinical presentation suggests diagnosis of acute pancreatitis.

Imaging of the liver, bile ducts and pancreas

Routine X-rays

Gallstones may be seen on routine abdominal X-rays (15% contain sufficient calcium to be radio-opaque).

- *Hepatic calcifications:*
  Echinococcus cysts
  Calcified haematomas
  Tumours: Haemangioma, hepatoma (very rare)
- *Pancreatic calcifications:*
  Chronic recurrent alcoholic pancreatitis
  Pancreatic stones in the ducts

Contrast radiology of the stomach and duodenum

A barium meal can show displacement of the stomach by pancreatic masses, pseudocysts or tumours. Barium in the duodenum can show a dilated loop suggestive of carcinoma of the head of the pancreas, or the inverted 3 sign, found in carcinoma of the ampulla of Vater.

Contrast radiology of the bile ducts

If the patient is not jaundiced, a cholecystogram or an intravenous cholangiogram can be performed.

- *Cholecystogram*
  This investigation is based on the fact that halogenated materials will be excreted from the liver via the bile. The gall-bladder concentrates halogen 8 to 10 times, so that it becomes visible on X-ray. Usually a double dose of biloptin tablets are given the night before, and X-rays are taken ten to twelve hours later. Supine and erect views are taken before and after a fatty meal, which causes the gall-bladder to contract. If the gall-bladder does not fill, this is usually an indication of an obstruction, with a stone in the Hartman pouch. If the gall-bladder fills, stones are seen as filling defects.
- *Intravenous cholangiogram*
  Biligraphin is given IV and is excreted by the liver into the bile ducts. Unfortunately, this stimulates water secretion into the bile, diluting the biligrafin. However, the bile ducts are clearly visible on X-ray and the size of the ducts and gallstones (filling defects) can be seen.

  Owing to the relatively poor opacification of bile ducts in this method, it has been largely replaced by methods of direct cholangiography, using the currently available injection methods.
- *HIDA scan*
  If jaundice is present, the bile ducts can still be demonstrated by the use of Tc^{99} marked imino-diacetic acid derivatives, the so-called HIDA scan. In normal patients, the HIDA concentrates in the liver within minutes of injection. Thirty minutes after the injection, the bile ducts and gall-bladder will have filled and thirty to sixty minutes after the injection it will have moved into the duodenum. A gall-bladder which does not fill is indicative of cholecystitis. In bile duct obstruction, it does not empty into the duodenum. There are also other similar radiopharmaceutical drugs such as PIPIDA and DISIDA.

Direct injection contrast cholangiography

- *Endoscopic retrograde cholangiopancreatography (ERCP)*
  Biligraphin is injected directly into the papilla via duodenoscopy. Ideally, one tries to fill both the bile and pancreatic ducts. Sometimes, for technical reasons, only the bile or pancreatic ducts are filled. The size, stenoses and filling defects of the ducts are clearly visible.
- *Percutaneous transhepatic cholangiography (PTC)*
  A thin needle (Okuda needle) is inserted into the bile ducts percutaneously and small amounts of biligraphin are injected until the needle hits a dilated duct and the entire ductal system fills with dye. The size, stenoses

and filling defects of the ducts can be clearly seen. If the obstruction cannot be relieved, bile can leak out of the needle wound from the liver into the peritoneal cavity.

Ultrasound

This is a very useful investigation. It is non-invasive and does not involve any irradiation. Dilated intrahepatic bile ducts, indicative of extrahepatic bile duct obstruction, can be well demonstrated. It is very useful for showing pancreatic tumours. It is usually the investigation of choice for diagnosing gallstones in the gall-bladder. It is also very reliable in the diagnosis of abscesses and cysts in the liver and pancreas.

Computer tomography

This is of particular value in the diagnosis of intrahepatic and pancreatic disease, tumours and abscesses.

Isotope pancreas and liver scans

Colloidal sulphur marked with Tc^{99} is commonly used. After injection, it is absorbed by the RE system and gives a good image of the liver and spleen. It is useful in the diagnosis of large space-occupying lesions, such as primary tumours, metastases, cysts and abscesses.

Biopsy

If a diagnosis cannot be made by means of imaging procedures, or if the biochemical tests cannot clarify the diagnosis, it becomes essential to obtain tissue for histological examination. Percutaneous needle biopsy of the liver tissue is the procedure of choice. This can be performed if the following contra-indications are not present:

- The prothrombin period must not be prolonged.
- The platelet count must not be lower than 40 000 ml.

Biopsy can also be taken laparoscopically under direct vision. If the prothrombin period and platelets cannot be corrected, the biopsy can be taken by inserting special biopsy forceps via the internal jugular vein, inferior cava and hepatic vein. Haemorrhaging will then take place into the venous system, which does not create problems.

Aspiration cytology can also be performed on a pancreatic mass by inserting a fine percutaneous needle for cell aspiration. Sometimes a direct biopsy can be taken of a carcinoma of the ampulla of Vater via an endoscope. Aspiration cytology can also be performed on cells aspirated from the pancreatic duct.

Collection of venous samples

Samples must be taken from various levels of the splenic vein and biochemical measurements made. It may be useful in localizing endocrine tumours of the pancreas.

Arteriography and splenoportography

Arteriography of the coeliac trunk can be useful in localizing tumours and in determining their size.

Splenoportography can be used to diagnose portal hypertension. Portal pressures can be measured simultaneously.

Practical classification of surgical conditions of the liver, bile ducts and pancreas

JAUNDICE

OBSTRUCTIVE JAUNDICE

Gallstones

Complications of gallstones

- Cholecystitits
- Gallstone ileus
- Stones in the bile duct
- Cholangitis
- Sclerosing cholangitis
- Benign stenosis
- Gallstone pancreatitis
- Acute pancreatitis

Malignant conditions causing obstructive jaundice

- Carcinoma of the gall-bladder
- Carcinoma of the hepatic bifurcation
- Periampullary carcinoma

Tumours of the pancreas

PORTAL HYPERTENSION

LIVER ABSCESSES

- Bacterial liver abscess
- Amoebic liver abscess

Swellings of the liver

Cysts

- Paracitic cysts (Echinococcus)
- Simple cysts
- Cysts of the intrahepatic bile duct

Benign tumours

- Haemangioma
- Adenoma
- Focal nodular hyperplasia

Malignant tumours

- Primary cancer of the liver
- Pathological liver cancer types
- Metastases in the liver

Trauma

This will be discussed in a separate chapter.

JAUNDICE

Bilirubin metabolism

Bilirubin is a byproduct of haemoglobin. An adult produces between 420 and 520 micromol of bilirubin per day, 80% of which is derived from breakdown of old red blood cells in the spleen, liver and bone marrow, and 20% from catabolism of other haem-containing proteins in the liver.

The unconjugated bilirubin, bound to albumin, is fat-soluble and gives rise to the indirect Van den Berg reaction. The unconjugated complex is conjugated with glucoronic acid in the hepatocytes, with the help of the enzyme glucoronyl transferase, produced by the smooth endoplasmic reticulum.

The conjugated bilirubin is water-soluble and gives rise to the direct Van den Berg reaction. Conjugated bilirubin is excreted via the bile ducts into the intestinal canal, where it is bacterially hydrolysed to unconjugated bilirubin and then reduced to urobilinogen, which is colourless.

Urobilinogen is absorbed to a certain extent and excreted by the kidneys in the urine and re-excreted by the liver in the bile. The majority of the urobilinogen is changed by bacteria into stercobilinogen, which gives stool its brown colour.

Jaundice arises

- If the volume of bilirubin is so large that the normal hepatic mechanisms cannot handle it. This is prehepatic unconjugated hyperbilirubinaemia.
- If there is an obstruction of the extrahepatic bile ducts. This is posthepatic unconjugated hyperbilirubinaemia.
- If there is liver disease associated with a degree of cholestasis. This is hepatic or combined conjugated and unconjugated hyperbilirubinaemia.

It is useful to present the classification of jaundice in two ways.

Classification I

A. Prehepatic jaundice

Increased breakdown of red blood cells

Haemolytic jaundice:

1. **Congenital conditions**
   - Spherocytosis
   - Sickle cell anaemia
   - Thalassaemia
2. **Auto-immune anaemia**
3. **Infections**
4. **Toxins**

B. Intrahepatic jaundice

1. **Congenital abnormalities**
   - Transport and storage of bilirubin (Gilbert disease)
   - Abnormalities of bilirubin excretion (Dubin-Johnson syndrome)
   - Abnormalities of uptake and storage of bilirubin in the liver (Rotor syndrome)
   - Abnormalities of glucoronyl transferase activity (Najar syndrome)
2. **Viral and other infections**
3. **Cirrhosis**
4. **Drugs**
5. **Toxic substances**

C. Posthepatic jaundice

- Obstruction of the bile ducts
- Gallstones
- Carcinoma

- Fibrotic stenosis
- Parasites

Classification II

A. Unconjugated hyperbilirubinaemia

Increased breakdown of red blood cells:

1. **Congenital conditions**
   - Spherocytosis
   - Sickle cell anaemia
   - Thalassaemia
2. **Acquired auto-immune anaemia**
3. **Infections**
4. **Chemical toxic agents**

Abnormalities of bilirubin transport and storage

1. **Congenital (Gilbert disease)**
2. **Drugs, especially antibiotics**
3. **Metabolic immaturity, jaundice of the newborn**

B. Conjugated hyperbilirubinaemia

Abnormalities of bilirubin excretion

1. **Congenital (Dubin-Johnson syndrome)**
2. **Intrahepatic cholestasis, cirrhosis**
   - Hepatitis (alcoholic and viral)
   - Carcinoma
   - Granulomatous hepatitis (this includes many diseases)
3. **Drugs**
   - Chlorpromazine
   - Sex hormones
   - Halothane
   - Antibiotics
4. Extrahepatic bile duct obstruction
   - Gallstones
   - Carcinoma (bile ducts and pancreas)
   - Stenosis (iatrogenic)
   - Sclerosing cholangitis
   - Parasites

C. Combined unconjugated and conjugated hyperbilirubinaemia

1. **Bile duct obstruction with secondary hepatocyte damage**
   - Secondary biliary cirrhosis and cholangitis
2. **Hepatocyte damage with intrahepatic cholestasis**

OBSTRUCTIVE JAUNDICE

If a patient presents with jaundice, it is very important to identify one suffering from obstructive jaundice and to relieve the obstruction as rapidly as possible.

Clinical presentation

A thorough history and a complete physical examination are important. Unfortunately, it is seldom possible to make a final diagnosis on clinical grounds alone. Nevertheless, the following positive and negative points are important:

- A history of previous attacks of pain in the right hypochondrium and jaundice, strongly suggests gallstones.
- Painless jaundice of slow onset which deepens rapidly, followed by mass loss and severe pruritis, strongly suggests obstructive jaundice, probably caused by a malignant tumour.
- Light stools and dark urine indicate obstructive jaundice.
- A palpable gall-bladder (positive Courvoisier's law) suggests obstructive jaundice caused by carcinoma of the head of the pancreas.
- Stigmata of liver disease and portal hypertension such as spider nevi, palmar erythema, visible collateral vessels, splenomegaly and ascites, suggest an intra-hepatic cause for the jaundice.

Side room investigations

The presence of bilirubin and the absence of urobilinogen in the urine suggests a total extrahepatic obstruction.

Special investigations

The final diagnosis is usually based on special investigations.

Liver function tests

- A raised conjugated fraction of total bilirubin and high levels of alkaline phosphatase, with a normal serum albumin are strongly indicative of obstructive jaundice. The transaminase enzymes are only slightly raised. Gamma GT is usually also raised.

- Intrahepatic jaundice can be suspected if the unconjugated fraction of bilirubin is raised. The transaminase enzymes are much elevated, alkaline phosphatase is normal or only slightly raised. Albumin is lowered and the globulin fraction is usually high.

There is so often a mixed picture, that imaging of the bile ducts is usually necessary for making a diagnosis.

Imaging of the bile ducts

The following approach can be applied rapidly to make a definitive diagnosis:

- The first investigation is ultrasound. This shows dilated bile ducts in the liver, confirming that obstructive jaundice is probably present. If stones can be demonstrated in the gall-bladder and/or bile duct, the diagnosis is gallstone obstruction. Unfortunately, examination of the bile ducts is not easy on ultrasound. If ultrasound shows dilated bile ducts, without stones, but with a mass in the head of the pancreas, cancer of the head of the pancreas can be diagnosed.
- The next investigation is ERCP. The papilla of Vater can be seen directly during duodenoscopy and, if there is an ampullary carcinoma, a biopsy can be taken. The bile and pancreatic ducts are cannulised and dye is injected. If there are gallstones in the duct, these appear as filling defects in dilated ducts. The pancreatic duct is then normal. If there is a carcinoma of the head of the pancreas, an irregular narrowing of the bile duct and pancreatic duct is seen, with proximal dilatation. Sometimes there is total obstruction and the bile ducts and pancreatic duct cannot be filled at all.

  If the obstruction is caused by a carcinoma of the bile duct, an irregular stenosis is found, with proximal dilatation of the bile ducts.
- If ERCP is not available and ultrasound shows dilated intrahepatic bile ducts, a percutaneous trans-hepatic cholangiogram (PTC) is performed. A thin, floppy Okuda needle (Chiba needle) is inserted percutaneously into the liver until it hits one of the dilated bile ducts and the bile ducts fill. The stenosis can usually be well defined. The complication of bile leakage into the peritoneal cavity is fortunately rare if the thin Chiba needle is used. If ultrasound does not show dilated ducts and there is doubt about the diagnosis, then ERCP is preferable, after virus markers have been shown to be negative.
- If ERCP shows normal bile ducts, a percutaneous needle biopsy of the liver is taken for histological diagnosis.
- If ERCP is not available and ultrasound shows no dilated ducts, a needle biopsy must be performed to confirm the diagnosis.

Special problems in patients with obstructive jaundice

Bleeding tendency

Malabsorption of fat and fat-soluble vitamins is often found in patients with severe cholestasis. Hypoprothrombinaemia with a resultant bleeding tendency is a common problem. Vitamin K must be given preoperatively to patients with obstructive jaundice.

Hepatorenal syndrome

This a well-known cause of postoperative death in patients with osbstructive jaundice. It is more common in patients with bilirubin levels of more than 170 micromol/litre and a period of hypotension is the most important precipitating factor. The renal lesion is tubular necrosis, but the mechanism is unknown. Factors which play a rôle include bilirubin, bile salts, hypotensive damage to the tubular epithelium and, very importantly, endotoxins from Gram-negative bacteria, especially in the gastrointestinal tract or bile ducts.

Prevention

Paticnts must be well hydrated. Intravenous fluids must be commenced the night before surgery, along with antibiotics such as gentamicin and metronidazole. Intraoperatively, the patient must be kept well hydrated and Manitol 10% (200 ml) must be given. If urine output drops to below 1 ml per minute, more Manitol can be given. The rôle of preoperative bile duct drainage is not fully clear at this stage.

Preoperative bile duct decompression

Obstructive jaundice is associated with depression of myocardial function, increased peripheral resistance, weakened left ventricular contraction and constriction of the renal vascular bed. The immune response is suppressed and wound healing is retarded. It is obvious that permanent resolution of the bile duct obstruction is essential.

The merits of temporary external drainage of the bile ducts are questionable. The concept of drainage to prepare the patient for surgery is very attractive. In retrospectively analyzed series, considerably improved results have been reported. In prospective random trials, no advantage could be shown. Technical factors often cause problems. Haemorrhage can occur and catheters do not remain in place in the liver. A higher incidence of cholangitis also contributes to morbidity.

If patients have already presented with obstructive jaundice and cholangitis, a period of drainage is probably very useful, but the permanent resolution of the obstruction remains urgent and essential.

Pruritis

This symptom can be very irritating. Although the pathogenesis is unknown, accumulation of bile salts plays a rôle.

Cholestyramine, a bile salt-binding resin in doses of 12–16 g per day, sometimes helps. If the obstruction is not total and bile salts are still flowing into the small intestine where they can be bound, the medicine can be helpful.

Phenobarbital, in doses of 120 to 250 mg per day, may also be useful. Histamine blockers are not really effective.

Gallstones

Gallstones are very common and are increasing in incidence. More than 20% of women and 10% of men over forty have gallstones. Factors influencing the incidence of gallstones include race, sex, age and obesity. Gallstones are more common in whites than blacks. Swedes get gallstones twice as often as British citizens, Americans and white South Africans. Red Indians have a very high incidence of cholesterol gallstones. Seventy per cent of Pima Indian women over forty already have gallstones. Gallstones are twice as common in women, and the incidence increases with age.

Obesity is directly related to the incidence of gallstones. There has been no proven link to diet, although it has been suggested that a high fibre intake protects people against gallstones. There is no relationship between the "pill" and gallstones.

The pathogenisis of gallstones

Gallstones arise when crystals form from ingredients normally found in bile. There are two main types; cholesterol stones and pigment stones. There is probably no such thing as a pure cholesterol stone.

Cholesterol stones also contain calcium bicarbonate and pigment and are thus actually mixed stones.

Normal bile contains bile acids, chenodeoxy bile acid, lecithin, cholesterol, bilirubin and other anorganic and organic ions.

Cholesterol and lecithin form 90% of the solid content of bile and are transported in micellas formed by bile acids. Cholesterol precipitates as crystals in bile if micella formation is disturbed by supersaturation with cholesterol if too little lecithin or bile acid are present in the bile. These crystals accumulate around other particles such as mucosal cells, calcium bicarbonate and dead bacteria.

Pigment stones consist of calcium bilirubinate. Predisposing factors include excessive haemolysis, as in spherocytosis or other acquired haemolytic diseases. Bacteria also play a rôle by hydrolysing conjugated bilirubin to a water-insoluble unconjugated bilirubin complex, which then tends to precipitate and form pigment stones. Stasis in the bile ducts also plays a rôle in the formation of gallstones.

The natural course of patients with gallstones

It has been calculated that more than 70% of patients with gallstones are never treated surgically. More than 60% of them remain asymptomatic or develop mild symptoms which never lead to surgery. In prospective studies of patients with asymptomatic gallstones, it has been found that only 10% will develop symptoms of complications, leading to cholecystectomy, within five years. In patients who have already had an attack of gallstone colic, there is a 30% chance of further attacks in the next two years and a 20% chance that complications will develop. If gallstones are thus discovered by chance, there is no urgent indication for cholecystectomy.

Clinical presentation

Patients present with intermittent attacks of pain in the right hypochondrium or epigastrium. The pain is usually called gallstone colic, but is actually a constant pain, sudden in onset, which becomes gradually worse for about an hour and then improves slowly during the next hour. The pain may be exacerbated by ingestion of food, especially of the fatty variety. The pain may radiate to other parts of the abdomen, or to the shoulder, scapula or back. The intervals may be days, months or years. Sometimes vague symptoms like fat dyspepsia, discomfort after meals and flatulence are reported. Nausea and vomiting may be associated with the pain. On clinical examination nothing is found, aside from right hypochondrium tenderness.

Special investigations

About 15% of gallstones are visible on routine X-rays. In the past, the diagnosis was made by means of an oral cholecystogram. No filling of the gall-bladder indicates its obstruction by a stone in Hartmann's pouch. Sometimes the diagnosis is made on the grounds of filling defects visible in the dye which concentrates in the gall-bladder.

To a large extent, ultrasound has now replaced the cholecystogram. If stones are clearly visible echographically, the diagnosis is easy. If the clinical presentation is typical and ultrasound is normal, a cholecystogram must be performed. If the two are used in conjunction, a diagnosis can usually be made.

Differential diagnosis

Conditions mimicking the symptoms of chronic cholecystitis must always be considered. They include:

- Peptic ulcer – especially duodenal
- Gastritis and reflux oesophagitis, following sliding hernia
- Chronic recurrent pancreatitis
- Diverticular disease of the colon
- Angina pectoris

Functional syndromes, particularly spastic colon, must be considered. This diagnosis must not be based only on elimination of other conditions by means of negative special investigations, but must always be borne in mind because it is very common in the same population which has a high incidence of gallstones.

Adenomyomatosis

In this common condition, the mucosa of the gall-bladder proliferates and herniates through the muscularis mucosae to form small diverticula, the so-called Rokitanski-Aschoff sinuses. This condition may occur segmentally, or it may affect the whole gall-bladder.

Adenomyomatosis is often associated with segmentation of the gall-bladder by folds or annular strictures. It is not known whether the segmentation precedes the adenomyomatosis or vice versa. Adenomyomatosis is sometimes associated with cholesterolosis.

Cholesterolosis is a condition where cholesterol esters accumulate in the epithelial cells and macrophages of the wall of the gall-bladder. This gives rise to the typical appearance of yellow raised spots on a background of red mucosa. It is rare to find gallstones associated with this conditon.

Stones are indeed found in adenomyomatosis. The small diverticula are usually seen on the cholecystogram. Septa and filling defects, particularly of the fundus, are also typical.

The importance of adenomyomatosis lies in the fact that it is sometimes the only possible cause of pain in the right hypochondrium or epigastrium. The question arises whether a cholecystectomy is justified. The golden rule is that this condition is very seldom exclusively responsible for symptoms.

There are some exceptions. Cholecystectomy should probably not be performed solely for this condition if symptoms cannot be provoked by a cholecystokinin-stimulated cholecystogram (CSC). After the gall-bladder has been filled with dye for the oral cholecystogram, CCK is given slowly IV. If the symptoms are elicited when the gall-bladder contracts, the diagnosis can be considered.

Management of chronic cholecystitis

The management of symptomatic gallstones is cholecystectomy. The question arises whether an operative cholangiogram should be per-

formed routinely with every cholecystectomy. The chances are less than 10% that gallstones have already moved from the gall-bladder into the bile duct in patients with chronic cholecystitis. If there are stones in the bile duct, there is usually a past history of jaundice. There is also a raised alkaline phosphatase on liver functions. Some surgeons do an operative cholangiogram on a routine basis, but others believe it to be necessary only when:

- *there is a history of jaundice*
- *the alkaline phosphatase is raised*
- *there are multiple small stones in the gall-bladder*
- *the bile duct is dilated or stones are palpable.*

A routine intra-operative cholangiogram is probably not necessary. If there is a single large stone in the gall-bladder and the other factors mentioned are not present, it is not a cost-effective investigation.

Techniques for cholecystectomy

- *Right paramedian incision.*
- *Operate from the left side of the table, as it is easier (most surgeons operate from the right-hand side).*
- *Be on the alert for anatomical abnormalities of the cystic artery, as these are very common.*
- *The safest method is to begin at the fundus and to dissect the gall-bladder out of its bed until the cystic duct and cystic artery hang loosely.*
- *The artery is ligated with silk and the duct with catgut.*
- *The gall-bladder bed is dried up using diathermy but is not sutured.*
- *A corrugated drain is placed in the gall-bladder bed.*

Complications of cholecystectomy

The operative mortality of cholecystectomy is lower than 0,5%.

Morbidity

Haemorrhage

Usually a postoperative haemorrhage will arise if the ligature slips off the cystic artery. Reoperation is essential.

Bile leakage

Bile leaks from the gall-bladder bed when there are small accessory bile ducts, linking the liver parenchyma directly to the gall-bladder, which are cut and not noticed. This usually resolves spontaneously. If the cystic duct ligature slips off, or if the bile duct is damaged, a large leak arises, necessitating re-exploration.

Patients present with shock, jaundice and leakage of bile from the corrugated drain. The condition must not be confused with post-operative coronary thrombosis, which can mimic bile leakage.

Infection

Wound sepsis is common following cholecystectomy, but especially following bile duct exploration. Patients with gallstones usually have *E. coli, Strep. faecalis* and *Klebsiella aerogenes* in their bile. Broad spectrum antibiotics should be given prophylactically.

Residual bile duct stones

This will be discussed later with the management of bile duct stones.

Post-cholecystectomy syndrome

Vague epigastric pain and dyspepsia sometimes follow cholecystectomy, especially if no stones have been found in the gall-bladder. A cause for this syndrome in the biliary tract is very rarely found. It would be more advisable to investigate other probable causes for the pain for which the cholecystectomy was erroneously performed. Such conditions include pancreatitis, peptic ulcer, reflux oesophagitis and hiatus hernia, diverticular disease and spastic colon syndrome.

Dissolution of gallstones

Chenodeoxycholic acid (Chendol) and ursodeoxycholic acid can dissolve certain gallstones by reducing the cholesterol saturation of bile to such an extent that the stones gradually dissolve. The following factors are regarded as contra-indications:

- Pigment stones
- Calcified stones
- Stones larger than 1,5 cm

- A gall-bladder that does not fill after cholecystogram
- Liver diseases
- Severe symptoms which do not allow for longterm conservative treatment
- Obesity
- If stones have not shown signs of shrinking after six months of treatment

Chendol causes side effects such as diarrhoea and abnormal liver functions.

If all the side effects are taken into account, then less than 15% of patients are suitable for this treatment. In prospective trials, the treatment was successful in approximately 20–30% of cases in two years. Unfortunately, stones recur when treatment is stopped. Maintenance doses may prevent this, but the safety of this approach is questionable.

Lithotripsy

Gallstones, just like renal stones, can be fragmented by shock waves. It is more difficult to do this successfully with gallstones, because focusing the waves is a problem. There are series reported with successful fragmentation of stones. Sometimes patients develop complications such as gallstone colic and gallstone pancreatitis when the fragments pass through the sphincter of Oddi. This procedure can be used in conjunction with Chendol or ursodeoxycholic acid to disolve the fragments. The same problem of stone recurrence has been encountered. This method is still being developed.

COMPLICATIONS OF GALLSTONES

Cholecystitis

Acute cholecystitis

Acute cholecystitis develops in 15% of patients with symptomatic gallstones. The incidence of this complication increases with age. Ninety-five per cent of patients with cholecystitis have an obstruction of the neck of the gall-bladder or cystic duct.

The natural course is as follows:

- A stone or stones from the gall-bladder impacts in the Hartmann pouch or in the cystic duct.
- The gall-bladder contracts against this obstruction, causing dilatation.
- An inflammation, with oedema, develops in the wall.
- As the dilatation increases, the stone can loosen and fall back into the gall-bladder with relief of the inflammation and oedema.

Sometimes the gall-bladder dilates and no severe inflammation develops. The bile pigments absorb and the gall-bladder content becomes a bright, slimy fluid, giving rise to a mucocele of the gall-bladder.

If the obstruction and inflammation persist, two things happen:

- the bile and the wall of the gall-bladder become secondarily infected with bacteria
- the tension in the wall presses on the blood vessels, causing ischaemia of the wall.

Necrosis and gangrene of the fundus can occur with perforation.

Clinical presentation

The disease is more common in elderly women. There is a history of chronic cholecystitis in 75% of patients. Pain arises in the right hypochondrium and, as the inflammation worsens, it spreads to the rest of the abdomen and to the back and shoulder.

On examination of the abdomen, there is tenderness and muscle spasm. If the patient takes a deep breath, and pressure is applied to the right hypochondrium, the patient will gasp if the finger touches the gall-bladder (Murphy's sign). A tender gall-bladder is palpable in 20% of cases. Jaundice occurs in 10%, even though there is no stone in the bile duct. There are two possible explanations for this:

- oedema of the cystic duct/bile duct junction
- inflammation of the adjacent liver in the gallstone bed.

Sometimes a large stone in the Hartmann pouch can cause pressure on the bile duct and result in jaundice (Mirizzi syndrome).

Special investigations

The white cell count is usually raised. A raised serum amylase level is not unusual, even if there is no gallstone pancreatitits.

An oral cholecystogram cannot be done because the patient is nauseous and vomiting and it takes too long. The diagnosis is usually confirmed on ultrasound, which shows a thickened gall-bladder containing stones.

A HIDA scan can also be performed. If there is dye in the bile duct and duodenum, but the gall-bladder does not fill, the diagnosis of acute cholecystitis is confirmed.

Differential diagnosis

The condition must be differentiated from pancreatitis, perforated peptic ulcer, a renal calculus, liver infections, acute appendicitis and coronary thrombosis.

Acalculous cholecystitis

In about 5% of adults with cholecystitis, no stones are found. In children, this figure is as high as 45%. This condition can develop completely spontaneously, but usually arises as a complication in:

- aged people who have undergone major surgery
- young people who have sustained serious injuries, especially if there was hypovolaemic shock and if there is a septic focus somewhere.
- It is also found quite commonly in patients in intensive care wards with generalized organ failure.

  It is more common in such patients who are also on hyperalimentation.

Although the actual pathogenesis is unknown, the following factors probably play a rôle:

Inspissation of bile, with thick, sticky bile in the gall-bladder and poor drainage. Dehydration and hyperalimentation may contribute.

Inadequte blood supply to the wall of the gall-bladder:

- The cystic artery is an end artery.
- Dilatation of the gall-bladder with increased tension in the wall, causes ischaemia.
- Hypovolaemic schock contributes to ischaemia.

Secondary infection arises from the septic focus.

The clinical presentation does not differ from that of gallstone cholecystitis. The problem is that these patients have other causes for pain and fever and are sometimes unconscious, or on respirators, making the diagnosis difficult. Also, no gallstones are visible and this may mislead the uninformed. It is important to consider this diagnosis in severely injured patients with organ failure. Because ischaemia and gangrene with perforation occur in 50% of cases, urgent surgery with cholecystectomy is essential.

The management of acute cholecystitis

Acute cholecystitis will resolve on conservative management in about 90% of cases. The other 10% will form an empyema of the gall-bladder, with or without perforation. The disease resolves when:

- *the obstruction is relieved because the gallstone either moves through into the bile duct or falls back into the gall-bladder*
- *the inflammation is limited by the body's defence mechanisms and isolated by the omentum. It then resolves very gradually, with fibrosis.*

The fact of the matter is that cholecystectomy is the treatment of cholecystitis. The only decision that needs to be made is the timing of the operation. This decision is based on clinical factors.

Group I

The patient is admitted with a tentative diagnosis of acute cholecystitis. While she is being resuscitated and investigated to confirm the diagnosis, the pain resolves and signs of inflammation disappear. In these cases, the stone has loosened, the inflammation will not worsen and surgery is not urgent. When the diagnosis has been made, a cholecystectomy can be planned for any future date, but preferably during the patient's admission.

Group II

The patient is admitted with a tentative diagnosis of cholecystitis. She is resuscitated, her diagnosis is confirmed and she is fit for surgery. A cholecystectomy is then performed on the next elective surgical list, as long as this falls within the next seventy-two hours. If this period is extended, the operation becomes more difficult due to increasing inflammation. The majority of patients fall into this group.

Group III

A very sick patient is admitted with a tentative diagnosis of acute cholecystitis. During resuscitation, it becomes clear that there is advanced cholecystitis, probably with an empyema of the gall-bladder. These are usually elderly patients, with high fever, signs of advanced abdominal peritonitis, severe tenderness, guarding and ileus.

After resuscitation and confirmation of the diagnosis, the patient must be operated on urgently. It is usually advisable to perform only a cholecystostomy, even under local anaesthetic if necessary.

Group IV

The patient is admitted with the history that she has already been ill for a few days at home. The patient is resuscitated and the diagnosis is confirmed. If there are no signs of abdominal complications, it is better to treat such a patient conservatively and to perform elective surgery three months later. After five days it is difficult to do a cholecystectomy, because inflammation makes dissection of the cystic duct and the cystic artery very difficult. The advantages of this approach are as follows:

- *The majority of patients will be admitted to hospital only once.*
- *Patients are not operated on in the middle of the night without a proper diagnosis.*
- *If there is an urgent complication, an emergency procedure is indeed performed.*
- *An operation is not carried out on a difficult case with advanced inflammation, who does not even have complications.*

Conservative management

- *Intravenous fluid*
- *Nasogastric suction*
- *Antibiotics, preferably a cephalosporin*
- *Regular monitoring of fever chart, pulse, clinical abdominal signs and white cell count.*

If the symptoms and signs exacerbate, surgery becomes an urgent priority.

Cholecystectomy

The operation is usually easy if it is performed early in the oedematous stage. The tissue planes are easy to find, facilitating dissection. A retrograde cholecystectomy is recommended because it is so safe. If there are normal indications for cholangiography during the operation, then this must be done. A corrugated drain is placed in the cystic duct area.

Subtotal cholecystectomy (Thorek operation)

If it is clear that the cystic duct-bile duct junction cannot be dissected out safely, the anterior wall of the gall-bladder is removed and the posterior wall is left in the gall-bladder bed. The cystic duct is ligated and closed inside the lumen of the Hartman pouch. The mucosa of the remaining wall on the liver must be destroyed by means of diathermy. A corrugated drain is placed in position. This is a very safe alternative.

Cholecystostomy

The gall-bladder fundus is opened through a pursestring suture and bile, pus and stones are suctioned out. Remove whichever stones are easily removable. **Do not perform the dissection in the region of the Hartmann pouch or attempt any manipulation which will prolong the operation time.** *Insert a tube into the gall-bladder and fix it to the abdominal wall by means of a pursestring suture. Later, when the patient is stronger, a Gram can be performed via the tube. If the bile ducts are patent and no stones are visible on the Gram, the tube is simply withdrawn. The fistula closes and the patient can go home.*

If she is fit, an elective cholecystectomy can be performed later. Elderly, weak patients can merely be followed up.

If there are stones in the biliary tree, a cholecystectomy must be performed (stones in the gall-bladder). If the stones are in the bile duct, then an endoscopic sphincterotomy can be performed. Cholecystostomy is a very good operation for these seriously ill patients.

Gallstone ileus

This condition will be discussed here, because it is regarded as a complication of cholecystitis. A large gallstone in Hartmann's pouch erodes through the wall due to chronic pressure necrosis. There is usually an inflammatory adhesion between the gall-bladder and the second section of the duodenum, where the fistula arises. A stone larger than 2,5 cm in diameter will move down the intestinal canal until it cannot move any further through the lumen. It then causes a mechanical obstruction. More than 70% of these obstructions occur in the distal ileum, but they have also been described in the jejunum. There have even been cases where the obstruction has occurred in the duodenum itself or in the colon, if the fistula develops between the gall-bladder and the colon. Only a very large stone will cause a colonic obstruction.

Clinical presentation

These patients are usually elderly women who present with small bowel obstruction. They have the usual symptoms and signs; colicky pain, abdominal distension and increased bowel sounds. Sometimes, but not often, there is a previous history of acute cholecystitis. A history of chronic cholecystitis is more common.

Special investigations

Abdominal X-rays show mechanical small intestine obstruction, with distended bowel loops and air-fluid levels. Sometimes (± 20%) a gallstone can be seen at a site other than the gall-bladder. The most important diagnostic finding is air in the biliary tree.

The fistula would show on barium meal. However, it is not advisable to do a barium meal because of obstruction of the small bowel.

Management

There is often confusion about the diagnosis. Initially, patients present with a partial obstruction and, because no obvious cause can be found, surgical treatment is delayed. It is important to correct the patient's fluid and electrolyte balance. At operation, the stone is milked backwards towards a segment of healthy, dilated bowel, and removed via an enterotomy. Make sure that there is no second stone in the intestine. **Do not try to crush the stone or milk it through to the caecum as an alternative to enterotomy, as this damages the intestine. Do not perform a cholecystectomy as part of the same operation.**

In the postoperative period, an elective cholecystectomy is recommended for younger, fitter patients. Older patients who are unfit are not operated on but only followed up, because a fistula between the gall-bladder and duodenum does not usually cause any further problems.

Stones in the bile duct

Ten per cent of patients with stones in the gall-bladder also have stones in the bile duct. Ninety per cent of these bile duct stones arise in the gall-bladder and reach the bile duct via the cystic duct. The other 10% arise primarily in the bile duct. Primary bile duct stones are usually oval, are found with gravel in the duct and can be crushed with one's fingers. It has been postulated that bile duct stones are more common in bile ducts where stasis is present. Pressure studies done on patients with primary bile duct stones have shown raised resting pressures. These findings have not been confirmed by all researchers.

Stones can stay in the bile duct for a long time without causing complications. Because the complications of bile duct stones are so serious, the mere presence of a stone in the bile duct is an indication for removal. The usual complications include obstructive jaundice, cholangitis and gallstone pancreatitis. There is sometimes a mild, chronic rise in bilirubin, which may not necessarily manifest clinically, but which can give rise to biliary cirrhosis after a few years.

Clinical presentation

Most patients with stones in the bile duct present with chronic cholecystitis and the bile duct stones are found at cholecystectomy, without having manifested any symptoms. Patients may present with obstructive jaundice, with or without upper abdominal pain. They sometimes present with infection and pain, rigors and jaundice (Charcot's triad). They can also present with gallstone pancreatitis. If the patient presents with obstructive jaundice, the usual signs of dark urine and pale stools are found, but the gall-bladder is impalpable (negative Courvoisier's law).

Special investigations

Conjugated bilirubin and alkaline phosphatase are elevated. Transaminase is only slightly raised and albumin is normal. Ultrasound shows dilated intraphepatic bile ducts. Gallstones may be visible in the gall-bladder and bile duct. It is difficult to evaluate the bile duct ultrasonically. If there is any doubt, the diagnosis must be confirmed on ERCP. If ERCP is not available, PTC can be performed.

Management

Patients with jaundice must be prepared for possible surgery by supplementing fluid and electrolytes and by giving Vitamin K, to prevent a bleeding tendency caused by a short prothrombin period.

There are two possible ways to remove bile duct stones:

- *Cholecystectomy and exploration of the bile duct, with removal of stones.*
- *Endoscopic sphincterotomy and removal of stones. If this is done, the gall-bladder, with its stones, can be left* in situ *or an elective cholecystectomy can be performed at a later stage.*

If the patient is at normal risk for his age, and the gall-bladder is filled with stones, the treatment of choice is a cholecystectomy with exploration of the bile duct. In a patient with bile duct stones who has undergone a previous cholecystectomy, the treatment of choice is an endoscopic sphincterotomy. If the patient is elderly and completely unfit, the treatment of choice is an endoscopic sphincterotomy.

Cholecystectomy and exploration of the bile duct

An operative cholangiogram must always be done, even if bile duct stones have already been diagnosed preoperatively. It offers the following advantages:

- *It provides information about the number of stones and where they are situated.*
- *It delineates the anatomy of the bile ducts, especially the junction of the cystic duct and the gall-bladder. It warns the surgeon of abnormalities, which are relatively common.*

The stones are removed from the duct using instruments, after which the duct is rinsed thoroughly. There are conflicting opinions as to whether Bakes sounds must be inserted through the sphincter. The placement of a 4 mm sound, just to calibrate the sphincter and to prove that it is patent, cannot do any harm. The intraoperative choledochoscope is useful for ensuring that all the stones have been removed. After exploration, a T-tube is placed in position and a T-tube gram is done to determine whether all the stones have been removed and whether dye can flow into the duodenum. If there is any doubt about filling defects, rinse the dye through and repeat the gram. Bring the T-tube out through the abdominal wall together with the corrugated drain, and make sure that the patient does not pull the T-tube out accidentally, while coming round from the anaesthetic. Cover it with bandages until the patient is fully awake. It can then be allowed to drain into a bag.

On the eighth day, the tube is clamped. If there is distal obstruction in the bile duct, the patient will develop pain and bile will leak past the tube. If this is the case, open the tube immediately. Do a postoperative T-tube gram on day 10. If this is normal, the tube can be removed.

Residual stones

T-tube in the bile duct

Despite all precautions, stones remain in the bile duct in about 30% of patients who have undergone exploratory surgery. If "stones" are seen on the postoperative T-tube gram, it must always be repeated, while taking every precaution to prevent air bubble formation. If a filling defect is still present, follow these steps:

- *Keep the T-tube in position.*
- *Do an endoscopic sphincterotomy. If the stone is situated distal to the T-tube in the bile duct, it can be rinsed out with the aid of the T-tube. If the stone is proximal to the T-tube, and there is no doubt that an adequate endoscopic sphincterotomy has been performed, the T-tube can be removed and the stone allowed to pass through on its own.*

The T-tube is left in position initially. Should an endoscopic sphincterectomy be impossible for technical reasons, the T-tube or its tract can be used to remove the stone.

Dissolving gallstones

Gallstones can sometimes be washed through the sphincter after glucagon has been administered to relax the sphinchter.

- **The use of mono-octanoin**
  Capmul 8210 (mono-octanoin) is a semisynthetic plant oil which dissolves cholesterol stones in about 60% of cases. The oil must be given through the T-tube at 3–5 ml per hour for four days. Unfortunately, it does not dissolve mixed stones successfully.

- **Extraction of the stone through the T-tube tract**
  The T-tube is left in situ *for six weeks to allow the tract to mature. Recheck whether the stone is still present in the tube. Using X-ray monitoring, a Burhenne pliable catheter is inserted through the tract past the stone. A Dormia basket is then pushed through the catheter to catch the stone and pull it out.*

  Other methods used similarly include a suction catheter to adhere to the stone and pull it out; and the use of a thin, pliable, fibre-optic choledochoscope.

  Mazzarielo, who developed this technique, reports a 90% success rate.

Re-operation

A follow-up operation must never be done in the first six weeks, as inflammation in the area will make it very difficult. If other methods do not succeed and there is no impaction or obstruction of the common duct, the T-tube can be removed and a second operation done much later, should the patient become symptomatic, or develop raised bilirubin and alkaline phosphatase. If there is obstruction, the T-tube is left in situ *and re-exploration is delayed for two months.*

Stones discovered in the bile duct long after cholecystectomy

If a patient presents with obstructive jaundice caused by bile duct stones months or years after a cholecystectomy, the question always arises as to whether this is due to residual stones or new primary bile duct stones. It is useful to re-evaluate all the previous clinical findings.

- Was there a history of jaundice before the cholecystectomy?
- Were there multiple small stones in the gallbladder?
- Was an operative cholangiogram performed? If so, re-evaluate the gram. Was the duct dilated?
- Was the bile duct explored?
- Were multiple stones found in the duct?

If the answers to the above questions are positive, it is probably a residual stone. If they are negative, and the duct is much dilated, or if a single oval stone and gravel can be seen, consider a primary bile duct stone.

Management

Do an ERCP and, if there is no long stricture at the distal end of the duct and the stone is not too big (smaller than 2,5 cm), do a sphincterotomy. If the duct is extremely dilated with large stones, or if the endoscopic sphincterotomy was unsuccessful, surgery is necessary.

Considerations concerning surgery

If the previous history and clinical findings and the appearance of the stones in the duct suggest secondary (i e residual) stones; and the duct is not very wide (less than 2 cm) with a sphincter which can be easily calibrated (never dilate) with a 4 mm Bakes dilator, then the stone can simply be removed. However, the previous history and clinical findings and the appearance of the stone (oval, soft and easily crushed between the fingers), could be indicative of a primary gallstone. Drainage procedure must then be considered. Choose between choledochoduodenostomy and transduodenal sphincteroplasty.

Indications for choledochoduodenostomy

- One or more previous explorations of the bile duct for stones.
- A duct wider than 2 cm.
- Multiple stones. It is difficult to be sure that all the stones have been removed.
- Stones in the hepatic duct.
- Benign obstruction of the distal duct. Stenosis of the sphincter, especially if it is a long stenosis.
- Malignant obstruction in the distal duct in an unfit patient.

Choledochoduodenostomy is a very safe operation and relatively non-invasive if the side-to-side technique is used. Two complications of this procedure have been described, namely stenosis of the opening with resultant cholangitis and accumulation of debris in the blind end of the bile duct distal to the opening, the so-called "sump" syndrome.

If the opening is made larger than 2 cm, stenosis is very rare. The "sump" syndrome is also rare and can be cleaned out endoscopically.

Cutting through the choledochal duct and end-to-side suturing prevents the "sump" syndrome, but this anastomosis is more inclined to leak and the procedure has a higher mortality.

Indications for transduodenal sphincteroplasty

- Impacted stone in the distal end of the duct.
- Stenosis of the sphincter of Oddi.
- Short distal benign bile duct stenosis.
- Primary bile duct stones with gravel, where the duct is thin-walled and not excessively dilated (smaller than 2 cm). Such ducts are not suitable for choledochoduodenostomy.

There are fewer indications for operative sphincteroplasty nowadays, as it can often be done more easily and safely endoscopically. Unfortunately, there are alwayd cases where endoscopy is not technically possible.

Cholangitis

In 1877, Charcot described his triad suggesting the diagnosis of cholangitis, namely rigors, jaundice and pain. At the time, he also postulated that bile duct stones or benign and malignant strictures of the bile ducts are responsible for this syndrome. Since then, it has been clearly established that the syndrome depends on the presence of bacteria and foreign bodies, usually gallstones, in the bile ducts and a partial or total obstruction of the tract.

Normal bile is almost always sterile. If gallstones are present, bacteria can be cultured in more than 70% of patients. In cases of malignant biliary tract obstruction without stones, bacteria are found only in 25% of cases.

E. coli (75%), *Klebsiella pneumonia* (40%) and *Streptococcus faecalis* (30%) are found most commonly in patients with cholangitis. Anaerobic bacteria, especially *Bacteroides fragilis,* are found in 20% of cases. The bacteria reach the biliary tract by various routes:

- Ascending infection due to duodenal reflux.
- Via the lymphatics.
- Blood spread, either arterial, or via the portal vein.

The most important cause is probably reflux and explains why cholangitis is rarer in cases of total obstruction with carcinoma. With the increasing use of biliary tract instrumentation such as ERCP and PTC, this has also been found to be an important cause of cholangitis.

Clinical presentation

Charcot's classic triad, rigors, jaundice and pain, is naturally well known. It must be borne in mind that the triad is not essential for making the diagnosis. When the disease is more advanced, septic shock and central nervous system depression are also found. The condition can present clinically in various ways, ranging from slight fever and jaundice to fulminating septicaemia and septic shock. On examination, fever, jaundice and tenderness in the right hypochondrium can be found.

Special investigations

- Leucocytosis is usually present.
- Liver functions indicate cholestasis.
- Bilirubin and alkaline phosphatase are elevated and raised transaminases indicate liver damage, usually due to cholangitis, which ascends into the smaller bile canaliculi and later forms intrahepatic microabscesses.
- Ultrasound will show dilated bile ducts and gallstones.
- If there are already abscesses in the liver, they will show up as less dense areas.
- CT may be useful, especially to identify smaller liver abscesses.
- If there is no urgent indication for bile duct drainage, it is essential to first demonstrate the anatomy of the bile ducts and the underlying obstruction by means of ERCP or PTC.

Differential diagnosis

It is sometimes difficult to differentiate cholecystitis from cholangitis. They may occur concurrently. Rigors and severe jaundice suggest cholangitis. ERCP can exclude biliary tract pathology. Other conditions which must be considered include viral hepatitis, liver abscesses, pancreatitis, appendicitis and diverticulitis.

Management

This depends on the nature and severity of the illness.

General measures

• Antibiotics

All patients with cholangitis must receive broad spectrum antibiotics. The antibiotic must preferably be excreted in the bile and must be effective against Gram-negative aerobic and anaerobic bacteria, as well as against Gram-positive aerobic bacteria. A good, cheap combination is penicillin, an aminoglycoside, e g gentamicin, and an antibiotic which is effective against bacteroides, such as metrani'dazole or clindamycin. Some of the newer penicillins, such as piperacillin and imipenem are well excreted in the bile and are very effective against biliary tract bacteria. However, they are very expensive. The third generation cephalosporins are also very effective, but remember that they are less effective against Gram-positive anaerobes.

Sick patients, especially those with septic shock, must be given intravenous fluids and nasogastric suction. A central venous pressure catheter, or even a Swan-Ganz catheter to measure pulmonary wedge pressures, is useful in these cases. It is essential that the patient be admitted to an intensive care unit for supportive management.

• Drainage of the bile ducts

A large group of patients will respond to antibiotic therapy and can then be throughly investigated to determine the underlying cause of the cholangitis. If the patient does not improve within hours, drainage of the bile ducts is essential. An emergency operation is performed and the bile duct is opened, suctioned clean and any obvious stones are removed. **Do not do an extended bile duct exploration with lavage in these very sick patients.** *The duct must be drained quickly and a T-tube placed in position. Remember that a cholecystostomy is not adequate for bile duct drainage. If the patient is fit enough, a cholecystectomy can be performed if there is associated cholecystitis, otherwise a cholecystostomy must be performed in conjunction with bile duct drainage.*

Palpate the liver rapidly and if an obvious abscess is felt, drain it.

Currently, endoscopic sphincterotomy can be considered in very unfit, sick patients. Some researchers suggest percutaneous transhepatic drainage. The most practical approach is probably the following:

- *Administer antibiotics.*
- *If the patient improves, examine the biliary tract with ERCP and treat electively according to the findings.*
- *If the patient does not improve on conservative treatment, do an endoscopic sphincterotomy.*
- *If it does not succeed due to technical reasons, or if the patient does not improve, drain the bile duct surgically.*

Prognosis

If patients are drained early and effectively because they have not improved on antibiotic therapy, the mortality is 10%. If septic shock has already set in, the mortality is as high as 50%, in spite of drainage. **It is thus vitally important to make an early diagnosis and to drain effectively before septicaemia and septic shock set in.**

Sclerosing cholangitis

This condition can also be called stenosing cholangitis. It can occur in isolation, or it can be associated with a number of other inflammatory, vascular or fibrosing conditions. It was previously known as primary sclerosing cholangitis and was identified by the following characteristics:

- thickening, by fibrosis, of the extrahepatic bile ducts or intrahepatic bile ducts, or both together
- without the presence of gallstones, viral- or drug-induced hepatitis and
- there was to have been no previous surgery to the tree.

Currently we no longer make a distinction between primary sclerosing cholangitis and secondary cholangitis. It has become clear that gallstones can arise secondary to stenoses of so-called primary cholangitis, due to stasis and infection.

Aetiology

The condition is regarded as an auto-immune disease or a hypersensitivity condition which may be dependent on the Schwartzman reaction in the bile ducts.

Pathology

The condition usually affects both intra- and extrahepatic bile ducts. The most pronounced lesions are often found at the bifurcation of the hepatic ducts. If the lesion is limited to this area, carcinoma must be strongly suspected.

Sometimes the disease is limited to the intrahepatic bile ducts and, very rarely, to the extrahepatic bile duct. It is found in association with other diseases, especially ulcerative colitis. It can also be associated with Crohn's disease, retroperitoneal fibrosis, pancreatitis, vasculitis and porphyria.

Clinical presentation

It is more common in men than in women, around the age of forty. It begins with pain, loss of appetite, loss of mass and later intermittent jaundice, with pruritis. Eventually, a total obstructive jaundice develops, which later leads to biliary cirrhosis, portal hypertension and bleeding varices.

Special investigations

Liver function suggests an obstructive jaundice with liver damage.

ERCP is essential to confirm the diagnosis. It shows multiple narrowings ("string of beads" appearance) and blunting of the smaller intrahepatic bile ducts ("pruned tree", "leafless tree" appearance).

Differential diagnosis

Carcinoma of the bile ducts

A Klatskin tumour, which causes a stenosis at the bifurcation of the hepatic duts, must be borne in mind. The diagnosis, which is made on histological grounds, is sometimes very difficult.

Chronic pancreatitis

This condition can cause a stenosis of the bile duct where it runs through the groove in the pancreas.

Primary biliary cirrhosis

The condition can also destroy the small intrahepatic bile ducts. The mitochondrial antibodies are positive, while the eosinophilia found in sclerosing cholangitis is absent.

Management

The use of steroids, with or without azothiaprine and antibiotics, can sometimes delay the progress of the disease temporarily.

Where possible, stenoses must be dilated and kept open by tubes. This is merely palliative. Sometimes, when it is limited to the extrahepatic bile ducts (rare), a bypass can be done, using a loop of intestine. This condition is progressive and patients eventually develop liver failure and portal hypertension. ***It has now become one of the most important indications for liver transplantation.***

Benign bile duct stenosis

This condition can develop as a complication of gallstones and recurrent cholangitis. The most important cause is injury to the bile ducts during cholecystectomy. There is usually a history of an easy cholecystectomy without any apparent problems, followed by jaundice and cholangitis. Sometimes there is a history of bleeding from the cystic artery, which was controlled with difficulty. There is also sometimes a history of so-called ectopic bile ducts and abnormal anatomy.

Clinical presentation of bile duct injury

Early presentation

It is unusual to notice the injury during the operation. The usual presentation is that of a cholecystectomy which apparently went well. In the postoperative period, there is bile leakage from the corrugated drain, or if no drain was inserted, a fluid collection in the abdomen. Jaundice sets in within days and fever, with signs of cholangitis, follows.

Late presentation

In these cases, the operation appeared to have gone well, but was followed by a mild fever and transient jaundice postoperatively. Months or years later, the patient presents with jaundice and cholangitis. A diagnosis is then made and the stenoses are usually only found on ERCP, often with proximal stones which have developed due to stasis.

Management

If injury is noted intra-operatively, a repair must be carried out immediately, as this yields the best results. If it is a clean cut, the duct must be sutured. Polyglycol absorbable sutures are preferable. If the bile duct is wide, a continous waterproof suture can be used. If the duct is narrow, interrupted sutures are better.

If more than 1 cm of the duct has been damaged, it is better to use a Roux loop of intestine for the anastomosis. If the injury is only discovered postoperatively, no rash action must be taken. Patients are usually jaundiced and there is almost always infection. If a reconstruction is attempted under these circumstances, it will almost certainfly fail. The infection must be drained and antibiotics administered. If there is a bile fistula without sepsis, a fistulogram must be performed and/or an ERCP to delineate the lesion anatomically. Six weeks after the sepsis has cleared, the repair can be done.

Late presentation

If the patient presents with jaundice or cholangitis, an ERCP must be done, after infection has been controlled with antibiotics. This usually shows exactly where the lesion is situated and whether there are any stones present. It is useful to do a PTC to demonstrate the proximal bile duct anatomy.

Four different types of lesions have been described (Bismuth):

Type I

The stenosis is in the common hepatic bile duct with a 2 cm stump distal to the bifurcation.

Type II

The proximal stump between the bifurcation and the stenosis is less than 2 cm.

Type III

No stump is available.

Type IV

The stenosis involves the bifurcation.

Management

Type I

It is very rarely possible to excise the stenosis and to do a direct end-to-end anastomosis of the bile duct. It is usually better to suture a Roux loop onto the stump.

Type II

Suture a Roux loop to the stump.

Type III

Split the bifurcation and suture a Roux loop to the splayed ducts.

Type IV

This is a very difficult problem. Usually it is situated so high in the hepatic parenchyma and there is so much fibrosis, that direct suturing is impossible.

Two methods have been described

1. **The Rodney Smith method:** *A Roux loop is brought up and part of the intestinal wall is cleared of the muscular wall so that only the mucosa remains behind. It is then lifted upwards by tubes brought from the intestine, through the bile duct to the surface, through the hepatic parenchyma up to the skin. No suturing is done and the intestinal mucosa is pulled into position next to the bile duct mucosa by means of the transhepatic tubes.*
2. **The Hepp-Couinaud operation:** *It is preferable to make a direct anastomosis between bile ducts, which are lined by mucosa, and a Roux loop. The left hepatic duct runs horizontally for about 4 cm near to the surface of the liver, between the caudate and quadrate lobes, covered only by the hilar plaque of the liver tissue. The duct can be approached from the right side from its junction with the right hepatic duct, by dilating it and placing a Desjardin clamp in it, so that the overlying liver tissue can be cut through.* **Be careful to avoid injuring the left portal vein.** A 3 cm mucosa-to-mucosa anastomosis to the Roux loop can be done. The left duct can also be approached by following the round ligament between the medial and lateral segments of the left lobe. The duct is

dissected open and an anastomosis is made, using a Roux loop.

Postoperative course

It is not usually necessary the splint the duct after a Hepp operation. After the Rodney Smith procedure, the transhepatic tubes must be left in position for four months and then are removed after a satisfactory gram. The Hepp operation yields better results than the Rodney Smith operation.

Gallstone pancreatitis

Although gallstones are not the most common cause of pancreatitis in South Africa, is is more convenient to discuss the whole subject of pancreatitis, including the more common alcoholic pancreatitis, here.

Aetiology of acute pancreatitis

The majority of cases of acute pancreatitis are caused by alcohol and gallstones (more than 80%). Other causes include:

- **Hyperlipidaemia.** Associated with familial type I and V in the Frederickson classification of familial hyperlipidaemia.
- **Drugs.** Immunosuppresants such as steroids, azothiaprine and cyclosporin A can cause pancreatitis. Other drugs include tetracyclines and oestrogen-containing preparations.
- **Viral infections.** The mumps virus and certain enteroviruses, such as Coxsackie B virus, cause pancreatitis.
- **Injuries.** Direct injuries, or surgery to the pancreas can cause pancreatitis.
- **Familial pancreatitis.**
- **Hyperparathyroidism.** Raised parathormone and raised calcium blood levels can both cause pancreatitis.
- **Idiopathic pancreatitis.**

Pathogenesis of gallstone pancreatitis

Opie first drew attention to a patient with pancreatitis who died and had gallstones impacted in the ampulla of Vater on postmortem examination. He then developed his common canal theory. This is based on the premise that if the bile duct and the pancreatic duct have a common opening into the ampulla of Vater, an impacted stone will cause bile reflux into the pancreatic duct. This leads to extravasation of enzymes, causing pancreatitis. Later, it became clear that patients can develop pancreatitis wihout such impactions. Even gallstones in the gall-bladder or bile duct can cause pancreatitis.

The work of Acosta, and later Kelly, showed that gallstones are often found in the stools of patients with gallstone pancreatitis, suggesting that the cause may be migration through the sphincter of Oddi. It has also been shown that patients with small stones (smaller than 3 mm) are the ones who develop pancreatitis.

Pathogenesis of alcoholic pancreatitis

The precise pathogenesis is unknown. It has been shown that alcohol causes an increased protein content in pancreatic juice. The proteins precipitate out and cause obstruction of the smaller pancreatic ducts. There are also indications that alcohol influences the function of the sphincter of Oddi. Sometimes it lowers pressure and sometime it increases it. It is not precisely clear how this influences the pathogenesis of the disease. There may also be a direct toxic effect in some people after a period of sensitization.

Pathology of pancreatitis

The disease is divided into:

- acute pancreatitis and
- chronic pancreatitis.

Both forms of the disease can present with recurrent attacks.

Acute pancreatitis

There are two main types, namely:

- oedematous interstitial pancreatitis and
- necrotizing pancreatitis.

Oedematous interstitial pancreatitis

Obstruction of the ducts probably takes place, with congestion, leading to oedema. If the condition improves and the obstruction clears, the oedema is reabsorb by the lymphatics and the pancreas recovers completely.

Necrotizing pancreatitis

If the condition does not resolve rapidly, necrosis will set in. The proteolytic enzymes of the pancreatic juice cause tissue necrosis. Collagenase breaks down the connective tissue between the lobules and thus helps spread the condition. Lipase affects the neutral fat in the fat cells. Elastase has a destructive effect on the walls of the blood vessels and contributes to the haemorrhagic picture which is found in association with necrosis. Later, the necrotic tissue can become secondarily infected. The necrotic tissue is later absorbed and replaced with connective tissue, especially if the process is recurrent. In recurrent alcoholic pancreatitis, calcification of the pancreas often occurs.

Clinical presentation

It is useful to compare and contrast the clinical presentation of gallstone- and alcoholic pancreatitis. Gallstone pancreatitis is found in older women and alcoholic pancreatitis in younger men. There is sometimes a history of previous cholecystitis, but often an attack occurs with no prior warning. In alcoholic pancreatitis, there is a long history of alcohol abuse. Spirits and wine are the main culprits. Alchololic pancreatitis is less common among beer drinkers. There is a history of a party on Saturday, with pain beginning on Sunday afternoon and becoming so severe that the patient is admitted to hospital on Monday afternoon. There is often a history of previous attacks.

The patient complains of severe abdominal pain, radiating to the back. He rolls around on the bed and tries to assume a position (often on all fours) which relieves the pain. He has a rapid pulse and may be shocked.

On examination, the abdomen is tender, with guarding and a doughlike consistency. He may have an ileus, with no bowel sounds. If there is haemorrhagic pancreatitis, the Grey-Turner sign (discolouration of the costovertebral angle) or the Cullen sign (discolouration periumbilically) may be seen. An epigastric fulness may be palpable (pseudocyst) and bowel sounds may be absent on auscultation.

Special investigations

Biochemical measurements

Serum amylase is raised in more than 90% of patients. Amylase may also be raised in other acute abdominal conditions such as cholecystitis and perforated peptic ulcer. Levels which are raised tenfold are pathognomonic of pancreatitis. Sometimes amylase is not raised in the serum, but urine amylase is raised. The amylase has thus already been cleared from the serum. The test to compare amylase clearance to creatinine clearance and to work out a ratio between them, can also be performed. The ratio is raised in patients with pancreatitis who have normal serum amylase levels. The reason for the increased amylase clearance in pancreatitis is not clear, but there may be increased permeability to amylase in renal tubuli. Currently, iso-amylase, which is more specific for pancreatic amylase, can also be measured.

Lipase is also raised in acute pancreatitis.

X-rays

X-ray abdomen: Gallstones may be seen, suggesting gallstone aetiology. A sentinel loop, which is a loop of dilated intestine in the left upper abdomen, can sometimes be seen. The colon cutoff sign, with gas in the hepatic and splenic flexures of the colon and a collapsed transverse colon, is useful if it is present.

Ultrasound: Increased density and oedema of the pancreas can sometimes be seen. If present, a pseudocyst can be seen on ultrasound.

Computer tomography: This is far more reliable than ultrasound for the diagnosis of acute pancreatitis. The pancreas appears swollen and there is obliteration of the peripancreatic fat layers. Later, fluid can be seen around the pancreas. A phlegmon, or diffuse necrotic inflammation of the pancreas and surrounding tissues, is observed as an irregular, dense mass. CT is also useful in the diagnosis of pseudocysts and abscesses. **An abscess can be distinguished from a pseudocyst by virtue of the fact that it contains high density areas in its centre, signs of breakdown of necrotic tissue.**

ERCP: Although ERCP can sometimes cause pancreatitis, experience has shown that there is no great risk associated with the use of this investigation during attacks of pancreatitis. If gallstones are found, a sphincterotomy can be performed.

Natural course of the disease

The majority of cases are not life-threatening and resolve spontaneously on conservative treatment. In a small group, about 5%, the disease follows a fulminant course with a very high mortality. Various methods are used to identify these severe cases, so that they can be treated more intensively.

Ranson's criteria

On admisison

- Age higher than fifty-five
- White cell count over 16 000
- Blood glucose higher than 11 mmol/l
- LDH greater than 350 IU/l

First 48 hours

- Drop in haematocrit of more than 10%
- Blood urea rise exceeding 10 mmol/l
- Calcium less than 2,0 mmol/l
- Arterial PO_2 less than 7,5 kPa
- Base deficit of more than 4,0 mmol/l
- Estimated fluid sequestration of more than 6 litres

If more than three of the above criteria are positive, the mortality is higher than 60%.

The criteria of Osborne, Imrie and Carter

- White cell count higher than 15 000
- Blood glucose more than 10 mmol/l
- Plasma urea greater than 16 mmol/l
- LDH greater than 600 IU/l
- AST greater than 200 IU/l
- Calcium less than 2,0 mmol/l
- Plasma albumin less than 32 g/l
- Arterial PO_2 less than 8 kPa

Again, if more than three criteria are positive, the patient has life-threatening pancreatitis.

McMahon's peritoneal lavage colour criteria

After ensuring that the stomach and bladder are empty, a catheter is inserted into the peritoneal space, in the midline just inferior to the umbilicus. Fluid is aspirated. One litre of warm saline is run rapidly into the abdominal cavity. After the patient has been turned, the fluid is allowed to run out again. Severe pancreatitis is present if:

- more than 20 ml of dark peritoneal fluid is aspirated
- the saline running out is straw-coloured or dark. It is usually compared to a McMahon colour chart.

If a severe illness is predicted on using one or more of these methods, the patients must be admitted to an intensive care unit and monitored for organ failure, especially pulmonary or renal failure.

Management

If the case is not serious, the patient must be kept nil per os and given intravenous fluids. Patients recover within a few days. If a diagnosis of gallstone pancreatitis is suspected, the biliary tree must be thoroughly investigated. If underlying bile duct pathology is found, the patient should undergo surgery during the same admission, usually a week to ten days after being admitted. A cholecystectomy and intraoperative cholangiogram must be done and the bile duct must be explored if gallstones are seen.

If the patient has alcoholic pancreatitis, the social workers must be consulted to try and help control the alcoholism. If the alcohol abuse persists, the patient will have recurrent attacks of pancreatitis and will eventually develop exocrine and endocrine inadequacy with diabetes.

Conservative management of severe pancreatitis

- *Pethidine is preferable to morphine for analgesia, as the latter causes spasm of the sphincter of Oddi.*
- *In severe pancreatitis, the patient must be put on nasogastric suction and given fluid and electrolytes via a central venous pressure line. Remember that severe fluid sequestration occurs. The patient must be given parenteral feeding to allow the pancreas total rest.*
- *Prophylactic antibiotics, preferably cephalosporins, should be given.*

Special drugs

- *Trasylol (Aprotinine). This drug prevents experimental pancreatitis in animals, provided it is given before or during the induction of the disease. In three prospective series where the drug was tested on patients, two yielded completely negative results and the third favoured Trasylol. The accepted opinion is that Trasylol has no rôle to play in acute pancreatitis.*

- *Glucagon. This hormone inhibits pancreatic exocrine secretion. In two prospective trials, no advantages were found.*
- *Calcitonin. This hormone also inhibits pancreatic exocrine secretion. Raised blood levels are usually found in patients with pancreatitis. Administration of additional calcitonin does not influence the course of the disease.*
- *Somatostatin. This is a powerful inhibitor of both exocrine pancreatic secretion and gastric secretion. No good prospective trials are available, but in the series where it was used, it did not appear to make any significant difference.*
- *Cimetidine. Because this drug inhibits gastric acid secretion, a few prospective trials were done in acute pancreatitis. The drug made no significant difference.*

Peritoneal lavage

Possible advantages of this method include:

- *The diagnosis is confirmed if dark straw-coloured fluid with a high amylase content is aspirated.*
- *It also helps in determining the severity of the disease (McMahon's criteria).*
- *It may remove some toxic substances and support the patient in renal failure.*

Method: Two litres of balanced warm electrolyte solution, with heparin added (antibiotics are controversial), must be run into the abdominal cavity. After a half an hour, the fluid is allowed to drain. The lavage is continued for seventy-two hours.

Results: The early reports, including one prospective trial, have shown positive results. Unfortunately, many patients who survive the initial critical period, contract infection. Two later prospective trials could show no advantages from peritoneal lavage. The current indication for this method is a patient with fulminant pancreatitis, with renal failure as part of the generalized organ failure. If a patient has undergone a laparotomy for diagnostic reasons and acute pancreatitis is found, catheters should be positioned and lavage carried out for seventy-two hours.

Endoscopic sphincterotomy

There are three series of patients with gallstone pancreatitis and with life-threatening disease according to Ranson's criteria, who improved dramatically with only slight mortality after an emergency endoscopic sphincterotomy. Neoptolemus has shown in a prospective study that endoscopic sphincterotomy improves survival and decreases complications.

Emergency pancreatic resection

Possible reasons for surgery in patients with acute necrotizing pancreatitis may include the following:

- *The progression of the disease can be prevented by removing the pancreas, which secretes proteolytic and lipolytic enzymes.*
- *The cardiovascular and metabolic complications can be limited if the toxic substances derived from dead tissue are removed.*

If these reasons are considered, early surgery seems to be indicated in seriously ill patients who do not respond to conservative treatment. A high mortality was reported in all the series where this was done. Beger of Germany reported good results with early surgery in infected necrotizing pancreatitis.

If patients deteriorate after good conservative treatment and CT examinations show necrosis, surgery is indicated. The retroperitoneal necrotic tissue can practically be lifted out by hand. Catheters are placed in the cavity and continuously lavaged until recovery is effected. If abscess develops, the abdomen must be re-explored.

Complications of acute pancreatitis

Pseudocysts of the pancreas

These are called pseudocysts because they are not true cysts, but collections of fluid and pancreatic juice in the retroperitoneal tissue encircling the pancreas. They are not situated in the lesser sac, as is often stated, but behind the lesser sac, obliterating the lesser sac and adhering to the posterior wall of the stomach. The wall of the cyst develops around the collection of fluid in the tissues.

Aetiology

This condition is associated with acute and chronic pancreatitis.

Prerequisites for pseudocyst (PC) formation

- An actively secreting pancreas
- Obstruction or partial obstruction of the pancreatic duct drainage
- Ductal rupture

The majority of pseudocysts (PC's) are found in acute alcoholic pancreatitis. It is much less common in gallstone pancreatitis.

Pathogenesis and natural course

In the past, this complication was found in about 12% of cases. If all patients are investigated with ultrasound or CT, the figure is as high as 50%. The cysts tend to resolve spontaneously in 50% of cases. This depends on the size of the cyst and the duration of the illness. Smaller cysts (smaller than 5 cm) are inclined to disappear within six weeks. Larger cysts which are still present after six weeks, do not usually resolve spontaneously and are inclined to develop complications.

The complications of PC

- Rupture: Free rupture can occur into the abdominal cavity, intrapleurally, or into a hollow organ. Free rupture into the abdominal cavity, with ascites, has a mortality of 20%.
- Haemorrhage: The splenic blood vessels, the gastric mucosa itself, or the spleen may be eroded with massive haemorrhage.
- The PC may become secondarily infected, spontaneously or following diagnostic ERCP.
- The cyst may compress the bile ducts or even the duodenum.

Clinical presentation

A patient with a serious attack of pancreatitis presents with severe pain and a palpable epigastric mass.

Currently, the diagnosis is confirmed by ultrasound or CT. On CT, distinction can be made between a pseudocyst, an abscess and a phlegmon with irregular dense areas.

Management

Always remember that a small PC resolves spontaneously within six weeks. Also, complications are rare in the first six weeks and the cyst wall takes six weeks to mature. For these reasons it is not usually necessary or wise to perform surgery in the first six weeks. If patients become much sicker, with pain, enlargement of the cyst and a deterioration in general condition, an emergency operation must be performed. Under these circumstances, external drainage must be carried out.

External drainage

The cyst is suctioned until empty and a tube is positioned for external drainage. About 50% of cases will resolve completely and others will develop a pancreatic fistula requiring surgical treatment.

Internal drainage

If the cyst is operated on after six weeks and it is situated behind the lesser sac, it is approached via the gastric lumen. The cyst is opened through the posterior wall of the stomach. The opening is undersewn and the anterior wall of the stomach closed. **Avoid injuring the splenic artery during drainage.**

If there is pus in the cyst, the same operation can be done, but a tube must be brought out from the cyst, through the gastric lumen to the skin, for internal/external drainage.

If the PC is not adherent to the stomach, drainage can be achieved with a Roux loop of intestine.

Percutaneous drainage

Success has been achieved with percutaneous ultrasound-guided positioning of drainage catheters. This can be considered in ill, unfit patients.

Excision of the cyst

It is sometimes advisable to excise part of the body of the pancreas and its tail along with the cyst, in longstanding symptomatic cysts which have arisen as a complication of chronic recurrent pancreatitis. A cystadenocarcinoma of the pancreas must be considered in such cases.

Prognosis

External drainage causes fistulae in more than 50% of cases and has a mortality of 15%. Internal drainage has a cyst recurrence rate of 10% and a mortality of 5%.

Pancreatic juice ascites

This is a relatively rare condition. It presents either as isolated ascites, or as ascites with a pleural effusion, or as an isolated pleural effusion. The ascites fluid contains high concentrations of amylase and more than 2,5 g/dl of protein. It arises from direct leakage from the pancreatic system into the abdominal cavity, or as leakage from a pseudocyst into the peritoneal cavity. Another factor which plays a rôle is lymphatic stasis due to retroperitoneal inflammation, which impedes the resorption of pancreatic juice. This is a complication of alcoholic pancreatitis and has not yet been described in gallstone pancreatitis.

Clinical presentation

It is twice as common in men as in women. The age group is usually around forty. Occasionally patients have no history of pancreatitis. Patients complain of abdominal distension which has either come on suddenly or, more commonly, has developed slowly. They also complain of weakness, loss of mass, anorexia and diarrhoea. They sometimes have a low-grade fever and hypotension. On clinical examination, there is ascites but no peritonitis. A pleural effusion may be found.

Special investigations

The ascites fluid has a high concentration of amylase and more than 2,5 g/dl of protein. Serum amylase levels are usually raised. X-rays may show pancreatic calcification. Ultrasound and CT show signs of pancreatitis or a pseudocyst. ERCP is the most important investigation. It will show whether there is a pseudocyst and where leakage is taking place.

Management

Conservative management

Conservative management can be attempted for four weeks. The patient is put on total parenteral alimentation. Somatostatin, a powerful inhibitor of exocrine secretion, is given. If the condition has not resolved after four weeks, surgery must be performed.

Operative management

If the leak is situated in the tail area of the pancreas, removal of the body and tail, together with the leaking duct or cyst, is indicated. If the leak is situated in the head, it is better to suture an intestinal loop to the fistula or cyst for internal drainage.

Irradiation

In very weak patients, irradiation of the pancreas can be considered. It is unpredictable, but sometimes the condition resolves.

Chronic pancreatitis

This is a chronic inflammatory condition of the pancreas, with permanent destruction of pancreatic tissue. The exocrine tissue is destroyed first, followed by the endocrine tissue. Eventually, when more than 85% of the pancreatic tissue has been destroyed, the patient presents with diabetes, malabsorption and steatorrhoea.

The majority of patients with chronic pancreatitis are alcoholics. Gallstone pancreatitis is an acute pancreatitis with total recovery of the pancreas between attacks. If the gallstones are removed, the whole syndrome resolves.

Aetiology of chronic pancreatitis

Alcohol

Patients begin with acute pancreatitis. Every time they take alcohol an acute attack recurs, until there is widespread tissue destruction with calcification in the majority of cases.

Obstruction of exocrine ducts

If the pancreatic dust is partially obstructed, chronic pancreatitis may follow. A number of conditions are found:

- Stenosis of the sphincter of Oddi. This occurs, but the aetiology is unclear. Gallstones are one possible cause. Chronic alcoholism may play a rôle.
- Stenosis of the pancreatic duct. Congenital stenosis, due to abnormal embryological development and the fusion of two ductal systems, has been described. Acquired stenosis of unknown origin can also occur.
- Pancreas divisum. This is an abnormality of the ductal development, where the ventral and dorsal ductal systems do not fuse and drainage thus takes place via the *minor papilla*. This anomaly is found in 10% of

the population, but is found in 25% of patients with chronic pancreatitis. It has been postulated that the greater part of the pancreas is thus inadequatedly drained, causing pancreatitis.

Miscellaneous conditions

Nutritional abnormalities, cystic fibrosis, coeliac disease and bile duct tumours are sometimes found. A number of patients have no obvious cause.

Clinical presentation

Patients present with attacks of severe pain. The pain can last for days, weeks or months. In time, the painfree periods shorten and eventually the pain can become persistent. The pain causes general debility, in that the patients do not eat well, do not sleep well and become dependent on analgesics. A large group become drug addicts. In some fortunate patients, the pain disappears spontaneously in time as the pancreas becomes totally replaced by fibrosis and calcification. These patients then develop impairment of exocrine function, with malabsorption and steatorrhoea and are generally emaciated and malnourished.

More than half of these patients also develop insulin-dependent diabetes.

On clinical examination, there are signs of malnutrition and mass loss. Nothing is usually felt on palpation, but a small percentage can present with a pseudocyst. Examination of the stools reveals pale, fatty stools that float on water.

Special investigations

- **Abdominal X-ray** will show calcification of the pancreas in more than 50% of patients.
- **Pancreatic function tests.** The juice is collected from the duodenum after stimulation with secretin and cholecystokinin. In advanced impaired exocrine function, a low volume, low bicarbonate and low enzyme secretion is found.
- **Examination of the stools.** Fat intake is limited to 100 g per day. Normal people will then lose less than 5 g of fat per day in their stools. These patients excrete more fat.
- **Endocrine function.** Glucose tolerance tests are done. Abnormal glucose tolerance and stool fats are strongly suggestive of chronic pancreatitis.
- **ERCP.** This investigation has provided many new insights into the evaluation of patients with chronic pancreatitis. The following are found:
  - Normal ducts in a very small percentage of patients.
  - Obstruction at the ampulla with a regular, dilated duct (rare).
  - Irregular, dilated ducts with areas of dilatation proximal to multiple stenoses ("chain of lakes" appearance).
  - Pseudocysts and cavities in the pancreas.
  - Pancreatic stones. These are calcified protein conglomerates in the ducts.
  - Double duct dilitation. Narrowing of the lower end of the bile duct with proximal dilatation, dilatation of the pancreatic duct and calcification of the pancreas, are strongly suggestive of chronic pancreatitis.
  - Pancreas divisum is sometimes found if the main duct does not fill from the ampulla, but can be filled from the *papilla minor*.
- **Ultrasound and CT.** They show calcifications in the pancreas and also confirm dilated ducts and pseudocysts.

Management

- *Because almost all patients are chronic alcoholics, it is very important to do everything possible to control the alcoholism.*
- *It has been found that all forms of treatment yield better results in patients who stop drinking. Certain surgeons refuse to even consider surgical intervention in patients who continue to drink.*
- *The nutritional status must be improved, by adding enzymes to meals. Enzyme combinations such as Cotazyme must be sprinkled over food.*
- *Attempts must be made to wean the patients from opiates.*

Surgical management

A number of procedures are available for the treatment of the pain of chronic pancreatitis. The true cause of the pain of chronic pancreatitis is not always clear. The following possible causes may play a rôle:

- *Attacks of acute inflammation in patients with chronic pancreatitis due to alcohol abuse.*
- *Pancreatic juice under tension in the ducts due to obstruction.*
- *Tension in the pancreatic cysts.*

Since ERCP has become available, certain researchers have shown that there is not much connection between the appearance of the ductal system and pain. In some cases of burnt out, calcified pancreatitis, there are severe deformities in the ductal system without much pain. Nevertheless, many cases with dilated ducts proximal to stenoses react well to drainage procedures. The operation of choice should relieve pain by correcting structural abnormalities and should have an acceptable mortality.

Drainage procedures

Sphincteroplasty

This is very seldom indicated. It is done if there is a stenosis in the sphincter of Oddi without any other stenoses higher up in the duct. It is also indicated at the minor papilla if a pancreas divisum is present, with a dilated duct. It has a lower mortality, but pain relief is disappointing.

Pancreaticojejunostomies

- *Caudal anastomosis (Duval). If a stenosis occurs deep in the duct, the tail can be amputated and a loop of jejunum can be anastomosed to the pancreas for drainage. This has a lower mortality, but disappointing results.*
- *Longitudinal anastomosis of a jejunal loop to the duct (Peustow). If there are multiple stenoses with dilatation ("chain of lakes"), the duct is opened lengthwise and a loop of jejunum is sutured along the length of the duct. This has a low mortality. It yields good pain relief in the majority of patients.*

Drainage of cysts by jejunal loops or the stomach

This gives relief from pain in most patients.

Resection

This gives relief in even more patients, but has a high morbidity and mortality.

Pancreaticoduodenectomy

A Whipple procedure, or total pancreaticoduodenectomy can be considered in patients with recurrent pain after drainage procedures, who have forsworn alcohol. A modification, where the pylorus is spared to reduce morbidity, has been described by Traverso and Longmire. The mortality is lower than when the same operation is performed for cancer (4% compared to 10%).

Partial pancreatic resections

- *Subtotal (Child). Only a small piece of the pancreas is spared to protect the distal bile duct.*
- *Distal pancreatectomy is performed when the disease affects mainly the body and tail.*

Patients with severe pain and definite calcification show the best improvement after surgical treatment. Patients who give up alcohol also improve more.

Other methods

- **Denervation:** *Bilateral splanchnicectomy can be considered, but the pain relief is disappointing.*
- **Injection of resin into the ducts:** *This method is simple, but the results are disappointing.*

Prognosis

Fortunately, the pain disappears spontaneously in some patients after a few years. Steatorrhoea will arise in all patients in time. Almost all patients develop impairment of endocrine function. The mortality of the disease is more than 50% in five years. Patients die of the complications of the disease, and also because of the procedures which are carried out on them. Malignant disease, cirrhosis and suicide are other causes of death.

Other complications of chronic pancreatitis

Bile duct obstruction

Stenosis of the distal bile duct develops in about 10% of patients with chronic pancreatitis. Sometimes there is obvious clinical jaundice, but often there is only a subclinical rise in bilirubin and marked rise in alkaline phosphatase. Patients later develop biliary cirrhosis and such patients must undergo bile duct drainage. **Do not do a cholecystenterostomy because they develop stones in the bile duct.**

Duodenal stenosis

Duodenal obstruction can sometimes develop, due to fibrosis and inflammation or pressure from pseudocysts.

Segmental portal hypertension

Splenic vein thrombosis is a complication of acute pancreatitis. Later, during the chronic phase, the patient can develop portal hypertension in the area drained by the splenic vein, with bleeding varices in some cases. The condition is treated by resection of the distal pancreas and spleen.

Malignant conditions causing obstructive jaundice

The malignant diseases of the external bile ducts can be divided into two groups:

1. Conditions related to the hilus of the liver

- *Carcinoma of the gall-bladder*
- *Carcinoma of the bifurcation of the bile ducts*

2. Conditions related to the ampulla of Vater

- *Carcinoma of the pancreas*
- *Carcinoma of the distal bile duct*
- *Carcinoma of the ampulla*
- *Carcinoma of the duodenum*

This classification is useful, because the clinical presentation and management are uniform for each area.

Carcinoma of the gall-bladder

This is the most common carcinoma of the biliary tree. It is almost always associated with stones, usually large gallstones. It is four times more common in women than men and occurs more frequently in older patients. It will be found in about 1% of all cholecystectomies for gallstones. In patients over the age of seventy, it is found in 5% of all cholecystectomies. More than 90% are adenocarcinomas and the rest are squamous and adeno-epidermoid tumours.

Staging

The tumours are staged according to their degree of spread through the wall of the gall-bladder.
Stage I: Confined to the mucosa.
Stage II: Infiltration into the muscular wall.
Stage III: Infiltration right through the gall-bladder wall.
Stage IV: Infiltration into the liver, with or without lymph node involvement.

Clinical presentation

The condition is associated, almost without exception, with gallstones. The presentation is thus that of gallstones and the tumour is only discovered at operation. The typical symptoms of carcinoma are pain, loss of mass and jaundice (more than 50%). Masses are sometimes palpable.

Management

Various circumstances can occur:

1. *The carcinoma is only discovered a few days postoperatively by the pathologist.*
   a) Confined to the mucosa or slight infiltration of the muscular layer (St I and St II): No further treatment necessary.
   b) Infiltration right through the wall: Go back and excise the gall-bladder bed and lymph nodes in the area, and follow with irradiation. Another alternative is simply to follow up with irradiation, without operating again.
2. *The carcinoma is discovered intraoperatively. The operation of choice remains the same as above for Stages I, II and III, namely cholecystectomy, with removal of the gall-bladder bed and lymph nodes, followed by irradiation.*
3. *An inoperable situation is very often encountered. Take a biopsy and irradiate. Insert a tube through the bile duct obstruction to relieve the jaundice. The prognosis of this disease is generally poor. Isolated cures have occurred in patients who have undergone cholecystectomy for Stage I carcinoma and are healed. Extensive liver resections are not indicated. The gall-bladder bed lies directly*

over the junction between the right and left lobes of the liver. Chemotherapy does not play an important rôle in the treatment of this disease.

Carcinoma of the hepatic bifurcation (Klatskin tumour)

This scirrhous adenocarcinoma of the bifurcation of the bile ducts, although a relatively rare tumour, is the most common bile duct tumour. It is found with equal frequency in both men and women. It is slow-growing, spreads relatively late and patients usually die of the complications of bile duct obstruction such as cholangitis.

Clinical presentation

The most important presentation is obstructive jaundice with pruritis, pain, anorexia and weight loss. On examination, the liver is palpable but the gall-bladder is not. Sometimes the patient presents with cholangitis, namely fever, pain and jaundice.

Special investigations

Liver functions are typical of obstructive jaundice.

Ultrasound and CT show dilated intrahepatic ducts and sometimes a mass in the liver hilus with collapsed distal bile ducts. The most important investigation is percutaneous transhepatic cholangiography. This shows dilated intrahepatic bile ducts and an irregular stenosis of the bifurcation of the bile ducts, a very typical lesion. ERCP will define the lower end of the lesion.

Management

Only resection of the lesion can heal this condition. The tumour is resectible in fewer than 10% of cases. If it is confined to the bile ducts, it is advisable to resect the lesion and to anastomose a Roux loop to the bile ducts at the liver hilus. Because the tumour is slow-growing and tends to cause death due to the complications of obstructive jaundice, the obstruction must be overcome. The following possibilities are available:

Bypass operations

Anastomosis proximal to the tumour of the bile ducts, by means of the Hepp-Couinaud and Soupalt-Couinaud approaches which have already been described, is preferable. This allows for good palliation without the complication of sepsis, which so often arises when tubes are inserted.

The transhepatic U-tube

If the patient is not suitable for an intestinal bypass, the tumour is dilated and a transhepatic U-tube is positioned to overcome the obstruction. If the U-tube becomes blocked, it can be replaced by a similar tube, which is drawn through the same tract.

Endoprosthesis

In unfit patients, an endoprosthesis can be placed in position transhepatically, through the malignant stricture. The tumour is then irradiated and may sometimes respond favourably.

Liver transplant

Although the disease tends to recur in the transplanted organ, it can sometimes be considered in a suitable patient.

Operation not indicated

In advanced, unfit cases, it is often better to leave the situation as it is.

Periampullary carcinoma

It is important to realize that a group of carcinomas, with varying characteristics as a group, cause the syndrome of obstructive jaundice of malignant origin. The group comprises:

- Adenocarcinoma of the pancreas
- Carcinoma of the bile duct
- Carcinoma of the ampulla
- Carcinoma of the duodenum

Clinical presentation

The presentation of obstructive jaundice is found in middle-aged patients, and is slightly more common in men than in women. The jaundice is progressive, but may vary, probably due to necrosis of the tumour, with temporary moderate relief of the obstruction. It may be painless, but more than 50% of patients complain of pain.

There is usually hepatomegaly. A palpable gall-bladder (Courvoisier's law) is an important sign suggesting bile duct obstruction of malignant aetiology. This sign is found in about half the patients. Cholangitis, which is common in bile duct tumours of the liver hilus, is relatively rare if the malignant obstruction is situated at the lower end of the duct.

Special investigations

Liver functions indicate obstructive jaundice. Ultrasound reveals dilated bile ducts and a mass in the head of the pancreas can sometimes be seen. CT can reveal the same signs, but is more reliable for showing the tumour itself. ERCP is an important investigation. A tumour of the ampulla can be seen and confirmed by biopsy. Cholangiogram shows a malignant stenosis of the lower end of the duct and obstruction of the pancreatic duct, with proximal dilatation. If ERCP is unsuccessful, a PTC can be done to demonstrate the obstruction.

Management

Because many periampullary carcinomas are inoperable, and because radical surgery has a high morbitity and mortality, it is questionable whether radical surgery has any advantages over a simple bypass procedure. There are no prospective series to compare palliative bypasses with resections. In retrospective studies, very little advantage could be found in resection. In one study, where an attempt was made to compare comparable patients who had had resections or bypasses, the mortality was 4% for bypasses and 8% for resections, while average survival was eight months for bypass and ten months for resection. However, if the various conditions, which together form the syndrome of periampullary carcinoma, are studied individually, a different picture emerges.

Resectibility varies from 10% for pancreatic duct carcinoma, through 50% for duodenal carcinoma, to 90% for carcinoma of the ampulla. The five year survival following resection varies between 5% for pancreatic duct carcinoma, and 40% for duodenal and ampullary carcinoma. It is thus essential to offer resection to patients with bile duct, duodenal and ampullary carcinoma. Because it is often impossible to recognize all the various carcinomas which fall within the periampullary carcinoma group, all resectible carcinomas must be removed, as long as this can be achieved with a mortality lower than 10%.

In the past, the mortality of the Whipple operation was between 20 and 30%. With increasing experience and the development of intensive care units, the mortality in recently reported series has dropped to less than 10%.

Partial pancreaticoduodenectomy (Whipple operation) versus total pancreatectomy

Some surgeons recommend a total pancreatectomy. Their reasons include:

- *If a total pancreatectomy is performed, no anastomosis is necessary between the pancreas and the intestinal canal. The anastomosis is actually the part of the Whipple operation which gives rise to most of the complications, namely leakages and haemorrhages, which result in morbidity and motality.*
- *In some cases the resection is done through the carcinoma, making the Whipple operation a less effective cure than a total pancreatectomy. Although there is no random prospective study for comparison, a retrospective study done by the Mayo Clinic is available. In this study the mortality of total pancreatectomy was 14% and that of the Whipple operation 4%. Nor was there an improvement in the five year survival rate after total pancreatectomy.*

Extended total pancreaticoduodenectomy (Fortner operation)

In this operation, not only are a total pancreatectomy and lymphadenectomy performed, but even the portal vein is excised and repaired if it is affected by the tumour. More cases are thus operable. This operation has a higher mortality and the cure rate is no better than that of the other procedures.

Retention of the pylorus (Traverso-Longmire operation)

A standard pancreaticoduodenectomy *is performed, but the pylorus is spared to decrease postgastrectomy complications. This operation must only be performed in ampullary carcinoma and benign conditions (chronic pancreatitis).*

Palliation by means of bypass procedures

If the patient is unfit, or if there are already signs of spread of the disease outside the ampullary area (liver, lymph nodes or portal vein infiltration), only a bypass must be done to relieve jaundice. There is controversy as to whether just a cholecyst-jejunostomy or also a gastric bypass, the so-called triple anastomosis, must be done.

If patients survive for a few months, 15% will develop a further duodenal obstruction due to local infiltration by the growing tumour.

Therefore in younger, fitter patients, especially those with large local lesions, a gall-bladder anastomosis, followed by gastro-enterostomy and an entero-enterostomy (triple anastomosis), to prevent later duodenal obstruction, should be done.

In older patients who are unfit, or where diffuse metastases are present, only a cholecyst-enterostomy should be performed.

Adjuvant therapy

Because the vast majority of these patients already have metastases to lymph nodes, adjuvant therapy should, theoretically, be very useful. However, trials with postoperative radiotherapy and adjuvant chemotherapy have thus far been disappointing.

TUMOURS OF THE PANCREAS

Classification

Benign tumours

Endocrine origin

- Insulinoma

Exocrine origin

- Cystadenoma
- Adenoma
- Fibroadenoma

Others

- Lipoma
- Fibroma
- Neurofibroma
- Lymphangioma

Malignant tumours

Endocrine origin

- Gastrinoma
- Glucogonoma
- Vipoma
- Somatostatinoma

Exocrine origin

- Adenocarcinoma

Ductal cell origin

- Acinar cell origin

Other tumours

Sarcomas

- Leiomyosarcoma
- Malignant fibrous histiocytoma
- Fibrosarcoma
- Malignant neurolemmoma
- Liposarcoma
- Malignant lymphoma

Benign tumours of the pancreas are very rare. The most common benign tumour is the insulinoma. This endocrine tumour of the pancreas will be discussed in the chapter dealing with endocrine surgery. Cystadenomas are the only other benign tumours which sometimes present clinically and must be differentiated from pseudocysts of the pancreas and cystadenocarcinoma.

Adenocarcinoma of the pancreas

The incidence of this disease has increased significantly during the past decade. The reasons for this are not clear, but cigarette smoking, high coffee intake and a high fat diet are all factors which may play a rôle. Unfortunately, the findings vary, so that no definite conclusions can be drawn. Pancreatic carcinoma is at present the fifth most common cause of carcinoma deaths in the western world.

Two-thirds of these tumours are found in the head of the pancreas, thus forming part of the malignant obstructive jaundice group already discussed earlier in this chapter.

Carcinoma of the body and tail

About a third of pancreas carcinomas are found in the body and tail. Jaundice only presents late or not at all. Metastases are almost always present by the time the diagnosis is made.

Clinical presentation

The diagnosis is often delayed because there is no jaundice. Patients complain of abdominal pain and weight loss. If the pain is severe and refers to the back, carcinoma of the pancreas must be strongly suspected. Sometimes patients get relief from the pain by bending forward and they tend to sleep in a sitting position, as they do with the pain of pancreatitis.

Nothing is usually found on clinical examination, but if thrombophlebitis is seen, or if diabetes has recently developed, carcinoma must be strongly suspected.

Special investigations

Because the diagnosis is so difficult to confirm, it is often necessary to consider a combination of special investigations. The two most reliable investigations are ERCP, which shows stenosis or obstruction of the pancreatic duct, and CT, which is more reliable than ultrasonography in showing a mass in the pancreas. The diagnosis can then be confirmed by fine needle aspiration and cytology. The method is safe and reliable. Arteriography is sometimes useful.

Tumour markers such as CEA, CA 19–9, pancreatic oncofoetal antigen (POA), galactotransferase iso-enzyme II (GT II) are not sufficiently sensitive to be really useful.

If the clinical presentation is very suspicious, but special investigations do not confirm the diagnosis, a diagnostic laparotomy must be considered.

Management

Because the diagnosis is often made at a late stage, it is seldom possible to perform a distal pancreatectomy. If the tumour can be removed, there must be no hesitation in removing the body and tail, together with the spleen.

Prognosis

Less than 1% of patients will still be alive after a year. The five year survival following resection is even poorer than that of carcinoma of the head of the pancreas.

Cystadenocarcinoma

This is usually a multilocular tumour lined with mucus-producing epithelium. It is more common in women between the ages of forty and sixty, than in men. It is found mainly in the body and tail of the pancreas. The tumour may arise in a benign mucinous cystadenoma. These benign tumours are definitely premalignant and it is thus very important to distinguish them from other pancreatic cysts. Cystadenocarcinoma presents with metastases in about 25% of cases. If the tumour can be removed *in toto*, the five year survival rate is higher than 50%.

Acinar cell carcinoma

This is a rare tumour which occurs particularly in elderly patients. It sometimes presents as a syndrome of subcutaneous fat necrosis, polyarthritis and eosinophilia. The prognosis following resection is very poor.

Sarcomas of the pancreas

These are very rare and have a poor prognosis.

Malignant endocrine tumours

Gastrinoma, glucogonoma, vipoma and somatostatinoma present as malignant tumours in the majority of cases. They will be discussed in the chapter on endocrine surgery.

PORTAL HYPERTENSION

This arises when there is a partial or total obstruction of the portal venous system. In rare cases, portal hypertension can also develop if the flow through the venous system is increased to the extent that it cannot be accommodated in the normal venous bed. This occurs when large arteriovenous fistulae of the portal system arise.

The obstruction in the system can develop prehepatically, intrahepatically or posthepatically.

Prehepatic obstruction

This occurs in the portal vein or in the splenic vein.

- **Thrombosis of the portal vein**
  This is rare. It usually follows neonatal umbilical sepsis. Trauma and pancreatic or hepatic tumours are very rare causes. Thrombosis sometimes follows catheterization of the umbilical vein for exchange transfusions in rhesus factor jaundice. It is found very rarely in women who are on the "pill". It is a rare complication of pancreatitis.
- **Congenital abnormalities of the portal system**
  This is a very rare cause of prehepatic portal hypertension. The patients do not have a single portal vein, but a network of smaller vessels. Most of these cases are not actually congenital, but are probably the result of umbilical sepsis. If there is no such history, the diagnosis is sometimes made by a process of elimination.

Intrahepatic obstruction

Obstruction of the intrahepatic portal system can be

- Presinusoidal
- A mixed picture of presinusoidal, sinusoidal and postsinusoidal
- Postsinusoidal only

Presinusoidal intrahepatic portal hypertension

The most important cause is schistosomiasis. This disease does not cause cirrhosis, only a periportal fibrosis which follows a granulomatous inflammation. Other causes include myeloproliferative and lymphoproliferative diseases such as myelofibrosis and Hodgkin disease. Sometimes sarcoidosis can also cause presinusoidal portal hypertension.

Mixed picture

The most common cause of portal hypertension is liver cirrhosis.

Liver cirrhosis

Causes of liver cirrhosis

Alcoholic liver cirrhosis (65%)

Alcoholism is the most common cause of liver cirrhosis and its incidence is still on the increase. Cirrhosis is a diffuse process in the liver characterized by fibrosis, which disrupts the normal architecture and causes nodules. The earliest change is fatty infiltration, with fibrosis developing gradually. As the fibrosis increases, the fat disappears and nodules develop, probably due to liver cell regeneration. The fibrosis increases and the portal tracts and veins are eventually caught up in fibrous scars.

Patients develop alcoholic cirrhosis during binges. Hepatocyte necrosis occurs and the damaged cells contain rough hyalinlike eosinophilic cytoplasm, which is known as Mallory alcoholic hyalin. During bouts of alcoholic hepatitis, patients often bleed, with development of hepatic failure.

In the past, there was often reference to nutritional cirrhosis, but it is now generally accepted that alcohol is the underlying cause of so-called nutritional cirrhosis.

Postnecrotic cirrhosis (10%)

Longstanding chronic hepatitis is usually the cause of this cirrhosis. There is a gradual progressive necrosis of hepatocytes, which are replaced by fibrosis. The cells attempt to regenerate and nodules eventually develop. Sometimes patients survive massive cell necrosis, which is followed by cirrhosis.

- **Chronic hepatitis:** Chronic active hepatitis is usually caused by the B-virus, or the non-A – non-B virus. The A-virus does not cause this complication.

  The condition is sometimes caused by an auto-immune disease. This auto-immune phenomenon can be activated by certain drugs such as oxyphenacetine, methyldopa, isoniazid and paracetamol.

  An auto-immune form of the disease has been described in menopausal women. A number of immune markers are found. Hypergammaglobulinaemia and antibodies against DNA and smooth muscle, and more specifically against actin, are found. The disease is common in women with HLA-

B_1 and HLA-B_8, which suggests a genetic predisposition. About 50% of patients have no history of viral hepatitis.

Some patients undergo progressive destruction of the liver parenchyma, with cirrhosis arising within a few years. The mortality is about 40% in five years. Some patients also develop hepatoma.

- **Fulminating hepatitis:** This is found in about 10% of patients with B-virus hepatitis. It is rare in A-virus hepatitis. It can also follow the ingestion of toxic substances such as carbon tetrachloride, the mushroom *Amanita phalloides*, chlorpromazine and other drugs. The liver develops massive cell necrosis and collapse of the reticulin network. If the patient survives, nodules of regenerating cells form. The liver can recover completely, but diffuse fibrosis with cirrhosis sometimes develops.

Biliary cirrhosis (10%)

- **Secondary biliary cirrhosis:** This follows obstruction of the extrahepatic bile ducts and/or cholangitis. The intralobular bile ducts are damaged by accumulated bile and this causes inflammation, with secondary fibrosis. Cholangitis can also be a cause. If the obstruction persists without relief, cirrhosis can eventually develop.
- **Primary biliary cirrhosis:** This is an autoimmune disease which progressively destroys small intrahepatic bile ductules in the portal triad. It is followed by fibrosis with regeneration and reduplication of the bile ductules in the fibrotic scars, and mononuclear cell infiltration. Eventually, obvious fibrous septa can be seen, with the development of micronodules.

  The disease is most commonly found in middle-aged women. It is sometimes associated with rheumatoid arthiritis, Hashimoto disease and pernicious anaemia. IgM levels are raised. Complement fixing antibodies are present and, almost always, antimitochondrial antibodies. Sometimes there are also antibodies to smooth muscle and cell nuclei. The patient eventually develops liver failure. Portal hypertension occurs, but not very commonly.
- **Primary sclerosing cholangitis:** This condition has already been discussed. Eventually, it also leads to cirrhosis and portal hypertension.

Metabolic causes of cirrhosis

- **Haemochromatosis:** This is characterised by excessive deposits of ferritin and haemosiderin in the liver parenchyma, with development of micronodular cirrhosis. There is also haemosiderosis of other cells. The typical condition of bronze diabetes consists of a triad of skin pigmentation, diabetes and liver cirrhosis.
  - *Primary idiopathic haemochromatosis* – This is a genetic disease characterized by increased iron absorption, despite abnormally increased iron stores.
  - *Iron overload* – This includes certain haemolytic anaemias, increased iron absorption in patients with pre-existing liver cirrhosis, excessive iron ingestion in the food of black people who use iron pots and parenteral administration of excess iron, e g repeated blood transfusions.

  Patients present with raised plasma iron levels, raised serum ferritin levels and lowered iron binding capacity. The poor prognosis of the disease can be avoided by dietary adjustment and repeated, regular phlebotomies. Unfortunately, 25% of patients develop hepatocellular carcinoma. The five year survival of patients who are treated is 90%. In untreated patients, the five year survival is only 30%.
- **Wilson disease:** This is a familial, autosomal recessive abnormality of copper metabolism. The main target organs are the brain and the liver. Patients develop lenticular degeneration of the brain, and liver cirrhosis.
- **Alpha-1-antitrypsin deficiency (A1AT):** The mechanism of development of cirrhosis is unknown in these patients. There is a deficiency in the protease inhibitor, A1AT. The disease is diagnosed in the early neonatal period as a cholestatic hepatitis. Patients who are severely affected later develop pulmonary emphysema and liver cirrhosis.

Cryptogenic cirrhosis (10%)

This term is used when no cause for the cirrhosis can be identified.

Postsinusoidal portal hypertension

The most common cause is portal vein thrombosis. Thrombosis can be associated with use of the "pill", polycythaemia and sometimes neoplasms of the liver. Constrictive pericarditis and occlusion of the inferior vena cava can sometimes be the cause. The disease is known as the Budd-Chiari syndrome and consists of portal hypertension, severe ascites and, later, liver failure.

Portal hypertension in black patients

Presinusoidal portal hypertension is the most common type encountered. Schistosomiasis and portal vein thrombosis cause about 50% of cases. Alcoholic cirrhosis causes about 30% and all the other causes, including cirrhosis following viral hepatitis, form the rest.

Posthepatic obstruction in black patients

Obstruction of the *inferior vena cava*, with obstruction of the venous outflow tract, and hepatic congestion, ascites and oedema of the legs, is commonly found in black patients. The obstruction of the vena cava can be caused by

- a web,
- a thrombosis of the vein, or
- total absence of the vena cava with only a few collaterals.

The patient develops portal hypertension and, ultimately, hepatocellular carcinoma. A number of these patients are positive for B-virus infection.

Clinical presentation of portal hypertension

Haematemesis and melaena

The majority of patients present with an acute haemorrhage. Large amounts of blood are vomited. If the haematemesis resolves, the patient can present with melaena. Portal hypertension is the cause of haematemesis in about 10% of cases with upper gastrointestinal tract haemorrhage. If a patient presents with haematemesis, portal hypertension must always be considered. The most common cause is alcoholic cirrhosis and the stigmata of liver disease must be sought:

- A history of alcohol abuse or previous attacks of jaundice or viral hepatitis.
- Jaundice
- Hepatosplenomegaly
- Ascites
- Large collateral veins on the abdomen, especially periumbilically *(caput medusae)*.
- The other signs of liver disease include spider nevi, palmar erythema and clubbed fingers.
- Signs of encephalopathy, including slurred speech, flapping tremor and an unpleasant ammonia odour to the breath.

Special investigations

- Liver functions show raised bilirubin and lowered albumin.
- The prothrombin time and partial thromboplastin time are abnormal.
- Anaemia on full blood count.

Endoscopy

This is the most important diagnostic tool. It is performed with a fibre-optic endoscope. The varices in the oesophagus are found first. They may be bleeding actively, or show signs of previous bleeding, such as a black spot indicating clotting. There may also be no signs of bleeding varices. Complete the endoscopy, which will indicate another cause of bleeding in a significant number of patients (20%).

Gastric erosions are important. They may be true erosions, caused by alcoholic irritation of the mucosa, or they may be due to seepage of blood from a congested mucosa caused by portal hypertension in the submucous veins of the gastric wall. **It is important to grasp this concept, since the bleeding is controlled by procedures which lower the portal pressure.**

Other causes of bleeding associated with varices are gastric and duodenal peptic ulcers. These conditions are more common in patients with liver cirrhosis.

Endoscopy must preferably be performed by someone who can proceed with sclerotherapy of the varices, if they are the cause of the bleeding.

Barium meal

This is a useful investigation if endoscopy is not available. The typical picture of tortuous filling defects is seen in the lower third of the oesophagus in most cases. It can also show whether a peptic ulcer is present, but will not be of use in determining the cause of the bleeding.

Management

- *The acute bleed must be controlled as rapidly as possible. Remember that the patient has a tendency to rebleed.*
- *The patient must be resuscitated. The longer the period of hypovolaemic shock, the greater the chances that the patient will develop liver failure.*
- *The electrolyte imbalance must be corrected. Hypokalaemic alkalosis is often present in patients with severely impaired liver functions. Hypo- and hypernatraemia can also uccur.*
- *Liver failure must be prevented.*
- *The bleeding tendency must be treated.*

Control of bleeding from varices

The control of the bleeding does not depend solely on local factors; the liver functions of these patients are also of cardinal importance. Patients can be divided into two groups. Those in the group with relatively good liver functions either spontaneously stop bleeding, or respond to simple methods of control. The second group of patients with poor liver functions is inclined to bleed repeatedly and the mortality in this group is more than 25%.

Simple methods

The patient is properly resuscitated. Fresh blood is preferably used. If there is any impairment in clotting factors, fresh frozen plasma and platelet concentrate must be considered. Vitamin K is given. The stomach may be treated with a cold lavage.

A group of patients stops bleeding spontaneously. These patients usually have good liver functions. If they do not stop bleeding, or rebleed, vasopressin is administered. Two possible methods are available. Twenty units of vasopressin in 200 ml saline, given IV over twenty minutes, is generally used.

Vasopressin can also be administered in a continuous infusion in a dose of 0,4 units per minute. Vasopressin lowers portal pressure by direct constriction of the splanchnic arterioles. Side effects include reduced cardiac output (it also constricts the coronary vessels) and reduced blood flow to the liver and kidneys.

These side effects can be limited to a certain extent by giving nitroglycerine. A synthetic vasopressin analogue, triglycylvasopressin (Glypressin) is also available and it has fewer cardiac side effects.

Vasopressin can be repeated after four hours.

If the simple methods do not stop the bleeding, or if the patient bleeds again, a Sengstaken tube must be used. Pass the tube in through the mouth. Fill the gastric balloon with 150 ml of water containing hypaque, so that its position can be radiologically monitored. Usually the gastric balloon controls the bleeding through pressure on the cardio-oesophageal junction. If this does not control the bleeding, inflate the oesophageal bubble to 40 mmHg with a sphygmomanometer. Sometimes the bleeding will then stop.

Dangers of a Sengstaken tube

The Sengstaken tube is effective, but has several dangers attached to it. Secretions or blood accumulate in the oesophagus and the patient may aspirate. It is therefore important that this device should preferably be used only in an intensive care unit, where its oesophageal and gastric tubes can be aspirated continuously. If the tube is kept inflated for too long, necrosis of the mucosa can result. The tube must be deflated for ten minutes every twelve hours. **Take care that the tube does not cause pressure necrosis of the nostril or the corner of the mouth.** *In an unconscious patient (in liver failure), it is wise to intubate the trachea to prevent aspiration.*

If the bleeding has stopped and the patient does not rebleed when the tube is deflated, the tube must be left in position for twenty-four hours before it is removed. If the tube does not control the bleeding, or if bleeding resumes, preparations must be made for endoscopic sclerotherapy.

Invasive methods for controlling bleeding

Endoscopic sclerotherapy

The balloon is reinflated while preparations are made for endoscopic sclerotherapy. As soon as everything is ready, the balloon is deflated and fibre-optic endoscopy is performed.

2–4 ml of ethanolamine is injected into each varix. After this, the balloon is reinflated in the stomach and left in position for a few hours, after which it is deflated and removed if the patient is no longer bleeding.

If the patient is still bleeding, the injections can be repeated. A week later the endoscopy is repeated and further injections are given. This is repeated weekly until the bleeding stops.

Other methods have also been described. Rigid endoscopies are performed by some. Other substances can be injected, such as STD (Sodium tetradecil).

The sclerosants can also be injected around the varices into the submucosa.

In most cases, sclerotherapy will control the bleeding after repeated injections. Complications such as ulceration, perforation and stenosis of the lower end of the oesophagus have been described. Once the bleeding has been controlled, the patient can be considered for possible "shunt" surgery, or the injections can be continued on a longterm basis. These options will be dealt with later.

Percutaneous transhepatic obliteration of varices

A catheter is inserted percutaneously into a branch of the portal vein in the liver, using X-ray monitoring. The catheter is threaded into the portal vein and then via the coronary vein of the stomach into the collaterals. Gelfoam dipped in sclerosing substances is then injected into the vessels to obliterate them. This method is used where injections have been unsuccessful. It can also be successful in acute bleeds, but the collateral vessels later recanalize, with recurrence of bleeding.

Direct procedures on the bleeding varices

- *An EA stapling instrument is placed into the oesophagus via a gastrostomy and the oesophagus is tied off between the male and female parts (head- and stapling parts) of the instrument. When the oesophagus is stapled, the full thickness of its wall, including the varices, is cut through at the same time.*
- *Direct undersewing of the varices, via a thoracotomy and oesophagotomy (Boerema procedure).*
- *Transection and suturing of the oesophagus.*
- *Ligation of the collateral vessels and section of the stomach with reanastomosis (Tanner procedure). Ligation of all the collaterals via a thoracotomy incision of the oesophagus with reanastomosis, followed by laparotomy with ligation of all the blood vessels adjacent to the upper two-thirds of the stomach, with vagotomy and pyloroplasty and splenectomy (Suguira operation).*
- *Undersewing of varices from inside the stomach (Ong operation).*

All these operations can control bleeding, but rebleeding often occurs in the short term. These patients usually have poor liver functions and the mortality is high.

Emergency decompressions ("shunts")

If other methods do not control the bleeding and the patient is not in liver failure, a portal decompression must be performed.

An emergency splenorenal bypass (Warren shunt) is preferred. If this is not possible, an interposition mesocaval decompression is done. If the bleeding cannot be controlled by simple measures, this usually means that the liver functions are poor and, as a result, the mortality is very high; in excess of 60%.

General supportive measures

Almost all patients with portal hypertension have impared liver functions. This condition manifests as a bleeding tendency due to inadequate clotting factor synthesis by the liver. The patient can also lapse gradually into a hepatic coma following a big bleed.

Factors playing a rôle include large protein meal comprising blood, in the patient's gastrointestinal canal due to the bleeding. The impaired liver cannot deal with a large protein meal. Bacteria synthesize large amounts of ammonia in the colon and hypokalaemic alkalosis is a further contributing factor.

If the clotting factors are disturbed, it is essential to resuscitate the patient adequately with fresh blood, frozen plasma and platelet concentrate. Daily gastrointestinal lavages must be done to remove excess blood in the intestinal canal. Magnesium sulphate must be given as a purgative and neomycin 0,5 g six-hourly and lactulose 30 ml three times daily to control bacterial action on the blood in the colon.

The prognosis of patients with portal hypertension who bleed

At least 30% of such patients die during the first acute bleed, despite all methods of treatment. Some die of hypovolaemic shock and its complications. The majority die of the complications of liver failure.

Two-thirds of the patients who survive the first bleed will rebleed. Child described a method of predicting prognosis in patients with portal hypertension who have bled:

The Child classification

Group	A	B	C
Serum bilirubin mmol/ℓ	<35	35–50	>50
Serum albumin g/ℓ	>35	28–35	<28
Ascites	None	Easily controlled	Pronounced
Encephalopathy	None	Mild	Pronounced
Nutritional status	Normal	Good	Poor

Patients in Child group A have an operative mortality lower than 2%; group B 10% and group C higher than 50%.

The Child classification was adapted by Pugh as follows:

Parameter	Numeric Score		
	1	2	3
Encephalopathy	None	Mild	Pronounced
Ascites	None	Mild	Pronounced
Prothrombin index	>70%	40–70%	<40%
Bilirubin mmol/ℓ	<35	35–50	>50
Albumin	>35	28–35	<28

Risk groups

A = 5–6
B = 7–9
C = 10–15

The importance of the Child risk groups is that patients in groups A and B can be considered for "shunt" surgery. It is also important to note that patients can improve on conservative treatment so that they move up from group C to group B, or from group B to group A.

Management of patients who have stopped bleeding

Two aspects must be borne in mind:

- *Patients with portal hypertension will bleed again, especially if they drink heavily and develop alcoholic hepatitis.*
- *"Shunt" surgery is the best way to prevent rebleeds, but patients are inclined to develop encephalopathy.*

A logical approach is that Child A patients undergo selective "shunt" surgery – the Warren operation.

Child C patients should preferably be treated in the longterm with repeated sclerotherapy, as their operative mortality and chances of developing encephalopathy are unacceptably high.

In a prospective randomisation series, Warren showed that the best results are achieved with the following treatment:

- *Risk group C must be treated with longterm endoscopic sclerotherapy.*
- *Risk groups A and B must also be treated with sclerotherapy, but the group which bleeds repeatedly in spite of the injections, must undergo the Warren distal splenorenal bypass. In this trial, he proved that such an approach yields better results than operating on the good risk group at the outset. He does not define what he means by "uncontrollable bleeding". One can thus conclude that the bypass must not be performed as an emergency procedure.*

Portasystemic bypass operations

The principle is to make a venous anastomosis between the portal system, with its high pressure, and the systemic venous system, with its normal pressure. A very large collateral vessel is thus created to effect decompression.

Total bypasses

Portacaval shunt

- *End-to-side. The portal vein is cut through and the distal open vessel is ligated. The proximal vessel is sutured end-to-side to the vena cava.*

- *Advantages: Easiest of the bypass operations. The largest "shunt", therefore achieves the best lowering of portal pressure.*
- *Disadvantages: No venous flow to the liver. High incidence of encephalopathy and liver failure.*

- *Side-to-side. The portal vein is sutured side-to-side to the* vena cava.
  - *Advantages: Causes an outflow tract from the liver, in that retrograde flow takes place in the portal vein. This is responsible for the control of ascites, which is especially effective after this operation. It is once again a large bypass and thus lowers the pressure well.*
  - *Disadvantages: Because the blood flows from the liver, through the portal vein to the low pressure vena cava, there is a high incidence of encephalopathy and liver failure.*

Mesentericocaval interposition shunt

- *A large dacron prosthesis is inserted between the superior mesenteric vein and the vena cava.*
  - *Advantages: Easy operation, often done on an emergency basis.*
  - *Disadvantages: The shunt is inclined to clot, with rebleeding from varices.*

Splenorenal shunt

- *The classical end-to-side splenorenal shunt with splenectomy.*
  - *Advantages: Not such a large shunt; encephalopathy and liver failure less common.*
  - *Disadvantages: It is technically a more difficult operation than the portacaval shunt. Because it is not such a big shunt, it is inclined to clot, with rebleeding from varices.*
- *The Warren selective distal splenorenal shunt. The splenic vein is dissected out inferior to the pancreas and cut through. The distal open part which drains the spleen is sutured end-to-side to the renal vein. The other open vein is ligated. The coronary vein of the stomach, which drains into the portal vein, is ligated. The right gastric vein and epiploic vein are ligated.*

  The end result of this operation is the selective drainage of the gastro-oesophageal junction's venous plexus via the short gastric vein and the spleen to the systemic renal vein. High portal pressure to the liver is maintained.
  - *Advantages: Selective decompression of the varices with maintenance of blood flow to the liver. The incidence of encephalopathy and liver failure is thus lower.*
  - *Disadvantages: This is a difficult operation. In time, collateral veins form between the high and low pressure areas with recurrence of the varices. This is the operation of choice in elective cases.*
- *Selective decompression of the varices via the coronary vein to the vena cava (Inokuchi).*
  - *Advantages: Selective decompression with maintenance of hepatic blood flow.*
  - *Disadvantages: A difficult operation; a venous graft must sometimes be used to reach the vena cava.*

Preparation for bypass procedures

- *The patient must be treated in hospital to get him up to the best possible risk category. Shunts must be considered only in risk groups A and B.*
- *The anatomy of the portal system and collateral vessels must be demonstrated, using either splenoportography or selective arteriography. Although preoperative pressures are not essential to the planning of the operation, they can be measured while the needle is in the spleen for splenoportography. Another method is to measure the wedge pressures in the hepatic vein. This is a reflection of portal pressure in sinusoidal and postsinusoidal portal hypertension.*

  The type of shunt performed will depend on which veins are patent.
- *Diagnostic liver biopsy. If Mallory hyalin is found, alcoholic hepatitis should be diagnosed. These patients are a poor operative risk.*

Management of patients with portal hypertension who have not already bled

Patients with varices have a 25% chance of bleeding within a year. If they bleed, 30% of them will die. The risk of patients who have not bled within a year, will gradually decrease with time.

The question arises whether it is wise to act prophylactically if there are varices which have not already bled. In a random trial, it was found that prophylactic portacaval shunt had no advantage over follow-up in a control group. Fewer patients bled, but the eventual mortality was the same. There were more deaths due to liver failure following the shunts.

Current trials with prophylactic sclerotherapy have also not shown any advantage. The use of beta blockade with propanalol which lowers splanchnic pressures, does decrease recurrent bleeding. Somatostatin is being tried at present, but preliminary results have been disappointing.

Portal hypertension and hypersplenism

Mild hypersplenism is a common finding in patients with portal hypertension. The platelets seldom drop to lower than 50 000 and the white cells to lower than 2 000/mm^3. Spontaneous bleeding is rare. If hypersplenism is sufficiently severe to warrent treatment, it is wise to perform a Warren shunt, even if the patient has not yet bled from the varices. If the spleen is to be removed, a Warren shunt is no longer possible.

Encephalopathy following portasystemic shunts

Encephalopathy is common in patients with portal hypertension, especially following bleeding from varices and portasystemic shunts. The clinical symptoms range from personality changes, through impaired cerebration, to coma.

The condition is caused by a combination of toxins, which are formed by bacterial action on protein in the colon and cross the blood-brain barrier because they are not detoxified in the liver. They do not reach the liver because of the collateral flow of the shunt. The following substances play a rôle:

- Amino acid neurotransmitters. Gamma-amino butyric acid is synthesized by bacteria in the colon.
- Ammonia levels in the blood and CSF are also raised in patients with encephalopathy.
- False neurotransmitters such as octopamine and phenylethanolamine inhibit natural functions.

All these toxins work synergistically to cause the syndrome. Hypokaliaemia and metabolic alkalosis push ammonia into the cells, exacerbating the effects of the toxins.

Management

- *Avoid precipitating factors such as sedatives and diuretics.*
- *Restrict dietary proteins.*
- *Administer soluble antibiotics and give lactulose 20–30 g three times daily. This inhibits bacterial enzymes, thus reducing toxin synthesis.*
- *The Warren shunt has the lowest incidence of encephalopathy and is therefore the operation of choice.*

Ascites

Ascites develop in portal hypertention patients as a result of:

- Increased lymph formation on the surface of the liver (sinusoidal hypertension)
- Increased lymph formation on the surface of the intestines (portal venous hypertension)
- Hypoalbuminaemia
- Salt and water retention by the kidneys

Usually the ascites can be controlled by medical means. Before treatment is commenced, the precise cause of the ascites must be established beyond doubt, by examining a specimen for a transudate. The fluid must contain less than 25 g/l protein, less than 250 white cells/mm^3 and the amylase level must be low.

Management

Medical management

Initially, spironolactone 200 mg/day is given. Add furosemide 200 mg/day if the ascites does not react to spironolactone alone. These dosages can be increased to 400 mg/day. In severe cases, it is also necessary to restrict salt intake.

Other methods

Infusion of peritoneal fluid

If the renal function is good, the fluid can be drained off into a plastic bag and then re-infused IV by elevating the bag. As soon as the bag is empty, the tube must be clamped and more fluid must be tapped from the peritoneal cavity, using gravity. The fluid can thus be tapped over a period of eight to twelve hours and administered IV, with diuresis, so that protein is not lost, as long as the cardiac and renal functions are normal. Medical treatment must be continued concurrently. Repeat of infusion may become necessary periodically.

The Le Veen (or Denver) shunt

A sialistic tube is inserted subcutaneously from the peritoneal cavity to the internal jugular vein. The apparatus contains a unidirectional valve which prevents retrogade flow of blood into the tube. The Denver shunt contains a small pump which can, when external pressure is applied to it, increase flow in the tube. Before these tubes are inserted, the fluid must be cultured to ensure that it is sterile. Antibiotics must be given perioperatively. The patient must receive simultaneous medical treatment.

Complications

The tubes and valves tend to block and must then be replaced. About half these patients develop disseminated intravascular coagulation (DIC). They present with low platelet counts and increased fibrin breakdown products. This seldom assumes serious proportions. The phenomenon can be prevented at the time of insertion of the tube by tapping off the ascites fluid and replacing it with Ringer lactate. If there is any infection in the fluid, septicaemia can arise.

Portal vein thrombosis

These patients present with bleeding varices at a relatively young age. Because the liver functions are usually normal, they tend to stop bleeding spontaneously. They often also show signs of hypersplenism. The diagnosis is made on splenoportography. Wedge pressures in the hepatic veins are normal.

A Warren shunt is the treatment of choice.

Splenic vein thrombosis

This is a rare complication of acute pancreatitis, pseudocysts or trauma to this area. Patients present with bleeding varices and a very large spleen. The diagnosis is made on splenoportography, or on the venous phase of elective splenic artery arteriography.

The treatment is splenectomy.

The Budd-Chiari syndrome

The patient presents with hepatomegaly and definitely pronounced ascites. Liver biopsies show large, distended central venous sinusoids and pericentral necrosis. Centrolobular fibrosis develops later.

Ultrasound shows occluded hepatic veins. Venography must be performed to confirm the diagnosis and to determine whether the *vena cava* is patent.

Management

If the obstruction is limited to the hepatic veins, a side-to-side portacaval shunt must be performed. If the obstruction is in the vena cava, the management depends on the type of obstruction.

- **Type I:** *A membrane in the* vena cava. *It can sometimes be perforated by instrumentation via the atrium of the heart. It can also be excised.*
- **Type II:** *Thrombosis of a segment, and*
- **Type III:** *Absence of the vein in the area. This is treated symptomatically. If varices bleed, a mesoatrial bypass, using a dacron prosthesis, can be considered. Patients with Budd-Chiari syndrome must also be considered for liver transplants.*

The prognosis of patients with portal hypertension and cirrhosis

Less than 50% of patients with alcoholic hepatitis are still alive after five years, regardless of treatment. The most important causes of death are liver failure (42%) and haemorrhage (27%). Child risk group A patients fare significantly better than those in risk group C.

LIVER ABSCESSES

Liver abscesses can be caused by bacteria, amoebae or fungi.

Bacterial liver abscess

The most common cause is sepsis in the biliary tree. Ascending cholangitis cause multiple micro-abscesses, which can in time develop into multiple liver abscesses. An abscess can also arise from direct spread from a gall-bladder empyema.

Bacteria may reach the liver via the portal system from a gangrenous appendix of diverticulitis. With the use of antibiotics, these complications have become rare. Sometimes bacteria reach the liver via the hepatic artery, from a septic focus elsewhere. In about 10% of liver abscesses, no septic focus can be located.

Clinical presentation

If the abscess develops secondary to cholangitis or another septic focus in the area drained by the portal veins, the patient will present clinically with the primary disease. His condition will then deteriorate considerably to include swinging pyrexia, jaundice, rigor and pain in the right hypochondrium. A painful enlarged liver may be palpable.

Liver abscess sometimes presents very insidiously with fatigue, fever and weakness. Hepatomegaly will be present in only half these patients. Jaundice is rare.

Special investigations

- X-rays may show that the diaphragm is displaced and that there is a pleural effusion.
- An air/fluid level can sometimes be seen in the liver.
- The diagnosis is usually confirmed on ultrasound. It shows whether single or multiple abscesses are present and where they are situated.
- CT will also provide this information.

Management

The organisms usually come from the gastrointestinal canal and they include Escherichia coli, *bacteroides and* Streptococcus faecalis. *On rare occasions, staphylococcus and haemolytic streptococci can be responsible.*

Broad spectrum antibiotics must be given at once. A good combination is an aminoglycoside, metronidazole and ampicillin. When cultures become available, it may be necessary to adjust the antibiotic therapy. Blood cultures may help in the identification of the bacteria.

The abscess must be drained. Usually, a laparotomy is necessary in any case, to treat the primary septic focus. The abscess is drained at the same time. It is important to know beforehand whether there are multiple abscesses and to be certain of their precise location. It is sometimes not possible to drain all the smaller abscesses.

An alternative method is percutaneous, sonar-directed placement of drainage catheters in the abscesses.

Before the drainage tubes are removed, contrast must be given to check whether the abscess cavities have filled up with granulation tissue.

Prognosis

Multiple abscesses, especially those which are secondary to cholangitis, have a poor prognosis. The disease can spread diffusely throughout the liver, with septicaemia and liver failure. It is practically impossible to drain so many small abscesses adequately.

The mortality is higher than 20%. A single abscess, which is properly drained, has a much better prognosis. The mortality is lower than 10%.

Amoebic liver abscess

The parasite reaches the liver via the portal system from the primary focus in the colon. The patient can develop amoebic hepatitis and a large single abscess can then form, usually in the right lobe.

Clinical presentation

The disease is mainly seen in black men. About half of them give a history of preceding colitis, but the abscess presents in association with acute amoebic colitis in only a third of the patients. They complain of pain in the right hypchondrium and a painful, enlarged liver is palpable. Jaundice is rare.

Special investigations

The indirect haemagglutinin titre is raised in more than 90% of cases. Amoebic parasites can sometimes be found in stools. X-rays show a displaced diaphragm and sometimes a pleural effusion. The diagnosis is confirmed on ultrasound. CT will also provide this information.

Management

The patient must be treated with metronidazole 800 mg three times daily for ten days. The majority improve within seventy-two hours. If patients do not improve, the abscess must be aspirated, using ultrasound direction. Typical dark red anchovy paste content is aspirated. This does not usually contain parasites, as these are usually in the abscess wall. If a large abscess is present in the left lobe, it must be aspirated immediately, as it can rupture into the peritoneal cavity, or sometimes through the diaphragm into the pericardium. Surgical drainage is necessary if the abscess becomes secondarily infected by bacteria, or if it ruptures. A drain is placed in the abscess cavity and is only removed if a sinogram confirms that the cavity has filled up with granulation tissue.

It is rarely necessary to use other drugs such as choloroquin or emetine if the disease does not respond to metronidazole.

SWELLINGS IN THE LIVER

A. Cysts

- Parasitic cysts (Echinococcal)
- Simple cysts
- Cysts of the intrahepatic biliary tract – Caroli's disease
- Cystadenoma

Echinococcal cyst

This disease is caused by the canine tapeworm, *Echinococcus granulosis.* The tapeworm is found in the dog's gastrointestinal canal. The ova are secreted in the dog's faeces and are then ingested per mouth by sheep, the dog, or humans, who then act as intermediate hosts. The embryo enters the portal venous system from the duodenum and lands in the liver, where it forms a cyst. The wall of the cyst consists of a laminated layer lined with germinal epithelium, in which the scolices develop into breeding capsules or endocysts. The cyst is surrounded by a fibrous layer and filled with clear fluid. The wall calcifies with time.

Clinical presentation

Patients usually come from an area where sheep are farmed. They may complain of pain in the right hypochondrium and they sometimes have hepatomegaly. Patients have an eosinophilia and abdominal X-ray may reveal an area of calcification in the liver region. Ultrasound or CT scan will confirm the diagnosis.

Haemagglutinin inhibition and complement fixation tests will be positive. About 60% of patients have only one cyst and the rest have two or more. About 25% also have pulmonary cysts.

Sometimes the patient presents with the complications of the disease. Rupture into the abdominal cavity can cause anaphylaxis. The cysts sometimes rupture into the biliary tree, with jaundice caused by obstruction by the scolices. If there are cysts in the lung, the patient presents with pain and dyspnoea. These cysts may rupture into a bronchus, with secondary infection and a fluid level on the X-ray.

Management

If the cyst is strongly calcified, the parasite is usually already dead. If it is asymptomatic, no treatment is necessary. The most important surgical principle is to remove the cyst without spilling any of its contents into the abdominal cavity. If this happens, multiple daughter cysts form.

Two principles hold:

The cyst can sometimes be excised in toto *without any of its contents escaping. This is often possible in the lung, but seldom in the liver.*

(a) Sterilization of the scolices, followed by aspiration and removal of the endocyst. Silver nitrate or hypertonic saline (20%) is usually used. After this, the cyst is packed carefully with swabs dipped into 0,5% formalin, the contents carefully aspirated and the endocyst removed.

(b) Freezing of the contents of the cyst. The cyst can be frozen using an ultralow temperature probe, or liquid nitrogen. It is then easy to find the tissue plane between the endocyst and ectocyst, because the contents are frozen solid and not in danger of spilling.

It is wise to treat the patient with Mebendazole or Albendazole postoperatively to destroy possible daughter cysts. These drugs can also be used in the inoperable patient. **Remember that**

these drugs are toxic and can cause bone marrow suppression.

Simple cysts

They are usually single, unilocular and asymptomatic. A large cyst can sometimes present as a mass or cause discomfort. Multiple cysts are sometimes associated with polycystic kidneys.

Aspiration is not helpful, as these cysts refill. Saucerization of a cyst or cysts containing clear fluid solves the problem. The cysts drain into the peritoneal cavity where the fluid is resorbed. Multiple cysts do not usually require surgical treatment. If necessary, multiple cysts can be opened and connected to each other.

Cysts of the intrahepatic bile duct – Caroli disease

There is segmental saccular dilatation of the intrahepatic bile ducts. This can be diffuse or restricted to one area. Sometimes the extrahepatic bile ducts are also involved. The condition is often associated with congenital fibrosis of the liver and ectasis of the renal tubuli.

Patients usually present with cholangitis and the diagnosis is made on ultrasound or PTC.

Antibiotics must be given to control the cholangitis. It is sometimes possible to drain large cystic dilatations into a Roux loop.

The prognosis is poor if the patient develops the complications of cholangitis. An increased incidence of cholangiocarcinoma has been reported.

Cystadenoma

Solitary cysts lined with cuboid epithelium or multilocular cysts must be assumed to be neoplasms. They must be excised, as malignant change has been described.

B. Benign liver tumours

Haemangioma

This is the most common benign liver tumour. Histologically, it is a cavernous haemangioma.

Clinical presentation

These are six times more common in women. They are usually found by chance on laparotomy. Leave them alone. **Do not take a biopsy, as problems with haemostasis will arise.** *Large tumours may cause pain and discomfort. They may rupture and present with hypovolaemic shock. If the tumour is very large, it may react like an arteriovenous fistula and cause cardiac failure. It is dangerous to take a biopsy. Fortunately, the diagnosis can be confirmed by noninvasive means.*

- *CT with contrast shows a vascular lesion with delayed clearance.*
- *Technesium-marked red cell scans will confirm the diagnosis.*
- *An arteriogram shows a vascular lesion with a blood pool that clears slowly.*

Management

Large or symptomatic haemangiomas should be operated on and removed by means of a lobectomy. If the patient is unfit for surgery, radiotherapy can be attempted.

Adenoma

This lesion is found in women who are on the "pill". The tumour is usually single, but multiple tumours are found in a third of patients. The tumours are yellow, well-defined masses, usually smaller than 10 cm in diameter. Histology shows well-defined masses with normal hepatocytes, but no bile ductules or central vein.

Clinical presentation

About half the patients develop pain. Rupture and haemorrhages, which often occur during the menses, are dangers. The diagnosis is made on sonar or CT, but these lesions cannot be distinguished from hepatomas. Aspiration cytology is useful, but needle biopsy can cause bleeding.

Management

- *Symptomatic adenomas must be removed due to the danger of bleeding.*
- *Sometimes a wedge resection can be performed, but a lobectomy is usually necessary for deep-lying adenomas.*

- *The "pill" must be stopped immediately in asymptomatic adenomas.*
- *Sometimes the adenoma regresses.*

Focal nodular hyperplasia

This lesion is twice as common in women as in men. The "pill" does not cause these lesions, but does encourage them to grow faster. The "pill" should be stopped in patients who have this condition. The mass is usually smaller than 5 cm in diameter and 80% are single masses.

- Liver isotope scans are normal, but the lesions can be seen on CT.
- Arteriogram suggests a vascular lesion.
- On transection the appearance is typical: there is a central stellate lesion with spokes formed by fibrous septa.
- Histologically, they consist of nodules of normal hepatocytes.
- There is no central vein or portal triad.
- There is wasting of the bile ductules in the lobules.

This lesion does not usually enlarge and is also not inclined to bleed. In rare cases, the lesion can be sufficiently diffuse to cause portal hypertension.

Management

- *Asymptomatic lesions need only be followed up.*
- *Symptomatic lesions must be removed, but this is seldom necessary.*

C. Malignant liver tumours

Primary hepatic carcinoma

These tumours are common in South African blacks. The incidence in the white population is similar to that in the rest of the world. The occurrence of hepatic carcinomas in young blacks is significant. The average age of rural blacks with hepatic carcinoma is thirty-four, that of urban blacks fifty-one, and whites, sixty-four.

Hepatic carcinoma is 500 times more common in blacks under the age of thirty-five than in whites of the same age group and fifteen times more common in blacks over the age of sixty than in whites of the same age group.

Aetiology

The most common predisposing condition in whites is alcoholic cirrhosis. In blacks, two factors play a rôle:

- Almost all blacks under the age of thirty-five with hepatic carcinoma, have hepatitis B-virus (HBV) infection or show signs of having had the disease in the past.
- More than 80% are surface antigen (HBS Ag) positive and 30% are e-antigen positive.
- 15% of blacks over the age of fifty, with hepatic carcinoma, are HBV negative. Most of these patients have alcoholic cirrhosis.
- With HBV infection, aflatoxin forms a co-carcinogen or may cause carcinoma on its own.

Clinical presentation

In blacks, it is six times more common in men. Patients present with pain in the right hypochondrium, with or without hepatomegaly.

They present with fever, loss of appetite and weight loss. Their condition usually deteriorates rapidly. They sometimes present with an acute abdomen due to rupture of the tumour, with haemorrhage.

They can present with the symptoms and signs of spread to bone or to the lungs.

White patients present with sudden deterioration in their general condition, or they are patients with a known diagnosis of alcoholic cirrhosis.

Special investigations

The most important test to confirm the diagnosis is measurement of alphafoetoproteins. This alphaglobulin is raised in 100% of young blacks with hepatic carcinoma and in more than 85% of patients over the age of fifty who have the disease.

Ultrasound, CT and radionuclide scans are used to confirm the presence and site of the lesion in the liver.

Pathological hepatic carcinoma types

Hepatocellular carcinoma (hepatoma 85%)

These tumours present either as single masses or as multiple nodules of diffusely infiltrating carcinoma. In the nodular and diffuse tumours, metastases are already present in 90% of patients. Hepatoma spreads to the lymph nodes, lungs and peritoneal cavity. The tumour is also inclined to spread to the portal vein and vena cava.

Fibrolamellar hepatoma

This tumour has fibrous septa between the malignant cells and it must not be confused with focal nodular hyperplasia. It is found in younger whites and is not associated with HBV or cirrhosis. Patients may be considered for liver transplant, as metastases are less commonly found at the time of diagnosis.

Cholangiocarcinoma (15%)

This is not usually associated with HBV or alcoholic cirrhosis. It tends to spread intrahepatically, but metastases are usually present by the time the diagnosis is made.

Angiosarcoma

This is a very rare, very malignant tumour. It is associated with exposure to vinyl chloride. It was also seen earlier in patients who have received thorotrast for diagnostic investigations. **This substance has now been banned.**

Management

Surgical excision offers the only hope of cure. In black patients it is seldom possible to consider resection. Preconditions for resection include:

- *The tumour is restricted to the liver, with no metastases.*
- *The lesion must be removable by local excision, lobectomy, or trisegmentectomy.*
- *If lobectomy is necessary, the rest of the liver must not be cirrhotic.*

At present early diagnoses are attempted in patients with a known predisposition to carcinoma, such as haemochromatosis. If an early, localized carcinoma is found on ultrasound and CT, the tumour can be excised, leaving a 1 cm free border. Other methods that can be employed include ligation of the hepatic artery and administration of chemotherapy, e g Doxorubesfine, intra-arterially. Results are disappointing.

Prognosis

Black patients usually die within three months. A number die due to rupture of the tumour. In whites, less than 10% of tumours are removable. If excision is possible, 30% will survive for five years.

Metastases in the liver

Metastases are twenty times more common than primary liver cancer. The primary lesion is usually situated in the gastrointestinal canal, but carcinomas of the female breast, uterus and ovary, as well as the kidney and lung, also often spread to the liver. It is important to remember that, in less than 10% of cases hepatic metastases are the only metastases.

Clinical presentation

All cancer patients should be staged, which includes investigations for liver metastases. Sometimes these are obvious with hepatomegaly, jaundice and ascites. LFT may be useful and a raised alkaline phosphatase is especially suspicious. Ultrasound and CT are useful.

Management

In the majority of cases, liver metastases imply that surgical treatment is unlikely to help the patient. In carcinoma of the colon particularly, an attempt must be made to remove the metastasis. About 5% of such cases are suitable and the five year survival of such suitable cases is 25%. A wedge resection or lobectomy must be performed if no other metastases can be identified and if the primary lesion has been removed completely.

It is sometimes possible to remove the metastases of a carcinoid tumour. This may be useful, even if the entire tumour cannot be removed. Chemotherapy, given via the hepatic artery or portal vein, yields disappointing results.

THE SPLEEN

Normal blood cells pass through the spleen without being damaged in any way. Old and abnormal cells are broken down in the spleen. About 20 ml of red cells are removed daily in this manner. In patients who have had a splenectomy, deformed red cells and cells which contain nuclear remnants (Howell-Jolly bodies) are found in the peripheral blood.

White cells and platelets, especially if they are covered with antibodies, are also destroyed. The spleen plays a rôle in both humoral and cellular immunity. It synthesizes immunoglobulins, particularly IgG. It also produces peptides, which play a rôle in phagocytosis. It is also involved in erythropoeisis in the bone marrow and can inhibit white cell and platelet formation.

Hypersplenism

This is an increase in the normal function of the spleen, namely removal of old cells, sequestration of normal cells and increased immunoglobulin production.

Primary hypersplenism

This is very rare and usually a diagnosis of exclusion, when no other cause can be found for splenomegaly and hypersplenism. It is usually caused by undiagnosed blood cell abnormalities or by the presence of antibodies to cells which cannot be identified. Underlying leukaemia or lymphoma are sometimes diagnosed only after the patient has undergone a splenectomy.

Secondary hypersplenism

This is hypersplenism due to splenomegaly of known aetiology. Portal hypertension is the most common cause. About 60% of patients with cirrhosis develop splenomegaly, but only 10% develop hypersplenism. The hypersplenism is seldom severe. Other diseases which can cause hypersplenism include Hodgkin disease, lymphoma and myeloid metaplasia. "Hairy cell" leukaemia often presents with splenomegaly and hypersplenism. Rheumatoid arthritis can present with splenomegaly and neutropaenia (Felty syndrome).

Clinical presentation

Patients usually present with the symptoms and signs of the underlying cause of the condition. Hypersplenism is usually found on blood investigations, without there being any symptoms and signs present due to leucopaenia or thrombocytopaenia. There is a normocytic, normochromic anaemia, leucopaenia of the granulocytes (2 000 to 4 000 per cubic millimetre) and thrombocytopaenia (50 000 to 100 000 per cubic millimetre).

The bone marrow shows generalized hyperplasia. The red cells can be marked with Cr51 and the platelets with Indium-111 and the rate at which radioactivity disappears from the bloodstream can be measured to determine the degree of destruction. A 2 : 1 ratio of radioactive accumulation in the spleen and liver is an indication that splenectomy will be successful.

Management

Splenectomy is often difficult and dangerous in these patients. The severity of the disease must be weighed against the operative risks. In portal hypertension, the most common cause of this condition, a portasystemic shunt should preferably be considered. Splenorenal bypass achieves both goals, namely decompression of the portal hypertension and splenectomy. If hypersplenism is not too severe, decompression of the portal hypertension with retention of the spleen (the Warren operation) is generally adequate. In the Felty syndrome, which presents with chronic lower leg ulcers, splenectomy will usually cause the condition to resolve.

Haemolytic anaemia

Hereditary conditions

Spherocytosis

This is an autosomal dominant genetic disease, caused by deficiency in spectrin, an important protein in the red cell membrane. The abnormality is a small red cell, which is not easily transformed and is thus delayed in its passage through the splenic capillaries. The cell membranes undergo fragmentation and the cells are broken down.

Clinical presentation

The patient develops anaemia, jaundice and splenomegaly. Spherocytes of varying size and shape, are seen on a Wright stain of the blood. The Coombs test is negative. Cr51-marked red cells have a shortened lifespan and are sequestered in the spleen. Pigment gall stones are found in more than 80% of adults.

Management

Splenectomy heals these patients. After removal of the spleen, the cells have a normal lifespan, despite the spherocytosis. A cholecystectomy must be performed for the gall stones. During the operation, accessory spleens must be carefully sought.

Hereditary nonspherocytic haemolytic anaemia

Several conditions with enzyme abnormalities have been described. These include pyruvate kinase deficiency and glucose-6-phosphate dehydrogenase (G6PD) deficiency. Anaemia, jaundice, reticulocytosis and bone marrow hyperplasia can already be found in young children. Splenectomy helps in pyruvate kinase deficiency, so that fewer blood transfusions are necessary. It does not help in G6PD deficiency.

Thallassaemia major

This is also an autosomal dominant genetic disease, with abnormality of one of the globin chains of the haemoglobin molecule. The homozygote form of the disease presents with anaemia, jaundice and hepatosplenomegaly. A blood smear shows target cells and red blood cells with nuclei. Foetal haemoglobin (HbF) is also present.

Splenectomy is useful to dispose of the large, uncomfortable spleen and patients also then need fewer blood transfusions.

Acquired haemolytic anaemia

This may be secondary to chemicals, drugs, infection and may even follow severe burns. Auto-immune acquired haemolytic anaemia is caused by an agglutination-gammaglobulin of complement. The macrophages of the spleen and reticulo-endothelial system have specific IgG receptors on their cell walls. These cells are responsible for the haemolysis. In some cases, IgM is bound to antigen on the red cells and these cells bind to macrophages in the liver. Splenectomy is thus not helpful in these cases.

Clinical presentation

For the most part, auto-immune haemolytic anaemia affects middle-aged women. They present with haemolytic crises against a background of chronic anaemia. The spleen is enlarged in most cases. The direct Coombs test is positive.

Management

Corticosteroids cause remission in 75% of cases, but only 26% will have permanent remission. Splenectomy is performed in cases

- *which do not respond to steroids*
- *where patients have a setback after an initial remission on steroids*
- *where steroids are contraindicated for medical reasons.*

The purpuras

Idiopathic thrombocytopaenic purpura

This condition may be idiopathic or secondary to lymphoproliferative diseases, drugs or infections. A circulating antithrombocytic auto-antibody is present and binds to platelets, making them more easily destructible. The spleen is most probably responsible for both the synthesis of the antibodies and the destruction of the red cells.

Clinical presentation

Attacks of petechiae, ecchymosis and gastrointestinal tract haemorrhage occur.

There are two types of clinical course:

- An acute type: This is common in children and often follows a viral infection. There is a high incidence of spontaneous remission and a good response to steroids and splenectomy.
- A chronic type: This is more common in women and can begin at any age. There may be a long history of bruising and menorrhagia. There is usually a weak response to steroids and the response to splenectomy is not very good either.

Special investigations

- There is a thrombocytopaenia.
- White and red cell counts are usually normal.
- Bone marrow contains many megakaryocytes.
- Bleeding time is prolonged, capillary fragility is increased and the clotting time is normal.

Management

The acute type must be treated with steroids. If there is a rapid response, the prognosis is good. If the patient does not react, splenectomy is recommended. Splenectomy is usually necessary in cases with the chronic type. Splenectomy should not be done in children, as they usually undergo spontaneous remission. Secondary thrombocytopaenia must be treated conservatively by removing the causative factors.

Idiopathic myelofibrosis

This condition is caused by an abnormal proliferation of mesenchymal tissue, with resultant fibrotic infiltration of the bone marrow, spleen, liver and lymph nodes. Extramedullary haemapoiesis takes place in the spleen, long bones and liver.

Clinical presentation

Spontaneous bleeding, bone pain, fatigue, weakness and dyspnoea occur. The spleen is large, hard and irregular. Patients often develop spontaneous hypertension.

Special investigations

The blood picture usually shows a raised white cell count, often associated with a raised platelet count. Later, hypersplenism occurs with decreased platelets and haemolytic anaemia.

Management

Splenectomy is indicated if:

- *there is severe haemolysis*
- *there is severe thrombocytopaenia*
- *there is a large spleen, causing pain and discomfort; splenic infarction is common*
- *there is bleeding from varices from portal hypertension.*

Cysts and tumours of the spleen

All the usual cysts can be found in the spleen, such as *Echinococcus* cysts, dermoid cysts and false cysts, which are probably caused by haemorrhages or infarctions. Tumours include haemangiomas and lymphomas. Spread to the spleen is seen in advanced cases of carcinoma, especially from breast and lung carcinomas.

Splenic abscess

Splenic abscesses can develop in haematomas. It is sometimes the terminal lesion in patients with abdominal sepsis. The diagnosis is usually made on ultrasound, but gas can sometimes be seen in the spleen on an abdominal X-ray.

Aneurysm of the splenic artery

Two types occur:

- in the elderly, who have aneurysms due to generalized atherosclerosis
- in young women, probably congenital in origin. The aneurysm is discovered during pregnancy. There is a danger of rupture.

Usually the aneurysm is discovered by chance on an X-ray of the abdomen and shows as a round calcified lesion in the left hypochondrium. In elderly people, surgical intervention is not necessary. If the aneurysm is symptomatic, or if it is found in young people, a splenectomy must be performed.

Splenic rupture

This topic will be discussed in the chapter dealing with trauma.

The abdominal cavity and intestinal tract 5

Many conditions of the intestinal tract present as an acute abdomen. Other conditions which must be considered in the differential diagnosis of an acute abdomen have already been discussed in previous chapters and will now be mentioned only when the differential diagnosis is discussed.

What does the patient complain of?

Abdominal pain

Localization

Pain in an organ usually arises due to distension, inflammation or ischaemia. If the disease process spreads through the wall of the organ to involve the visceral or parietal peritoneum, it becomes better localized and is known as parietal or somatic pain.

Visceral pain

The pain is poorly localized and is experienced mainly in the central abdomen. It is vague and persistent. The sympathetic nerves responsible for visceral pain arise from segments T5 to L2 and their nerve ends are situated in the muscle layer of the intestinal canal. The patient therefore experiences pain in that part of the abdominal wall which is innervated by spinal nerves of the same segmental origin as the visceral sympathetic nerves. The patient will therefore experience foregut pain in the epigastrium (T5–T9), midgut pain at the umbilicus (T9–T11) and hindgut pain in the hypogastrium (T11–L2).

If the patient has had previous attacks of the same pain, he may have learnt to localize it more accurately. If severe intestinal distension takes place, with powerful contraction of the intestinal muscle layers to overcome the obstruction, a severe, diffuse, deep-seated pain arises in the midabdomen, and comes and goes as the muscle layers relax. This is known as colic.

Somatic or parietal pain

This pain is usually well localized, but can sometimes be referred to another area. The pain is sharp and severe and can be exacerbated by movement. It can usually be localized precisely to one of the four abdominal quadrants, or to the epigastrium, or periumbilically. Pain sensation is carried by the somatic afferent fibres of only one side. The pain is referred to the part of the abdominal wall which is supplied by the same nerves; there is therefore often guarding and underlying skin hyperaesthesia in this area.

Referred pain

This is usually caused by irritation of the central part of the diaphragm, which is supplied by the phrenic nerve. The pain is thus referred to the shoulder. Irritation of the periphery of the diaphragm is referred to the costal margins via the thoracic spinal nerves and irritation of the pelvic peritoneum is referred to the perineum via the sacral nerves.

Shifting pain

This phenomenon is important in the diagnosis of acute intestinal conditions. The pain begins as visceral pain and is therefore poorly localized to the midabdomen. As inflammation spreads and involves the parietal peritoneum, the pain shifts to the true site of the affected organ and overlying muscle tension and skin hyperaesthesia set in. As the irritant expands or spreads in the abdominal cavity, pain can also shift or spread to involve other areas of the parietal peritoneum. The pain of a perforated peptic ulcer, which is first felt in the epigastrium, is a good example. If the gastric contents spill into the Morrison gutter in the right abdomen, the pain spreads to the right iliac fossa.

Onset of pain

- **Very sudden onset or severe pain**

This is usually caused by perforation of a viscus, eg perforation of a peptic ulcer. This can occur without any preceding pain, or it may be preceded by vague, poorly localized pain. Sometimes there is a history of being wakened in the middle of the night by the sudden, severe pain.

- **Severe pain which develops rapidly**

This is initially poorly localized and vaguely experienced in the midabdomen. It then becomes worse within a few hours and localizes to one of the quadrants, with overlying muscle tension. It is caused by leakage from or inflammation of a viscus, which rapidly becomes worse and involves the surrounding parietal peritoneum, e g cholecystitis, appendicitis, or pancreatitis.

- **Pain which develops slowly**

The pain is vague and poorly localized, but heightens gradually within days and eventually becomes persistent and well localized in an abdominal quadrant. This is caused by inflammation which develops slowly.

The nature of the pain

It is important to listen carefully to the patient's description of the nature of the pain. A sharp, stabbing, superficial pain usually suggests peritoneal irritation by fluid such as gastric content, bile, pus or blood.

A deep, dull pain, which is difficult to pinpoint, is caused by ulceration or infiltration by a malignancy. A severe, intermittent cramping pain which is described as colicky pain, indicates obstruction of a hollow viscus containing muscle. This is caused by intestinal or ureteric obstruction. Although the colic of intestinal obstruction can be very severe, it is usually more bearable than that caused by ureteric obstruction. This pain is described as unbearable and the patient often cries out with pain. So-called gallstone colic is not true colicky pain, as there are not any intervening periods of relief from the pain.

What relieves the pain

- **Analgesics**

Colicky pain and pain caused by inflammation are readily relieved by analgesics. Pain caused by ischaemia (incarcerated bowel or infracted bowel) and pain caused by chemical inflammation (pancreatitis) respond less readily to analgesics.

- **Movement**

Pain caused by peritonitis and ureteric colic is exacerbated by movement. Even the movement of the abdomen during respiration exacerbates the pain of peritonitis. Patients with pancreatitis roll around and assume a sitting or crouched position to relieve the pain.

- **Vomiting**

This relieves the pain of a peptic ulcer. Antacids also relieve this pain.

- **Flatus and stools**

These relieve the pain of partial bowel obstruction or functional conditions of the colon (spastic colon syndrome).

Vomiting

This is a sign found to a greater or lesser extent in most conditions of the intestinal canal. The nature of the vomiting can give an indication of the underlying condition, but it is of especial use in the diagnosis of bowel obstruction.

A high bowel obstruction causes blue-green bile-coloured vomiting, which presents in the early stages of the illness. In lower small bowel obstruction, the vomiting is brown and later becomes foul-smelling. In colonic obstruction, vomiting is a late sign caused by gradual distension of the small intestine. This vomiting is preceded by long episodes of nausea.

Constipation and obstipation

Constipation is found in partial colonic obstruction and intestinal ileus. Obstipation (no stools or flatus passed) is indicative of an absolute mechanical obstruction of the intestinal canal. One is sometimes misled by the history that flatus was passed until very recently. This may be due to flatus that was already present in the colon at the time of the large bowel obstruction.

Diarrhoea

Watery diarrhoea suggests a medical cause. This diarrhoea is usually divided into:

- **Osmotic diarrhoea**

This is caused by excessive water being drawn into the intestinal lumen by excess water-soluble molecules in the intestinal canal, e g excess carbohydrates in malabsorption diseases.

- **Secretory diarrhoea**

In this case, the mucosa of the small or large intestine is irritated by something, e g infection in the intestinal canal.

Diarrhoea containing blood often indicates an underlying surgical condition. Sometimes alternating diarrhoea and constipation are found. This is suggestive of a partial mechanical obstruction of the colon.

Blood in the stools

This is often an indication of gastrointestinal disease which will require surgical treatment.

What else does the clinician wish to ascertain?

Previous illness and history of surgery

Thorough enquiry as to previous illnesses and abdominal surgery is essential before making a diagnosis.

Family history

A history of hereditary diseases which can cause acute abdominal pain and which may mimic acute intestinal conditions is sometimes very useful. Such conditions include acute intermittent porphyria and hereditary blood disorders such as spherocytosis, haemophilia and sickle cell anaemia.

A hereditary condition such as familial polyposis may also be an underlying factor.

Drug intake

This may be causative, e g inhibition of nerve transmission (ileus), irritation of the mucosa (pills containing potassium), anticoagulants (intestinal wall or intraperitoneal haemorrhage) or they may mask the true clinical presentation (corticosteroids or analgesics).

Travel history

Exposure to malaria, amoebiasis, or typhoid can be deduced from a recent history of travel.

What does the clinician find on examination?

General signs

The position in which the patient prefers to lie may help in the diagnosis. Is he feverish and is he sweating? If the patient is feverish and sweating, infection is indicated. He may sweat from sheer pain. Low grade fevers are found in most inflammatory conditions. The absence of fever does not exclude infection. High fever, swinging pyrexia and rigors indicate septicaemia secondary to peritonitis.

Shock is an important sign. Severe abdominal pain and shock suggest a catastrophe in the abdomen. Consider hypovolaemia secondary to blood loss, or fluid losses into the distended intestinal canal or interstitial tissue in the retroperitoneum or peritoneal cavity. Fluid losses also occur with vomiting.

Septic shock must be borne in mind if there is underlying sepsis, and shock with a hyperdynamic circulation, a rapid bouncing pulse and warm periphery.

Abdominal signs

Inspection

Scars from previous surgery can give a clue to the underlying condition, but they are especially suggestive of the possibility of small bowel obstruction caused by adhesions. A distended abdomen suggests a distended bowel, indicative of obstruction. Consider the five F's – foetus, flatus, faeces, fat and fluid.

Visible peristalsis suggests bowel obstruction. A mass can sometimes be seen. A tumour, an abscess, a distended bowel loop and an enlarged organ can present in this way.

Auscultation of the abdomen

Intermittent increased bowel sounds indicate mechanical obstruction of the intestinal canal. These increased bowel sounds often precede the onset of the colicky pain. Later, if the bowel becomes badly distended, the bowel sounds decrease in frequency and volume. Bowel sounds are usually absent if there is an ileus. The heart sounds are then audible over the abdominal cavity, due to conduction of the sounds by distended bowel loops. If a vascular murmur is heard, consider an aneurysm or embolus to the blood vessels supplying the bowel.

Palpation of the abdomen

This must be undertaken with care, especially if there is an acute abdomen. In acute abdominal conditions, warm hands must be laid on carefully. If pressure is then carefully and gradually applied, muscle tension can be elicited if present. This tension may be generalized or localized.

A distinction must be drawn between guarding and rigidity. Guarding relaxes if the patient is asked to breathe deeply or if his attention is distracted by a reassuring conversation. Rigidity persists throughout respiration. In severe rigidity, the abdomen can be extremely hard or even boardlike.

Abdominal tenderness can be diffuse or localized. Inflammation causes the most severe tenderness. Generalized diffuse inflammation of the peritoneal cavity (peritonitis) causes generalized tenderness. Localized inflammation, e g appendicitis, causes localized tenderness. Bowel obstruction causes vague, poorly localized tenderness.

Rebound

If pressure is applied gradually to the abdomen and then suddenly relieved, the patient will experience a sharp pain if there is peritonitis. This sign can also be elicited by asking the patient to cough. Localized peritonitis can be diagnosed by eliciting localized rebound on percussion.

If a mass is palpable, its characteristics must be determined. Tenderness, anatomical site, boundaries, surface and consistency are all important diagnostic signs.

Percussion of the abdomen

Resonance indicates air or gas. Loss of liver dullness may mean free air under the diaphragm. Shifting dullness means fluid in the abdominal cavity; ascites, blood or urine.

Examination of the inguinal region

This is absolutely essential to exclude a strangulated inguinal or femoral hernia. A Richter hernia (partial incarceration of the abdominal wall) through the femoral canal is a well-known pitfall. A fat patient presents with partial small bowel obstruction. No obvious cause can be found. Beware of the occult mass of a strangulated Richter hernia in the inguinal fold.

Rectal examination

This is absolutely essential in abdominal conditions. Tenderness in one of the iliac fossae, pelvic and rectal masses, faecal impaction, or a mass (carcinoma of the wall) can confirm the diagnosis.

Vaginal examination

This can supply additional information about the female genital system and thus confirm the diagnosis.

Special investigations

Laboratory tests

- Full blood count: A high white cell count, especially with a shift to the left on the smear and a rising white cell count, are indicative of significant infection. A low white cell count may be indicative of viral infection or typhoid.
- Serum electrolyte and urea measurements give an indication of dehydration and fluid losses.
- Blood gases: These must be measured in patients with acute abdomen. A pronounced metabolic acidosis and raised serum anorganic phosphate are found when there is dead bowel.
- Examination of the stools: Bacterial cultures must be done and amoebae must be sought in warm stools.

Radiological examination

This is extremely important in the diagnosis of an acute abdomen and a definitive diagnosis is often only made on X-ray.

X-rays

- Chest X-ray: This may show thoracic pathology which presents with referred abdominal pain. A pleural effusion and raised hemidiaphragm indicate subphrenic sepsis. Air under the diaphragm is best seen on a standing chest X-ray and implies perforation of a viscus. An air/fluid level under the diaphragm is suggestive of a subphrenic abscess. Lateral photos will indicate the position of the air/fluid level in relation to the liver.
- X-ray abdomen: It is important to take supine and standing views. The supine photos will show distended bowel loops. Standing photos show air/fluid levels.

  It is normal to find gas in the stomach (swallowed air) and in the colon and rectum (flatus). An air/fluid level is normally found in the stomach (stomach bubble). Although air is sometimes found in the small intestine, it can, for practical purposes, be considered abnormal.
- Supine view: Distended gas-filled bowel loops can be seen. Colonic loops (normal) must be distinguished from small bowel loops (abnormal).
- Colon: This is anatomically situated on the periphery of the abdominal cavity. Wide bowel loops with haustrations are characteristic.
- Small bowel: This is centrally situated, the loops are narrower and many transverse folds (*valvulae conniventes*) are characteristic.

Standing view

- Air/fluid levels in dynamic loops. The two air/fluid levels in the same loop are not at the same level due to peristalsis. In practice, this means a mechanical bowel obstruction.
- Air/fluid levels in dynamic loops. In practice, multiple loops, fluid levels shallower and at the same level, because fluid levels are present in dynamic loops, indicate paralytic obstruction. Gas can be seen up to the rectum.
- An air/fluid level in a closed loop. A very large, distended loop with a large air/fluid level, smaller air/fluid levels proximally in the bowel and collapsed distal bowel indicate obstruction in a closed loop.
- Localized air/fluid levels (sentinel loops). Air/fluid levels are found in a certain area without associated distended bowel loops. This is usually suggestive of localized infection. Loops in the RIF suggest appendicitis.

X-rays with contrast

The acute abdomen

- The small intestine: Barium studies can be done to differentiatc between an ileus and a mechanical small bowel obstruction, provided there is relative certainty that there is no dead bowel (danger of perforation) or mechanical obstruction of the colon.
- The large intestine: An emergency barium enema must be administered on suspicion of a large bowel obstruction without signs of peritonitis. It is especially useful in distinguishing the common condition colonic ileus (pseudo-obstruction) from true mechanical colonic obstruction. It is also sometimes necessary for the diagnosis of a volvulus of the sigmoid colon or caecum.

Radiogical examination of the small and large bowel

The small bowel can be examined by inserting contrast and air via a long tube (Miller-Abbott type). Barium enema is a useful investigation. Filling defects in the lumen, mucosal ulceration and partial colonic obstruction (applecore sign) can be seen. Diverticula present as barium-filled sacs bulging out from the bowel wall.

Arteriography

- If intestinal ischaemia is under consideration, selective emergency arteriography will demonstrate thrombosis or embolism of the blood vessels.

  It is also useful in localizing intestinal bleeding, especially in the colon.
- Localization of chronic bleeding or abdominal tumours. Selective arteriography may be useful in localizing a vascularized intestinal lesion. It may also demonstrate the increased blood supply of a tumour (tumour blush).

Radionuclide scanning

This is a noninvasive alternative to arteriography for localizing bleeding points in the colon. Technesium scanning may also demonstrate a Meckel diverticulum as the cause of the intestinal bleeding.

Ultrasound and computer tomography

These are not very useful in the diagnosis of intestinal conditions. They are extremely useful in determining the nature of an intraperitoneal mass and in diagnosing abscesses of the peritoneal cavity.

Endoscopy

Sigmoidoscopy is performed in suspected cases of colorectal obstruction. Tumour obstruction or sigmoid volvulus can be diagnosed in this way.

Parasynthesis

This is indicated if there is fluid in the abdominal cavity and the diagnosis is uncertain. The nature of the fluid often helps in the diagnosis. Blood, bile, pus or infected ascites all suggest specific underlying causes.

Classification of conditions of the abdominal cavity and intestinal canal

A. OBSTRUCTION OF THE INTESTINAL CANAL

The small intestine

Mechanical obstruction

Causes

(a) Adhesions in the peritoneal cavity
(b) Incarcerated hernias

Less common causes

(a) Volvulus
(b) Tumours
(c) Obturator obstruction
(d) Inflammation of the bowel wall
(e) Haemorrhage

Paralytic ileus

- Postoperative
- Electrolyte imbalance
- The effects of toxins or drugs
- Inflammation with peritonitis

Large bowel obstruction

Common conditions

- Faecal impaction
- Colonic ileus
- Volvulus
- Carcinoma of the colon

Rarer conditions

- Ischaemic colitis
- Ulcerative colitis
- Crohn disease
- Diverticulitis

B. INFLAMMATORY CONDITIONS OF THE INTESTINAL CANAL

Bacterial infections

The small intestine

- Non-specific infections
- Specific infections
  - Yersinia infections
  - Typhoid
  - Tuberculosis

The appendix

- Appendicitis
- Appendix mass
- Thrombophlebitis suppurativa

The colon

Inflammatory conditions

- Bacillary dysentery
- Pseudomembranous enterocolitis
- Tuberculosis
- Diverticular disease of the colon
- Free perforation
- Colovesical fistula
- Massive rectal bleeding

Parasites and viruses

- Amoebiasis
- Amoebic granuloma
- Schistosomiasis of the colon
- Lymphogranuloma venereum

Inflammatory conditions of unknown aetiology

- Crohn disease
- Ulcerative colitis

C. Ischaemia of the intestinal canal

- Acute mesenteric vascular insufficiency
- Bowel ischaemia without clotting of mesenteric vessels
- Ischaemic colitis
- Chronic ischaemia of the intestinal canal
- Compression of the coeliac artery

D. Radiation damage in the intestinal canal

- The small intestine
- The rectum

E. Tumours of the intestinal canal

The small bowel

Polyps and benign tumours

- Peutz-Jeghers syndrome
- Benign tumours

Malignant tumours

- Adenocarcinoma
- Carcinoid syndrome

The colon

Polyps

- Inflammatory polyps
- Hyperplastic polyps
- Hamartomas
- Neoplastic polyps
- Familial polyposis

Malignant tumours

- Carcinoma of the colon
- Rectal carcinoma

F. Functional conditions of the colon

- Spastic colon syndrome

G. Rare conditions of the intestinal canal

- Pneumatosis cystoides intestinalis
- Idiopathic ulcer of the small bowel
- Duplication cysts of the intestinal canal
- Endometriosis

H. Rectal conditions

- Rectal prolapse
- Giant rectal ulcer
- Rectal pain

I. Anal conditions

- Haemorrhoids
- Perianal haematoma
- Thrombosis of the external plexus
- Fibrous polyps and anal papillae
- Fissure-in-ano
- Peri-anal abscesses and fistula
- Tumours of the anus
- Pruritis ani
- Pilonidal sinus

J. Intestinal Fistulae

K. Abscesses of the abdominal cavity

- Intraperitoneal abscesses
- Retroperitoneal abscesses

A. OBSTRUCTION OF THE INTESTINAL CANAL

Small bowel obstruction

Mechanical obstruction

This can be divided into high and low small bowel obstruction. It may be acute, subacute or acute on chronic obstruction. Mechanical obstruction occurs as a result of external pressure, or kinking of the wall (adhesions), infiltration with stenosis of the wall (tumours), or obturator obstruction (which is intraluminal, e g worms, gallstone ileus or food residue).

In mechanical obstruction, it is essential to differentiate between simple mechanical obstruction without ischaemia; and mechanical obstruction with inadequate blood supply to the wall with ischaemia, necrosis and perforation. Strangulated bowel with ischaemia requires urgent surgical intervention.

Closed loop obstruction, where both ends of the bowel are occluded, e g volvulus or strangulated hernia, tends to cause the bowel to distend massively, with ischaemia of the wall and, often, perforation. The bowel proximally above the obstruction distends due to air in the lumen. Some of this air is swallowed and some is produced by bacteria in the lumen. As the bowel distends, the vessels in its wall are stretched and this results in relative ischaemia, leading to fluid and electrolyte leakage into the lumen. The patient loses large amounts of electrolytes and fluid and develops hypovolaemic shock. It can be accepted that the patient has lost at least six litres of fluid.

If the bowel becomes strangulated, blood stagnates in the bowel wall, causing oedema and eventual necrosis of the bowel wall. There are massive fluid losses and a bacteraemia arises, because bacteria and toxins leak through the dead bowel wall into the peritoneal cavity, where they are absorbed. This causes hypovolaemic and toxic shock.

Causes of mechanical obstruction

- Adhesions: This is by far the most common cause of small bowel obstruction. Adhesions can follow any previous abdominal surgery, but are especially common after appendectomy. They may also result from previous peritonitis. Adhesions can cause bowel loops to adhere to each other, with kinking, or they can cause pressure on the bowel by means of bands, which can cause strangulation, with bowel necrosis.

If a patient has presented previously with obstruction caused by adhesions and he presents again with mechanical obstruction, the chances are good that this is due to further adhesions.

- Strangulated hernias: This is the second most common cause of mechanical small bowel obstruction. The strangulation can take place in inguinal hernias, femoral hernias or incisional hernias. Internal fossae are present, particularly in the region of the ligament of Treitz and the caecum, and they can cause internal strangulation.

Less common causes

- Volvulus: Spontaneous small bowel volvulus is rare. There is usually an underlying cause, such as a peritoneal adhesion or a remnant of the vitelline duct with a Meckel diverticulum.
- Tumours: Carcinoma of the small bowel is rare. The condition, when it does present, often manifests as small bowel obstruction. It can also sometimes form the lead point for the development of intussusception in adults.

Carcinoid is usually a small tumour and seldom causes obstruction. Lymphoma of the small bowel can cause obstruction.

- Obturator obstruction: Food residues, especially oranges, can accumulate in the bowel and cause obstruction. Patients usually have a history of a previous Bilroth II gastrectomy, have false teeth and have eaten oranges recently.

Gall stone ileus has already been discussed in a previous chapter.

Roundworms (*ascaris lumbricoides*) sometimes cause small bowel obstruction when they form a ball. This is common in young black patients.

- Inflammation of the bowel wall: Crohn disease is rare in South Africa, but now and then it is the cause of small bowel obstruction, due to fibrous stenosis. Although rare, fibrous stenosis is sometimes caused by idiopathic ulceration of the small bowel, fistula formation and ischaemia.
- Haemorrhage into the bowel wall of patients on anticoagulants.

Clinical presentation of mechanical obstruction

It is extremely important to differentiate between simple mechanical obstruction and mechanical obstruction with incarceration and ischaemia.

Pain

Patients complain of colicky pain. This is a very severe intermittent pain associated with increased bowel sounds. If the pain becomes severe and persistent, more localized and is associated with tenderness and guarding, it can be assumed that incarceration with ischaemia has occurred and that urgent surgical intervention is essential.

Vomiting

This is found early in high obstruction, but can be mild and only occur late in low obstruction.

Abdominal distension

This is found principally in patients with low obstruction, usually in those who begin vomiting late.

Constipation and obstipation

Flatus and faeces are often passed from the colon in the earlier stages, but later no stool or flatus is passed.

Special investigations

Laboratory investigations

A high white blood cell count, if present, favours the diagnosis of ischaemic bowel. There is often an electrolyte imbalance due to fluid losses caused by vomiting and leakage into the distended bowel lumen. If severe metabolic acidosis is found, especially in association with high blood phosphate levels, dead bowel must be strongly suspected.

X-rays

The diagnosis of bowel obstruction is, to a large extent, based on X-ray findings. Standing and supine views of the chest and abdomen must be taken. The supine views show distended bowel loops, characterised by a central position and transverse folds (*valvulae conniventes*) in the mucosa. There is usually no gas in the colon or rectum (total mechanical obstruction). The standing views show air/fluid levels. The air/fluid levels are not at the same height (dynamic levels), in contrast to the multiple air/fluid levels found at the same height in the loop (adynamic loops) of a paralytic ileus.

If there is any doubt as to whether one is dealing with a mechanical obstruction or paralytic ileus, barium can be given per mouth. In an ileus, the barium will flow through into the colon.

A rectal examination and sigmoidoscopy must always be performed. In small bowel obstruction, the rectum is usually empty.

Differential diagnosis

Firstly, a distinction must be drawn between a mechanical obstruction and paralytic ileus. The main points of difference are the absence of bowel sounds and the presence of gas in the colon on X-rays in paralytic ileus.

To determine the cause of mechanical obstruction, the following must be noted:

- Previous operations suggest adhesions.
- Examine the groins for an incarcerated hernia. A Richter hernia of the femoral canal must always be borne in mind.
- If there have been no previous operations and all the hernial sites are intact, consider the rarer causes, which will only be diagnosed at laparotomy.

Management of mechanical obstruction of the small bowel

- *The management is operation after resuscitation.*
- *A nasogastric tube must be inserted for suction.*
- *Fluid and electrolytes are measured, but must be replaced in the meantime.*
- *There is usually a deficit of at least four or more litres of fluid.*
- *If there are signs of strangulation, resuscitation, which may include blood transfusion, must be rapid, as an urgent operation is necessary. The nature of this operation will depend on the cause of the mechanical obstruction and the condition of the bowel after this obstruction has been relieved.*

Simple mechanical obstruction

Adhesions

Loosen the adhesions carefully and reposition the bowel. There is no reliable method to prevent further adhesions.

Hernias

If the small intestine is viable, replace the bowel and repair the hernia.

Incarcerated incisional hernias

Incarceration in incisional hernias usually occurs in patients who are seriously overweight. Firstly, the obesity contributes to the development of the hernia and secondly, to the incarceration of the hernia. Omentum and/or bowel is forced through the opening in the hernia because of a lack of space in the abdominal cavity due to the obesity. The bowel distends further and, because there is no space in the abdomen, it does not reduce spontaneously and impedes respiration and venous return to the heart. It presses on the diaphragm and vena cava. *The surgeon is often confronted with a large, obese, shocked patient in respiratory distress. Surgery may be urgent, but certain precautions must be taken:*

- *Restore fluid and electrolyte balance.*
- *Support respiration mechanically.*
- *Deliver the incarcerated bowel. If it is necrotic, a resection must be performed.*
- *If it is viable, the hernial orifice must be enlarged and the hernia must not be repaired. Simply close the skin so that more space is created in the abdominal cavity, otherwise respiration will be further impeded.*
- *Continue with mechanical support of respiration.*

When the patient has recovered, and if he loses weight, the hernia can be repaired later as an elective procedure.

Obturator obstruction

Orange fibre

If the diagnosis is made preoperatively, conservative management, which includes nasogastric suction and fluid replacement, can be attempted. If the diagnosis is only made at operation, break up the bolus and milk it towards the caecum.

Worms

If the diagnosis is made preoperatively, in that worms are visible in the distended loops on X-ray or on a barium study, conservative management with deworming agents such as Piperazine or Mebendazole can be attempted. Usually the worm bolus breaks up and the patient passes worms. It is sometimes postulated that worm treatment precipitates obstruction by causing paralysed worms to clump together. This is theoretically possible, but in practice patients who have never received any worm treatment present with this phenomenon.

Carcinoma

The carcinoma, with its lymphatic drainage in the mesentery, is removed in a large wedge and an end-to-end anastomosis is performed.

Mechanical obstruction with strangulated bowel and inadequate blood supply

Dead bowel must be resected. It is sometimes difficult to decide whether incarcerated bowel is viable and can be preserved. **Do not judge too hastily.** *Wrap the dark, discoloured bowel in warm, wet swabs and wait for half an hour. If the bowel becomes pink and peristalsis is present, the bowel is viable. Sometimes there are small, black, suspicious-looking areas. It is safer to tuck them in and cover them with serosa-to-serosa sutures. If there is any doubt, resect.*

Sometimes incarcerated bowel reduces from a hernia before it can be properly inspected during the operation. The bowel must be pulled out through the hernia for proper inspection. If there is any doubt, a laparotomy must be performed.

Conservative management of mechanical small bowel obstruction

Conservative management can be considered only if there are no signs of bowel ischaemia.

Adhesions

If a patient has had several previous episodes of adhesion obstruction and if there are no signs of bowel ischaemia, conservative management can be considered. Nasogastric suction and fluid replacement are given until the obstruction resolves. If this does not occur within a reasonable period of time, operation is preferable.

Multiple metastases

It must not be accepted that a patient with cancer has an inoperable abdominal condition. *If there is any doubt, an operation must* *be performed, even if only to create a shortcircuit. It is often clear that there is advanced spread of the cancer and conservative treatment is preferable for such patients.*

Crohn disease

This disease is rare in South Africa. If a diagnosed Crohn patient develops obstruction, conservative treatment must be attempted. The management of obstruction in Crohn disease will be discussed later.

Paralytic ileus

This condition is caused by impairment of splanchnic nerve stimulation of the muscle wall of the bowel. This condition is caused by:

- Handling of the bowel intraoperatively
- Electrolyte imbalances resulting from abnormal fluid and electrolyte losses
- The effect of toxins or drugs which inhibit nerve conduction
- Inflammation with peritonitis – haemorrhage into the retroperitoneal tissues

Clinical presentation

A bowel obstruction which is secondary to one of the underlying precipitating factors already mentioned, is present. The important characteristics of a paralytic ileus are:

- **The absence of colicky pain** Sometimes cramps may be present if there is a localized ileus with peristalsis in the proximal bowel. Pain from the underlying cause may be present.
- **Absent bowel sounds** Loud heart sounds are heard in the abdomen, conducted by the distended, gas filled bowel loops.
- **Pronounced vomiting** is characteristic.
- **Patients can still physically pass diarrhoea and flatus**, but are often constipated.
- **Abdominal distension** is found.

Special investigations

Laboratory investigations are often useful in diagnosing the cause of the ileus. Raised amylase can suggest pancreatitis. Abnormal electrolyte levels, especially low potassium levels, are usually found in patients with ileus.

X-rays

Distended loops are seen and there is gas in the colon and rectum. Adynamic air/fluid levels can be seen on standing views. If there is any doubt, barium can be given, and will flow through to the colon without demonstrating a mechanical obstruction.

Management

The most important elements in the management of paralytic ileus are:

- *Effective nasogastic suction to prevent further distension of the bowel.*
- *Restoration of fluid and electrolyte deficits.*
- *Management of the underlying cause of the ileus. Usually the fluid and electrolyte imbalance can be calculated by drawing up a balance sheet of what the patient has received daily and what his daily requirements are. There is often a surprising deficit.*

There must be absolute certainty that there is no mechanical obstruction. *This is especially difficult in postoperative patients who develop prolonged ileus. If there is any doubt, it is better to operate.*

The Neely-Catchpole regime is sometimes used in persistent cases of ileus. This consists of blockade of both the alpha and beta receptors with guanethidine and subsequent stimulation with very small doses of prostigmine. This is very seldom used.

Recurrent adhesion obstruction

A small percentage of patients have such frequent recurrences following freeing of adhesions, that procedures must be considered to prevent obstruction. The Nobel plication was the first operation performed for this condition. Loops of bowel were sutured to each other in an orderly fashion so that adhesions would form in such a way that kinking and obstruction did not take place. Currently, various operations based on the same principle are used. A tube is threaded through the small bowel so that it is concertinaed on the tube. Thus the small bowel forms a shortened straight line between the ligament of Treitz and the caecum. The bowel then adheres in this position and the tube is removed after a few weeks. Naturally, the mucosal surface area of the small bowel remains unchanged.

Large bowel obstruction

Obstruction of the large bowel occurs mainly in older patients. The obstruction is usually caused by one of four conditions: carcinoma of the colon (most commonly the sigmoid colon), faecal impaction, colonic ileus and volvulus of the sigmoid colon.

Strangulated hernias containing colon are rare. Adhesions seldom cause colonic obstruction. Rarer causes include diverticulitis, Crohn disease, ulcerative colitis and amoeboma of the colon. Fibrous stenosis, a late complication of ischaemic colitis, is a rare cause.

Diverticulitis can cause small bowel obstruction due to adherence of the small bowel to the inflammatory mass, or a pericolic abscess can cause colonic obstruction.

Clinical presentation

Elderly patients present with a severely distended abdomen and only moderate abdominal cramps. Vomiting is not a prominent feature. There is a history of obstipation.

On auscultation, bowel sounds are increased or sometimes absent. If a mass is palpable, carcinoma must be suspected, but it must be differentiated from faecal material or a diverticular abscess. On rectal examination, a large, hard, round mass of faeces is found in faecal impaction.

Carcinoma of the rectum is sometimes palpable. In sigmoid volvulus, the rectum is usually empty. If normal faeces are palpable in the rectum, colonic ileus must be considered. If the rectum is empty, a sigmoidoscopy must be performed to exclude a carcinoma of the rectum or rectosigmoid junction. It is also possible to see the rotated mucosal folds of a sigmoid volvulus.

Special enquiries

Patients with carcinoma obstruction sometimes give a history of a change in bowel habit and bleeding per rectum. Patients with faecal impaction and colonic ileus often come from institutions, are on treatment for cardiac failure and/or hypertension and have experienced similar episodes previously. Patients with volvulus may also have experienced previous episodes.

Abdominal X-rays

Volvulus of the colon usually has a very typical radiological presentation. A large, kidney-shaped distended bowel loop can be seen on the abdominal X-ray and a very wide air/fluid level on the standing view. A distinction must be drawn between the more common sigmoid volvulus and a caecal volvulus. The closed, distended, kidney-shaped sigmoid colon loop is situated in the right hypochondrium. The kidney-shaped, distended caecum is in the left hypochondrium, with an empty RIF.

If any doubt remains, a limited barium enema must be performed. Barium will not reach further than the rectosigmoid junction and the bird beak appearance is seen in a volvulus of the sigmoid loop. In volvulus of the caecum, the transverse colon fills, but the ascending colon shows the occlusion of the twisted bowel.

It is sometimes difficult to differentiate between colonic ileus and a carcinoma obstruction. Both cause distended colon with air/fluid levels, but in colonic ileus there is air throughout the entire colon up to the rectum. Colonic ileus must never be assumed to be the cause of an obstruction unless a carcinoma obstruction has been excluded on emergency barium enema.

Management of large bowel obstruction

Faecal impaction

If a diagnosis of faecal impaction has been made, the faecal plug must be removed. Enemas can be attempted, but manual removal is often necessary. Fluid and electrolyte balance must be restored, because there is often dehydration. As soon as the obstruction has been relieved, a barium enema should be performed to exclude carcinoma. Carcinoma sometimes plays a rôle in the aetiology of faecal impaction.

Colon ileus

Most of these patients have fluid and electrolyte imbalance. Drugs such as diuretics often play a rôle. Patients may also be on drugs, such as alpha and beta receptor blockers, which inhibit peristalsis.

Restore the fluid and electrolyte balance and adjust the drug dosage as far as possible. Enemas are useful for emptying the bowel. If the ileocaecal valve is competent, massive distension of the caecum can sometimes take place and impair the blood supply to the wall and lead to perforation. It may be necessary to perform a colonoscopy to decompress the proximal colon. If this is unsuccessful, a caecostomy may be necessary. Once the colonic ileus has resolved, a barium enema must be done to exclude underlying carcinoma.

Volvulus of the colon

Sigmoid volvulus

Remember that a volvulus of the sigmoid loop causes closed loop obstruction and that the axis rotation interferes with blood supply. Both factors contribute to the development of ischaemia of the bowel wall and can lead to perforation, with faecal peritonitis. One must therefore ascertain whether there are already signs of bowel ischaemia. The important symptoms and signs are:

- severe, localized continuous pain
- tenderness with positive rebound, indicating peritonitis
- the patient has a tachycardia and may be shocked

If there are signs of ischaemia, an emergency operation must be performed. If the bowel is viable at operation, it must be untwisted, but no emergency resection must be carried out.

Volvulus of the sigmoid colon is also found in young black men. In these patients, resection and anastomosis of the bowel can be performed as an emergency procedure, with good results.

If the bowel is gangrenous, the loop must be resected and the proximal loop must be brought out as a colostomy. If possible, the distal loop can be brought out as a mucus fistula, otherwise the distal open loop of bowel must be closed (Hartmann closure). When the patient has recovered from this operation, the colon can be sutured in an elective procedure.

If no signs of ischaemia are found at the original examination, a sigmoidoscopy is performed and a flatus tube is passed carefully via the sigmoidoscope through the rotated bowel to decompress the volvulus. The tube must be left in position for at least forty-eight hours.

If the patient is sufficiently fit, the bowel can be prepared and the sigmoid loop can be resected electively a few weeks later, with immediate anastomosis. If patients are totally unfit (many are aged patients in a poor general condition), they can merely be followed up. If the volvulus recurs, it can be decompressed repeatedly, using a flatus tube.

In a patient who is unfit, an extraperitoneal tunnel is sometimes made, and the sigmoid loop is placed into the tunnel to prevent further rotation. This is safer than resection.

Caecal volvulus

The management is operation. If the caecum is gangrenous, it must be resected and an ileotransverse colostomy performed. If the bowel is viable, it must just be untwisted. There are three possible approaches to prevent recurrence:

- If the patient is fit, resection and ileotransverse colostomy
- If the patient is unfit, a pexis of the caecum to the lateral peritoneum must be considered. This has a recurrence rate of about 25%.
- It is probably better to perform caecostomy. This serves a dual purpose: It decompresses the bowel and fixes the caecum to the abdominal wall.

Carcinoma of the colon

This obstruction occurs most often in the left colon. The proximal bowel is distended and if the ileocaecal valve is competent, a closed-loop obstruction results, with caecal distension and an impaired blood supply, which can cause perforation. If the valve is not competent (80%), the small bowel will distend, acting as a kind of safety valve. There is also a danger that the carcinoma may perforate as it penetrates the wall.

Management has two aims: decompression of the proximal bowel and resection of the carcinoma. Currently the achievement of both goals is attempted. If a proximal colostomy alone is performed, there is often no opportunity of removing the tumour. Patients are elderly and tend to develop complications.

Carcinoma of the right colon

Do a right hemicolectomy and an ileotransverse colostomy. If the patient is totally unfit, resect but do not do an anastomosis. Bring an ileostomy out onto the abdominal wall. It may then be possible to do an elective anastomosis. In very rare circumstances if a patient is very ill and unfit, only a caecostomy may be considered.

Carcinoma of the left colon

Resect the tumour but do not do an anastomosis, because the proximal bowel is massively distended and the bowel has not been prepared. The colostomy and mucus fistula are brought out onto the abdominal wall. If the distal bowel is too short, a Hartmann closure is performed.

Methods of restoring continuity by means of emergency procedures

- **Intraoperative colonic lavage:** *Some researchers suggest that the bowel must be prepared intraoperatively and primary suturing must be performed in suitable patients. After the tumour has been resected, a tube must be inserted through a caecostomy and a second tube into the distal open end. The bowel is now washed out until it is clean and then sutured. This method is difficult and time-consuming. The peritoneal cavity may become contaminated and the operation may be delayed for too long in unfit patients.*
- **Subtotal colectomy and ileorectal anastomosis:** *This method allows for elimination of the distended, contaminated colon. The ileum is then sutured to the rectum. It is unlikely that such an anastomosis will break down. The disadvantage of this method is that old patients experience problems with continence of the liquid stools. This does improve in time.*

Partial obstruction

Sometimes patients present with obstruction, because faeces impact above a carcinoma stenosis. This obstruction can be temporarily relieved by enemas and an elective resection can be performed after the bowel has been prepared. These patients form the minority and the majority still require an emergency procedure.

The three stage operation

In the past, a transverse colostomy was often performed on patients with carcinoma of the left colon. After preparation of the bowels, the tumour was then resected electively in a second procedure, with restoration of continuity and preservation of the proximal colostomy to give the suture line a chance to heal. The colostomy was then closed in a third operation.

The disadvantage is that three operations have to be performed and sometimes progress is never made beyond the transverse colostomy, with the result that the patient still has a carcinoma in place. This method must be used solely when the patient is totally unfit for an anaesthetic and can only tolerate a procedure performed under local anaesthesia. The other steps can then be completed when the patient's general condition has improved.

Prognosis of carcinoma obstruction

The mortality of caecal perforation is 40%. The prognosis of carcinoma obstruction is poor, as the tumour has already reached an advanced stage.

Rare causes of colonic obstruction

Unexpected causes of colonic obstruction are sometimes encountered. Ulcerative colitis and Crohn disease of the colon can cause stenosis. Ischaemic colitis can present later as stenosis of the colon. The pericolic inflammation of diverticulitis can present as obstruction.

Amoebiasis occasionally presents as an inflammatory mass causing obstruction in the region of the rectosigmoid colon.

B. INFLAMMATORY CONDITIONS OF THE INTESTINAL CANAL

Bacterial infections

The small intestine

Nonspecific infections

The small intestine normally has a relatively low bacterial count due to the continuous flow of its contents, the rôle of gastric acid and the presence of immunoglobulins. Any factor causing stasis can result in bacterial overgrowth. Such bacterial overgrowth causes diarrhoea, steatorrhoea, malnutrition and megaloblastic anaemia. This anaemia is caused by malabsorption of Vitamin B12, because anaerobic bacteria destroy it. These bacteria deconjugate bile salts and cause malabsorption, leading to steatorrhoea. This condition is known as the blind loop syndrome.

Causes include:

- bowel short-circuit operations
- bowel stenosis

- fistulae and
- diverticula, especially of the jejunum.

The diagnosis is usually confirmed by the Schilling test and hydrogen levels in exhaled air. The Schilling test confirms reduced absorption of Vitamin B12 administered per os. Hydrogen in exhaled air comes from bacterial fermentation of carbohydrates in the intestinal canal. Early pronounced hydrogen peaks after administration of lactulose indicate bacterial overgrowth in the small intestine.

If the patient has a condition which can be repaired operatively, this must be done. Resection of jejunal diverticula or repair of a blind loop will have the desired effect. If these cannot be repaired surgically, the patient must be treated with antibiotics and drugs to control the diarrhoea. Nutritional deficiencies must also be supplemented by dietary means.

Specific bacterial infections

Yersinia enteritis

Yersinia pseudotuberculosis usually causes a clinical syndrome which is difficult to differentiate from appendicitis. One distinction is that it is often associated with diarrhoea. At operation, the appendix is usually normal, but mesenteric lymph nodes are enlarged and inflamed and the terminal ileum is red, swollen and oedematous. In the past, the condition was confused with Crohn disease of the ileum.

The true diagnosis is confirmed by isolation of the bacteria in the blood and lymph nodes and a rising antibody titre. The condition follows a benign course and resolves spontaneously.

Yersinia enterocolitica presents with pain, fever, nausea, vomiting and diarrhoea. Sometimes septicaemia, erythema nodosum and arthritis are associated with the intestinal syndrome, but fortunately this is rare. If the disease does not resolve rapidly, or if complications arise, tetracyclines must be administered.

Typhoid

This disease is caused by *Salmonella typhi.* This bacteria is transmitted in water or food which has been contaminated by infected stools. Flies may also carry it from stools to food. The salmonella reaches the small intestine, where it penetrates the mucosa, affects the Peyer patches and involves the lymph nodes. It also spreads throughout the body, affecting the spleen, liver, kidneys, bone marrow, lungs and other tissues.

Clinical presentation

The disease can present in three stages:

Stage I

The patient feels ill, with headaches, myalgia, nausea and vomiting. He may also have abdominal pain and diarrhoea.

Stage II

The patient is now much sicker, with a high fever, dehydration and abdominal pain. Patients are confused and toxic and may develop cardiac failure.

Stage III

The abdomen is tender and there is hepatosplenomegaly. It is during this stage that the dreaded complication of perforation can occur. The patient's condition deteriorates, with a rapid pulse rate (it is usually slow), a raised white cell count (there is usually leucopaenia) and air is seen under the diaphragm on X-ray in most cases.

The diagnosis has, by this time, usually been confirmed by blood cultures and a raised titre on the Widal test.

Perforation occurs in about 3% of cases. Bleeding from the Peyer patches occurs in about 20%, but only 5% of these cases are serious.

Management

If a diagnosis of perforation is made, an operation must be performed. In the past, it was postulated that such patients could be treated conservatively and the perforation would seal spontaneously. This approach is no longer acceptable, except where there are no proper surgical facilities whatsoever.

General measures

Restore fluid and electrolytes. Administer antibiotics. A combination of ampicillin, 100 mg/kg/day, and chloramphenicol, 50 mg/kg/day, must be given. Cotrimoxazole is also effective against S. typhi.

The operation

A perforation of the antimesenteric surface of the distal ileum is usually found. The Peyer patches ulcerate and sometimes perforate. This perforation must be excised and the opening closed with interrupted polyglycol sutures. Examine the rest of the bowel, as other patches may already have perforated and become sealed with necrotic tissue. Suture serosa-to-serosa to seal off suspicious areas. It is seldom necessary to resect bowel. Ensure that no intraperitoneal abscesses have been missed. Other broad spectrum antibiotics may be necessary to treat peritonitis.

Haemorrhage

Although haemorrhage occurs in 20% of patients, it usually resolves on conservative treatment. If a life-threatening haemorrhage occurs, the distal ileum must be resected.

Typhoid carriers

More often than not this condition resolves on a three week course of ampicillin and chloramphenical. In resistant cases, it may sometimes be necessary to do a cholecystectomy, as this may be the source of the S. typhi.

Tuberculosis

This is common in black patients. It affects the distal ileum. Large circumferential ulcers arise and penetrate down to the submucosa. They heal by fibrosis and cause stenoses. Limited excision must be performed, so as not to remove bowel unnecessarily. If there are multiple stenoses, plasties can be performed, thus preserving bowel.

The appendix

About five out of every hundred of the white population will develop appendicitis during their lives. The disease is very rare in blacks, but its incidence is on the increase in urban blacks. Appendicitis is usually due to stasis in the appendix. Obstruction in the lumen may arise as a result of swelling in the wall, caused by viral infections with secondary bacterial infection, or due to objects in the lumen, such as faecoliths, worms, or foreign material ingested with the food.

In a small group, external pressure, e g fibrous bands, may play a part. In another small group, no evidence of obstruction is found.

The appendix swells, the blood supply is impeded and perforation takes place. This causes peritonitis, or, if it is limited by the body's defence mechanisms, an inflammatory mass or abscess.

Clinical presentation

Patients present with vague pain in the periumbilical area, followed by nausea and loss of appetite. The pain is not very severe at first, but it is persistent. Later, the patient may vomit. After a few hours, the pain shifts to the iliac fossa, where it becomes more localized. The pain is exacerbated by movement or coughing.

On examination, there is tenderness and guarding in the RIF. Rebound may be found. Rectal examination is usually normal.

If the appendix is situated in the pelvis, there will be consistent tenderness on the right side on rectal examination. If the appendix is situated retrocaecally, the classical presentation is not found. The pain is vague and does not shift. Tenderness may be found in the flank. If the appendix lies on the ureter, urinary symptoms may present.

Special investigations

A leucocytosis is usually found, with 75% leucocytes on the differential count. A leucocytosis is not always found; neither is there always pyrexia. Urine is usually normal, but it may contain leucocytes if the inflammation involves the ureter or bladder.

X-rays may be normal, or a few air/fluid levels may be seen in the RIF. Sometimes a faecolith is seen in association with these air/fluid levels. If the appendix has perforated, there may be air under the diaphragm, although this is a rare sign.

Ultrasound may be useful in confirming the diagnosis. A thickened, rigid appendix may be visible.

Appendicitis in children and the elderly

The classical presentation is usually absent. Patients present with loss of appetite, nausea and vomiting, and mild abdominal signs. In all too many cases, the diagnosis is delayed until perforation occurs.

Appendicitis in pregnancy

The incidence of appendicitis in pregnancy is the same as that in women of the same age group who are not pregnant. Pain, anorexia, nausea and vomiting occur. The patient is febrile and has a leucocytosis. Because the uterus displaces the appendix upwards, the localization of the pain is atypical and the diagnosis is thus often delayed. It is very important that the appendix be removed early, as it will not be sealed off by omentum if it perforates, because the enlarged uterus prevents this. The prognosis worsens if diagnosis is delayed. The foetal mortality rate is 10%.

Differential diagnosis of appendicitis

RIF pain in young women is one of the most difficult diagnostic dilemmas. Appendicitis must be differentiated from:

- **Salpingitis**

There is usually no history of nausea and vomiting. Pain is more often bilateral and the adnexae are very tender on pelvic examination. If a white vaginal discharge is found, it contributes to the correct diagnosis.

- **Urinary tract infections**

These are very common in women.

There is often a history of dysuria and frequency. Patients may be tender over the bladder area and lumbar region. The diagnosis rests on microsopic findings in the urine, which should display a pronounced pyuria. If many red cells are present, a stone must be considered and an excreting urogram performed.

- **Mittelschmertz**

Some young women experience pain on ovulation and tenderness and even guarding can occur due to irritation of the peritoneum by blood that may escape into the abdominal cavity. There is usually a history of recurrent similar episodes and it typically occurs in the middle of the menstrual cycle.

- **Mesenteric adenitis**

This is found in young patients and usually follows an upper respiratory tract infection. The fever is disproportionately high when compared to the relatively mild abdominal signs. Tenderness varies in position, and shifts if the patient is turned on her side.

The cause of the condition is not usually evident. *Yersinia enterocolitica* or *Yersinia pseudotuberculosis* are sometimes responsible. Viruses may also play a rôle.

- **Gastro enteritis**

Diarrhoea is usually a prominent sign and abdominal X-rays may show multiple small air/fluid levels.

Rare conditions to be considered

Crohn disease, Meckel diverticulum and caecal carcinoma must be borne in mind. Conditions above the diaphragm such as pneumonia, pleuritis and angina pectoris must also be considered.

Bornholm disease (Cocksackie virus pleuritis) can sometimes be misleading.

Differential diagnosis of a patient with acute peritonitis

The most common cause of acute peritonitis is still a perforated appendix. Bearing this in mind, other conditions must also be considered and differentiated from appendicitis. Although generalized tenderness, guarding and rebound are present, the point of maximum tenderness will give one a clue as to the cause of the peritonitis.

- Tenderness mainly in the RIF: appendicitis
- Tenderness mainly in the right hypochondrium: cholecystitis
- Generalized pressure tenderness without localization and a boardlike abdomen: perforation of a peptic ulcer
- Generalized tenderness with increased bowel sounds: small bowel obstruction
- An elderly patient with very severe, continuous pain and few signs on abdominal X-rays: consider mesenteric adenitis

Laboratory investigations can sometimes help in making a diagnosis. Raised amylase indicates acute pancreatitis. Remember that it is also raised in cholecystitis, perforation of a peptic ulcer and dead bowel. A tenfold rise is pathognemonic of pancreatitis.

Pronounced metabolic acidosis indicates bowel necrosis. The X-ray findings, which have already been discussed, may be decisive. Air under the diaphragm means that there is a perforated viscus. The most common cause is perforation of a peptic ulcer. Perforation of diverticulitis or appendicitis can also cause air under the diaphragm, but these are much rarer causes.

Management of acute appendicitis

The appendix must be removed before it perforates. In realizing this ideal, it is unavoidable that a certain percentage of normal appendices will be removed. A good rule of thumb is that at least two out of ten appendices removed will be normal. If less than 20% are normal, the surgeon is not sufficiently circumspect. If more than 20% are normal, he operates without sufficient consideration.

Antibiotic administration has further reduced the mortality of appendicitis; it is currently 0,1%. If perforation has already taken place, the mortality rises to 5%, i e fifty times higher.

Management of acute peritonitis when a definitive diagnosis has not yet been made

If a patient has acute peritonitis and the diagnosis is not known, a laparotomy must be performed after resuscitation of the patient and broad spectrum antibiotics must be administered. There is controversy about which approach should be used. If there is pressure tenderness in the RIF, a diagnosis of perforated appendix can be accepted and a Rutherford-Morrison approach (RIF incision, cutting through the muscle layer) must be used. This facilitates removal of the perforated appendix. Those who advocate the midline incision maintain that this offers better exposure and access to other organs and allows one to lavage the entire abdomen. It can be very awkward to remove a perforated appendix in the RIF through a midline incision and it is better to perform a smaller operation on patients who are so ill. If the diagnosis is incorrect, which happens exceptionally rarely, the RIF approach is closed and a midline approach used.

If there are absolutely no localizing signs, a midline approach must be used ab initio.

If a normal appendix is found

The appendix must still be removed, because there may be confusion later if there is an appendicectomy incision and the patient presents with an acute abdomen. Macroscopically the appendix may also appear normal, but may show inflammation on histological examination. Before the appendix is removed, 2 metres of the small intestine must be pulled out to exclude a complication of a Meckel diverticulum. If the diverticulum is inflamed, it must be resected. If it is a normal diverticulum with a wide opening, it must be left as it is.

If there is free fluid in the abdomen, especially if it is cloudy, the female genitalia must be examined and a hand must be inserted to feel for cholecystitis or a perforated peptic ulcer.

Also take a swab of the fluid and send it for culture to exclude primary peritonitis. If a swollen distal small bowel and large mesenteric nodes are found, everything must be left as it is. Investigate further for Yersinia infection. **Do not resect an acute ileitis**.

Chance appendectomy

Some surgeons remove a normal appendix when they open the abdomen for another procedure, e g cholecystectomy. **This should not be done.** *Appendicectomy is still the most important cause of band obstruction due to adhesions. Removal of a normal appendix, with the possibility, however slight, of complications, is therefore not justifiable.*

Appendix mass

Patients present with symptoms and signs of appendicitis, with a palpable mass in the RIF. Such a mass is caused by either an abscess surrounding the appendix, or omentum and bowel which have sealed off an incipient perforation of the appendix.

It is important to differentiate between the two conditions, because of the difference in treatment. Ultrasound is very useful in confirming an abscess. An abscess may rupture into the peritoneal cavity, causing generalized peritonitis; and it must therefore be drained. There are two possible ways of doing this:

- A catheter can be inserted into the abscess percutaneously under sonar guidance, for drainage.

- Surgical extraperitoneal drainage is a safer and more reliable method. An incision is made over the McBurney point, but the peritoneum is not opened. A tissue plane must be developed laterally between the peritoneum and the abdominal wall, until the abscess is reached. A drainage tube is then inserted.

If the mass is threatened perforation of the appendix which has sealed off, it can be treated conservatively. Put the patient on nil per os and replace fluid and electrolytes via an intravenous infusion. Give broad spectrum antibiotics. An aminoglycoside, penicillin and metronidazole constitute a good combination.

The patient's general condition and abdominal status must be monitored twice daily. If the patient improves, continue with conservative treatment. If his condition remains unchanged or exacerbates, an emergency appendicectomy must be performed.

An appendicectomy can be performed six to eight weeks after an abscess has been successfully drained, or after an inflammatory mass has been treated conservatively with success.

The advantage of this treatment is that the possible complications of peritonitis and wound sepsis are usually avoided and an elective appendicectomy can be performed with a very small chance of mortality.

Some surgeons prefer to operate on an inflammatory mass as an emergency procedure. They maintain that the total duration of the disease is shortened and the complications can be prevented by appropriate antibiotic therapy.

Management of the appendix with a mass in the wall

Patients sometimes present with symptoms and signs of appendicitis and, on operation, a tumour, rather than inflammation, is found in the wall of the appendix. The tumour is usually a carcinoid. These tumours are smaller than 2 cm and seldom metastasize. An appendicectomy is all that is required. If the tumour is larger than 2 cm, and/or the lymph nodes are enlarged or the caecum has been infiltrated, a right hemicolectomy must be performed. This is seldom necessary. If a mucocoele of the appendix is found, the appendix must be removed carefully so that its contents do not spill into the abdominal cavity. Most cases are caused by simple obstruction with mucus accumulation in the lumen. A small minority may be cystadenomas. Pseudomyxoma peritonei is a rare complication in such cases.

Thrombophlebitis suppurativa

This is a complication which is very rare these days, probably due to antibiotic usage in the treatment of acute appendicitis. This is an infective thrombophlebitis of the portal vein. It causes multiple liver abscesses and has a very high mortality.

Patients present with rigors, sweating and mild jaundice. Abdominal X-rays may show gas in the portal venous system. CT shows thrombosis of the portal vein and multiple gas-filled abscesses.

Management comprises removal of the septic focus (appendicectomy) and intensive treatment with broad spectrum antibiotics, including those effective against anaerobes.

The colon

Inflammatory conditions of the large intestine

The colon contains more than 400 different organisms. More than 90% of the normal flora comprise anaerobic bacteria. The most common anaerobes found are *Bacteroides fragilis*. A variety of *Clostridia* and cocci are also found. Aerobic bacteria include *E. coli, klebsiella, proteus* and *enterobacter. Streptococcus faecalis* is the enterococcus most commonly found. These bacteria function in normal physiological processes such as deconjugation of bile salts and synthesis of vitamin K and ammonia. Certain other circumstances play a rôle in the development of inflammation of the intestinal canal and peritoneal cavity.

Bacillary dysentery

This is caused by the genus *Shigella*. The bacteria are transmitted in contaminated food and water. After a short incubation period, the patient develops fever, diarrhoea and colicky abdominal pain. In time, the stools contain blood and mucus and the diagnosis is usually made on stool cultures.

Less severe infections resolve spontaneously. If the patient has a severe attack, he must be treated with an antibiotic to which the bacteria is sensitive. Such antibiotics include tetracycline, ampicillin or even sulphonamides. The surgical importance of this condition is that it must be differentiated from a surgically acute abdomen.

Pseudomembranous enterocolitis

There is a spectrum of conditions in adults, which are known as pseudomembranous colitis. They are characterized by fever, watery bloody diarrhoea and abdominal pain. Dehydration and hypotension may follow.

A patchy white exudate (pseudomembrane) can be seen on sigmoidoscopy. If the exudate is removed, an underlying granular bloody surface can be seen.

The condition follows a major surgery, especially of the gastrointestinal tract and there is usually a history that the patient was given clindamycin, lincomycin or ampicillin.

Sometimes an overgrowth of staphylococci can be cultured in the stool, and the condition is then known as staphylococcal colitis. It has recently become clear that only the minority of these cases actually have staphylococcal overgrowth. An overgrowth of *Clostridium difficile* is more often found. This organism produces a toxin which damages cells. The diagnosis is usually confirmed by measuring this toxin.

Management

All antibiotics must be stopped immediately. Fluid and electrolyte imbalances must be corrected and parenteral feeding may be necessary for a few days.

Vancomycin can be given in a dose of 500 mg six-hourly for two weeks. Metronidazole is an alternative.

The condition tends to recur if treatment is stopped. A second course of Vancomycin must then be administered.

Tuberculosis of the colon

Gastrointestinal tuberculosis is caused by the bovine and human tubercle baccilli. Bovine tuberculosis is rare in South Africa. Pulmonary tuberculosis is very common among black people, yet gastrointestinal tuberculosis is rare. It most commonly affects the ileocaecal area and presents as hypertrophic, ulcerative and ulcerohypertrophic types.

The hypertrophic type can sometimes be difficult to distinguish from carcinoma. Multiple ulcers can arise, causing stenosis. Patients sometimes present with anorectal abscesses or fistulae-in-ano.

Management

All patients must be treated with anti-tuberculous drugs. If obstructions arise, local segmental resections must be performed.

Diverticular disease of the colon

Diverticula are found more commonly in the colon than in any other part of the intestinal canal. In 95% of cases, the sigmoid colon is involved. The diverticula can also affect the descending, transverse and ascending colon. Very rarely, only the right colon alone is affected. Diverticulosis restricted to the right colon is especially common in orientals.

A single caecal diverticulum is a congenital abnormality and these diverticula are true diverticula which involve all the layers of the caecal wall.

Sigmoid diverticula are acquired, false, pulsion diverticula caused by raised intraluminal pressure, with protrusion of mucosa through a relatively weak point where the blood vessels enter the bowel wall. The cause of the increased intraluminal pressure is uncertain. It may be related to a low fibre diet, leading to hypertrophy of the circular muscle layer, with segmentation of the sigmoid colon and functional obstruction with raised pressure. This condition is rare in groups such as blacks, who eat a high fibre diet.

The concept that spastic colon syndrome is a predisposing factor for diverticulosis is attractive. Unfortunately, it has become clear that the motility patterns of the two diseases differ. Extremely high pressures are found in some patients with diverticulosis.

Not all patients with diverticulosis have circular muscle layer hypertrophy or raised intraluminal pressure. There may therefore be two types of diverticula, namely:

- hypertrophic muscle with high pressure, which presents with pain and constipation. This type is more inclined to develop complications;
- multiple diffuse diverticula without muscle hypertrophy and normal pressures. These patients are asymptomatic and complications occur less frequently.

In whites, diverticula develop in more than 60% of people before the age of eighty.

Clinical presentation

The majority of patients with diverticulosis are asymptomatic. A small group present with pain in the LIF, constipation and/or diarrhoea. There is no fever or leucocytosis. A tender sigmoid colon is palpable.

Special investigations

A sawtooth appearance is seen on barium enema. This was always accepted as a prediverticular phase. These days, it is believed to be typical of the contractions found in the spastic colon syndrome. Sometimes this functional bowel syndrome is found in conjunction with diverticula and the two are difficult to differentiate from each other.

Management

Patients respond to reassurance, support and a high fibre diet.

Diverticulitis

Acute inflammation of diverticula arises most often in patients who have had no previous symptoms. Diverticulitis can present in various ways:

- The diverticulum itself can become inflamed and then drain into the intestinal canal. This resolves spontaneously or on conservative treatment.
- The diverticulum may perforate. If it does, the perforation may be small and restricted to the bowel wall and it may form a peridiverticular inflammation or abscess. The perforation can seal off or the abscess can drain into the bowel lumen spontaneously, with subsequent resolution.
- A large perforation may leak into the peritoneal cavity and lead to generalized peritonitis.
- If the perforation is sealed off by adjacent small bowel loops, a small bowel obstruction may develop.
- An abscess can break through into an adjacent organ, with fistula formation. This usually happens between the sigmoid colon and the bladder.
- Inflammation in the neck of the diverticulum can erode a blood vessel, giving rise to a large rectal bleed.

Clinical presentation

Patients with diverticulitis present with pain in the LIF. The pain is gnawing and persistent. The patients are often constipated. A low grade fever and leucocytosis are present.

On palpation there is tenderness and guarding in the LIF. If the diverticulum perforates, the symptoms and signs become worse. Tenderness and guarding become more pronounced and a vague mass may be palpable.

If a free perforation occurs in the abdominal cavity, the patient develops a high fever, becomes very ill and shows signs of generalized peritonitis. The abdomen is distended and very tender, with rigidity. An ileus develops, and bowel sounds are absent. Abdominal X-rays may show air under the diaphragm.

If the inflammation involves the bladder, there will be symptoms of urinary tract infection.

Special investigations

Sigmoidoscopy cannot contribute much to the diagnosis. Barium enema should be avoided in the acute phase, as barium may leak into the peritoneal cavity. If there is doubt, a gastrografin enema may be attempted.

Colonoscopy should preferably be avoided in the acute phase, as leakage into the peritoneal cavity could develop. Ultrasound is useful in diagnosing a localized abscess.

Differential diagnosis

It is sometimes difficult to differentiate between the various causes of acute generalized peritonitis. Conditions that must be considered include perforation of an appendix, perforated peptic ulcer and a perforated gall bladder. Acute generalized peritonitis of unknown origin must be treated surgically and the diagnosis is often only made at laparotomy.

Management

If the patient has diverticulitis only, without complications, he can be treated conservatively. Bed-rest, nil per os, nasogastric suction, and fluid and electrolyte replacement are required. Broad spectrum antibiotics, such as ampicillin, an aminoglycoside and metronidazole, are given in combination.

As soon as the acute phase has passed, a barium enema must be performed to confirm the diagnosis and to exclude carcinoma. If a suspicious lesion is noted, colonoscopy must follow.

Peridiverticular abscess without peritonitis

Treat conservatively as for diverticulitis. If there is a palpable mass in the LIF, it can be drained. Usually the perforation seals off spontaneously and the condition resolves. In very weak patients, insertion of a drainage catheter under ultrasound guidance can be considered.

Free perforation with generalised peritonitis

When the abdomen is opened, a variety of situations can be encountered. There may be an obvious perforation, with faecal peritonitis. If this is so, the affected piece of bowel must be resected and the proximal colon must be brought out as a colostomy. The distal bowel is closed (Hartmann procedure). The wound must be well lavaged.

Sometimes no perforation can be found and only a mild peritonitis is noted. In the past, it was recommended that a proximal colostomy be brought out with a drain in the area of inflammation. It is probably just as satisfactory to insert a drain, close the abdomen and threat with broad spectrum antibiotics. If there is any doubt and the patient is a relatively good operative risk, a resection and colostomy must be performed.

Certain American workers recommend resection and primary anastomosis, but this is not usually advisable in distended, oedematous, unprepared colon.

Prognosis

Less than a quarter of patients with acute diverticulitis require surgical treatment. The operative mortality is about 5%. The mortality with generalized peritonitis is still in excess of 20%.

Elective surgery for diverticular disease

It is very seldom necessary to operate if patients do not develop complications. Almost all patients respond well to a high fibre diet. An elective sigoidectomy may become necessary only when patients suffer recurrent attacks of acute diverticulitis. Young patients under the age of thirty are more inclined to develop complications and must undergo elective resection, even if they have had only one episode of diverticulitis.

Mystomy of the sigmoid colon (Reilly operation)

Because segmental intraluminal raised pressure is largely responsible for the clinical presentation and origin of diverticula, it has been suggested that a myotomy of the hypertrophied circumferential muscles of the sigmoid colon ought to be done. The muscles are incised through an antimesenteric taenia, so that the mucosa bulges outwards. The same principle applies as in the Ramstedt operation. The operation yields good results, but complications are common and the mortality due to colon leakage is too high.

Colovesical fistula

This is three times more common in men. The fact that the uterus lies between the bladder and the sigmoid colon is probably the reason for the low incidence in women. Diverticulitis is the most common cause, but carcinoma must always be borne in mind.

Clinical presentation

Sometimes the fistula develops without any clinically apparent case of diverticulitis. Patients complain mainly of urinary tract symptoms, dysuria, frequency and pneumaturia. They sometimes notice faeces in the urine.

On examination, a mass is sometimes palpable in the suprapubic area, but more commonly, nothing is palpable.

Special investigations

Sigmoidoscopy is not usually of much assistance. Cyctoscopy shows oedema and inflammation of the bladder, and the fistula is often visible. A barium enema may demonstrate the fistula.

Management

There should be no hurry to operate, as patients do not have many symptoms. After the bowel has been prepared, the sigmoid colon is resected, the hole in the bladder closed, and a urinary catheter left in situ *for ten days.*

Remember the possibility of carcinoma. If carcinoma is found, the mass must be widely resected, the defect in the bladder closed and colon continuity restored.

Massive rectal bleeding

In the past, it was accepted that a heavy rectal bleed which presented in an elderly person, usually over the age of seventy-five, was probably due to a diverticulum. Currently, it has been shown that about 40% of such bleeds arise from other lesions, predominantly angiodysplasia. The overriding problem in the past was the assumption that, if there were diverticula in the sigmoid colon, they were probably the cause of the bleeding. Bleeding often recurred after a left hemicolectomy.

Clinical presentation

An elderly patient, without any signs of diverticulitis, presents with a heavy rectal bleed. Often the bleeding stops spontaneously for a few hours and then resumes. More often, it stops and does not recur. A rectal examination and sigmoidoscopy must be performed to exclude other local lesions which may be bleeding, such as haemorrhoids, polyps or even carcinoma.

If the patient stops bleeding, a barium enema is performed a few days later. Diverticula are usually found, but one must remember that they are not necessarily the cause of the bleeding. If no other lesions are found, the patient is merely followed up. Very few return with recurrence of bleeding.

Management of patients who continue to bleed

A small minority of patients continue to bleed. If more than three units of blood are required for resuscitation, it can be assumed that surgical intervention may become necessary. The most important problem is to determine whether the bleeding comes from the right- or the left colon.

A radionuclide scan is the most useful non-invasive investigation. If this investigation demonstrates the location of the bleeding point clearly and the patient continues to bleed, half the colon can be resected. If a radionuclide scan is either unavailable, or unsuccessful, selective arteriography can be considered. Unfortunately, this does not often show the bleeding point if the radionuclide scan is negative. If the bleeding point cannot be identified by investigations and the patient continues to bleed massively, a total colectomy with an ileorectal anastomosis must be performed.

Angiodysplasia is usually the cause of bleeding in the right hemicolon. It is an acquired condition found in patients over sixty. It is sometimes associated with cardiac valvular lesions.

The submucous venous plexus is dilated, but the veins outside the muscle layer are normal. It would appear that ectasis of the submucus venous plexus develops as a result of a relative obstruction at the site where the veins penetrate the muscle layer. Angiography shows a vein which fills quickly, with a submucous venous blush and then empties slowly through the muscle layer.

Patients with angiodysplasia bleed less heavily and stop bleeding sooner, but are inclined to recur more frequently than those who bleed from diverticula. Colonoscopy may be useful to demonstrate the lesion and it can also be coagulated colonoscopically. If this is unsuccessful, a right hemicolectomy must be performed.

Parasites and viruses

Amoebiasis of the colon

Although *entamoeba histolitica* infection is very common in some parts of South Africa (Natal), amoebic colitis is relatively rare. Most patients with chronic amoebic colitis present with diarrhoea and are then treated by medical gastroenterologists. Acute amoebic colitis often presents as an acute abdomen and the patient is admitted to a surgical ward.

Patients sometimes develop an amoebic granuloma in the caecum or at the rectosigmoid junction, mimicking the signs and symptoms of carcinoma.

Acute amoebic colitis

Clinical presentation

Patients present with bloody diarrhoea. The abdomen is distended and may show signs of acute peritonitis, due to colonic perforation. Proctoscopy shows large ulcera in the rectum. Sigmoidoscopy must preferably be avoided, because the bowel can easily be perforated.

Special investigations

X-rays show dilated colonic loops (toxic megacolon) and often free gas in the abdominal cavity. Examination of warm stools shows amoebae. Only the haematophagous form of *A. histolitica* proves the presence of active disease.

Management

The disease often follows a fulminating course. Patients are dehydrated and very toxic. Fluids and electrolytes must be replaced aggressively. A central venous line is useful to measure the fluid required to maintain the blood pressure. Metronidazole must be given immediately intravenously, in doses of 500 mg eight-hourly.

Indications for laparotomy

- *Signs of perforation. Acute peritonitis and air in the abdominal cavity.*
- *If the patient does not respond rapidly to resuscitation and metronidazole.*

The operation

There are many opinions as to what constitutes the best treatment for amoebic colitis. The greater part of the colon is usually involved and the bowel wall is either necrotic, or as fragile and friable as blotting paper when handled. Researchers in Natal have shown that thrombosis takes place in blood vessels and that the lesion is an ischaemic necrosis of the wall.

• Standard approach

If a localized segment is affected, with necrosis, it is excised and the two ends of the bowel are brought out as a colostomy and mucus fistula. If there are multiple lesions throughout the greater part of the colon, which is usually the case, a total colectomy must be performed with an ileostomy and Hartmann closure of the rectum. Later, when the patient has recovered, an ileorectal anastomosis is performed.

• The Natal approach

An ileostomy is constructed and the colon is irrigated, without any resection of the colon. This approach is based on the principle that bowel contents are diverted from the affected colon (ileostomy) and infected contents are washed out. If a perforation is noted during irrigation, it is closed by means of an omental patch. The omentum is pulled around the affected bowel so that it can seal the bowel off and hopefully bring a new blood supply to the ischaemic tissue by means of adhesions.

Prognosis

The mortality of fulminating perforated amoebic colitis is nearly 100% if it is treated conservatively. The mortality is higher than 40% if it is treated surgically.

Amoebic granuloma (amoeboma)

A large mass develops in the region of the caecum or rectosigmoid junction. The patient presents with partial or total obstruction. At the rectosigmoid junction, the mass must be differentiated from carcinoma; and at the caecum from a carcinoma, an appendix mass, or Crohn disease of the caecum.

Sigmoidoscopy and colonoscopy can confirm the diagnosis. If biopsies are negative and haemagglutinin tests are also negative, it is still advisable to give patients who may have amoeboma a trial of metronidazole therapy. An amoeboma resolves rapidly. If this does not happen, a right or left hemicolectomy must be performed to exclude carcinoma.

Schistosomiasis of the colon

The disease is caused by *Schistosoma mansoni*. Bowel disease is relatively rare. It can lead to fibrosis, with stenosis and obstruction. The diagnosis is usually made on rectal biopsy. The condition must be treated with antischistosomal drugs.

Lymphogranuloma venereum

This is caused by a *Chlamydial* infection, usually sexually transmitted. The primary lesion is on the penis or the vagina, and patients develop enlarged inguinal lymph nodes. In women the disease spreads to the rectum lymphatically. A proctitis, granulations, ulcerations and mucosal oedema arise. Later fibrosis develops, with rectal stenosis. Carcinoma can also develop secondary to this condition.

The diagnosis is made by means of a complement fixation test. The treatment of choice is tetracycline and erythromycin.

Inflammatory conditions of unknown aetiology

Crohn disease and ulcerative colitis

Because these two diseases are often confused if the lesion is confined to the colon, it is better to discuss them together. Both diseases are relatively rare in South Africa and even rarer in the black population.

The incidence of Crohn disease is on the increase in Europe and the USA, whereas that of ulcerative colitis has reached a plateau and now remains constant.

Crohn disease

Aetiology

The cause of this disease is unknown. The old milk sensitivity theory and the rôle of the psyche no longer enjoy any support. The presence of various infective agents such as viruses, microbacteria, chlamydia and Yersinia probably play more of a contributory rôle than a causative one. The latest thinking is that Crohn disease has a genetic background and that certain environmental factors contribute to this. The disease runs in families and also sometimes in families where other members have ulcerative colitis. The HLA-B27 antigen is common in patients with Crohn disease and ankylosing spondylitis. Immunological phenomena are also strongly under the spotlight. Granulomas are an indication of cell-mediated hypersensitivity and the systemic manifestations of arthritis and skin reactions are also suggestive of immunological phenomena. A lowered T-cell count is found in some cases. Antibodies to RNA are found, suggesting possible autoimmunity. The current findings suggest a genetically determined hypersensitivity reaction, probably initiated by infective agents.

Pathology

The disease can affect any area of the gastrointestinal canal, from mouth to anus. The skin is sometimes affected and granuloma of the eye has been described.

The distal ileum is most commonly affected - either alone or in conjunction with the colon. Ileitis alone is found in 25% of cases. Simultaneous ileal and colonic involvement occurs in 50% of cases and colonic involvement alone in 25%.

Lesions are occasionally found in the oesophagus, stomach and duodenum. If random biopsies are taken of apparently normal areas of the intestinal canal, subtle histological changes can be found. This suggests that the disease probably affects the whole intestinal canal.

Granulomas are found in the bowel wall in 60% of cases and in the lymph nodes in 25% of cases. The earliest lesion is involvement of the Peyer patches, followed by ulceration. Deep, fissurelike lesions and elongated, tortuous ulcers then develop with oedema of the mucosa lying between the ulcers. This gives rise to the macroscopic "cobbled" appearance. Eventually, the inflammatory process spreads throughout the bowel wall. The bowel is thickened and shortened. The mesentery and mesenterial fat spread across the bowel wall. There may be multiple lesions with normal areas interposed (skip lesions). Later, fibrosis, with stenosis, occurs.

Clinical presentation

Diarrhoea is found in 90% of patients. The watery stools do not contain blood if the small bowel only is affected, and only 25% of patients with colonic involvement have bloody diarrhoea. Colicky lower abdominal pain following meals is a common symptom. This can probably be ascribed to a partial chronic bowel obstruction. This is associated with weakness, fatigue, loss of weight and fever.

A mass is sometimes palpable in the RIF. Anorectal lesions are found in about 20% of cases. Fissures, fistulae and abscesses can occur.

Later, patients develop anaemia. Both iron deficiency and macrocytic anaemia can occur. Vitamin B12 uptake is impaired by an inflammatory process in the distal ileum. Sometimes the disease presents like acute appendicitis. If acute ileitis is found at operation, it must not be resected; only the appendix must be removed. The majority of such cases do not have Crohn disease at all, but conditions such as Yersinia ileitis. Even if it is Crohn disease, it should be treated conservatively.

Special investigations

Laboratory investigations

Anaemia and hypoalbuminaemia are common.

X-rays

A small bowel barium enema (barium inserted into the small bowel via a long tube) usually shows typical signs. These include a thickened distal ileum with a stenosis (string sign). Long tortuous ulcers and deep fissures can be seen in the mucosa and bowel wall. A cobbled appearance is usually visible. Multiple segments (skip lesions) strongly support the diagnosis. Deformity of the caecum or fistulae can also occur. The diagnosis can be histologically confirmed by means of colonoscopic biopsy.

Complications of Crohn disease

Free perforation of Crohn disease seldom occurs. Abscesses and fistulae to other organs are fairly common. Patients also develop bowel obstruction. The systemic complications will be described with and compared to ulcerative colitis.

Differential diagnosis

The important differences between Crohn disease and ulcerative colitis will be discussed later. The bowel lesions must be differentiated from tuberculosis, lymphoma and carcinoma.

Management

The management will be discussed with that of ulcerative colitis to draw comparisons.

Ulcerative colitis

Aetiology

The cause is unknown. As in Crohn disease, a combination of factors comes into play. The patient apparently becomes sensitized to a variety of antigens such as viruses or dietary factors. Any factors which cause increased permeability of the mucosa can lead to an inflammatory condition if the bowel is exposed to the same antigens again. The nature of these antigens will determine whether the patient develops Crohn disease or ulcerative colitis. There also seems to be an abnormality in the composition of mucus in these patients.

Pathology

Abscesses arise in the crypts of Lieberkuhn. The inflammation tends to spread horizontally and cause necrosis of the underlying mucosa. Ulceration occurs and shreds of mucosa hang loosely in the lumen and are called pseudopolyps. In contrast to Crohn disease, there is no normal mucosa between the ulcers and the inflammation does not spread throughout the bowel wall. The serosa and mesentery of the bowel appear normal. Ulcerative colitis is a disease of the mucosa, while Crohn disease affects the mucosa, the bowel wall and the mesentery.

If ulcerative colitis exacerbates and toxic megacolon arises, the blood supply of the colonic wall becomes impaired and necrosis of the wall, with perforation, can occur.

Ulcerative colitis always affects the rectum and extends proximally. In about 30% of cases, the entire colon is involved. In 50% of cases only the rectum is affected. In Crohn disease the rectum is spared in 50% of cases.

Anal fistulae are found in 10% of cases.

Clinical presentation

Patients present with bloody diarrhoea; copious watery stools containing blood, mucus and pus. They complain of tenesmus and discomfort, abdominal pain, nausea and vomiting. On examination, weight loss, fever and dehydration are found.

Sometimes the patient presents with an acute, fulminating attack with acute abdominal pain and distension. A small percentage present with systemic complications such as arthritis and pyodermia.

Sigmoidoscopy shows a granular, friable mucosa which bleeds easily on contact. The mucosa is red and velvety. In the healing phase, the mucosa has a granular surface with fine telangiectasis.

Special investigations

Laboratory investigations

Anaemia, leucocytosis and hypoalbuminaemia occur.

X-rays

A barium enema must be avoided during an acute attack. It can precipitate an attack of toxic megacolon or perforation. Barium enema shows an irregular mucosa with fine ulcers or large, underlying, irregular ulceration. Other signs are loss of haustrations (lead pipe appearance) and pseudopolyps in the mucosa.

Colonoscopy

This investigation must not be performed during an acute attack, as perforation may take place. Later it is very useful to determine the extent of colonic involvement and to perform multiple biopsies. The diagnosis is usually made on histological findings.

Differential diagnosis

Bacillary dysentery and amoebic colitis must be excluded, using stool cultures and serological tests. The most important differential diagnosis is between Crohn disease and ulcerative colitis. Aside from the clinical presentation, which may be useful, the diagnosis is usually made on X-ray differences and histological characteristics.

RADIOLOGICAL CHARACTERISTICS

Ulcerative colitis	Crohn disease
• Continuous	• Segmental
• Distal bowel and rectum involved	• Rectum spared in 50%
• Small, superficial ulcers	• Deep ulcers
• Rough mucosa with pseudopolyps	• Longitudinal, tortuous ulcers
• Bowel shortened	• Shortening less noticeable
• Loss of haustrations	• Cobbled appearance
• Lead pipe appearance	• Haustra preserved
• Small bowel not involved	• Local stenosis
• Mild distal ileitis sometimes	• Small bowel involved with colon 50% of cases

MICROSCOPIC CHARACTERISTICS

Ulcerative colitis	Crohn disease
• Inflammation confined to mucosa and submucosa	• Inflammation penetrates throughout bowel wall
• Crypt abscesses common	• Crypt abscesses rare
• Paneth cell metaplasia common	
• Granulomas rare	• Granulomas common

Complications

Systemic lesions

- Skin and mucosal lesions include *pyoderma gangrenosum* and aphthous stomatitis. These lesions are also found in Crohn disease.
- Uveitis is found in both diseases.
- Arthritis and ankylosing spondylitis are found in both diseases.
- Pericholangitis, sclerosing cholangitis and gall stones are associated with both diseases.

Carcinoma of the colon

There is an increased incidence of carcinoma of the colon in ulcerative colitis. Factors playing a rôle include:

- Early onset of the disease
- Total involvement of the colon
- Aggressive course of the disease

It is currently accepted that the incidence of malignant transformation was overestimated in the past. Dysplastic changes in the mucosa (Morson criteria) are accepted to be premalignant phenomena in the colon. Patients with total involvement and a ten year history should have an annual colonoscopy, with multiple biopsies and an experienced pathologist's opinion to identify dysplastic lesions early so that a colectomy can be performed. In such cases, early carcinoma is found in 30% of specimens.

Carcinoma of the colon is more common in patients with Crohn disease than in the general public. There is also an increased incidence of carcinoma of the small bowel in this disease. The lesions are found in the affected distal ileum in patients younger than the usual age group who contract small bowel carcinoma. The lesions are sometimes multifocal. The tumour is not usually diagnosed and is found in bowel which has been excised because of obstruction.

Toxic megacolon

This is found in both ulcerative colitis and Crohn's disease, but it is more common in ulcerative colitis. Precipitating factors include barium enema and anticholinergic drugs. Patients are very ill and toxic with a distended, acute abdomen. X-rays show distended colonic loops, usually more than 7 cm in diameter.

Perforation of the colon

This occurs most commonly during the first severe attack of acute ulcerative colitis. Perforation of the sigmoid colon and splenic flexure are the most common types. It can also be a complication of toxic megacolon. The caecum is then a common site.

Perforation is less common in Crohn disease.

Haemorrhage

Massive haemorrhage is rare, but is more common in ulcerative colitis than in Crohn disease.

Stenosis

This is found in both conditions. Carcinoma must always be borne in mind, especially in ulcerative colitis.

Management of Crohn's disease and ulcerative colitis

Conservative management

Because Crohn's disease probably affects the entire intestinal canal, it is wise to treat conservatively where possible.

Dietary adjustment

A low residue diet with high protein and milk content must be given. It sometimes becomes necessary to give parenteral feeding to catch up on nutritional backlogs. Iron, vitamin B12 and other vitamins must be given.

Corticosteroids

Oral corticosteroids must be administered in daily doses of 40–60 mg of prednisolone. In patients who are seriously ill, hydrocortisone can be given intravenously. Trials have shown that although steroids are of use in acute attacks, they do not reduce recurrence rates or the incidence of surgery. Corticosteroids are thus equally effective against acute attacks of Crohn's disease or ulcerative colitis, but do not reduce recurrence of either disease.

Sulphasalazine (salazopyrin)

This drug is useful in acute colonic Crohn's disease, but does not help if the disease is confined to the small bowel. Salazopyrin promotes remission in acute attacks of ulcerative colitis and also reduces the recurrence rate.

Azothiaprine

Azothiaprine (Imuran), or its metabolite, mercaptopurine, is used in chronic active Crohn's disease. It is useful in inducing remission and reduces the quantities of steroids needed.

Azothiaprine is less effective in ulcerative colitis.

Metronidazole

This drug is useful in the treatment of Crohn's disease. It is especially useful in resolving anal sepsis.

The rôle of surgery

Crohn's disease of the small intestine

The rôle of surgery must be regarded as palliative, since recurrent lesions in the remaining bowel are to be expected in the natural course of the disease. Thus, at all times, as much bowel as possible must be preserved. The quality of life of patients with Crohn's disease of the small intestine who are treated with optimal surgery when this is indicated, is significantly better than those where only conservative treatment has been applied. Surgery is indicated for fistulae, abscesses, perforation and obstruction. It is also indicated if patients do not respond to conservative measures. This happens especially frequently in disease of the distal ileum.

If surgery is to be performed, only the affected bowel must be resected. Wide excision must be avoided. The incision must be made as close as possible to the affected bowel, but must go through macroscopically normal bowel. There is no longer any justification for bypass operations. Recurrence is less frequent following excision and patients are better of.

If the patient develops obstruction and fibrous stenoses are found, a plastic can be performed on the stenosis, without resection.

Prognosis of Crohn's disease of the small intestine

Eighty per cent of patients with this disease will require surgery during their lives. Forty per cent will require further surgery within ten years, due to recurrent disease. Recurrence usually occurs at the anastomosis, or just proximal to it. The longer it takes for recurrence to develop, the better the eventual prognosis. Patients with Crohn's disease have a mortality rate twice that of the general population. In patients younger than forty, this figure is four times that of the general population of the same age group.

Surgical management of Crohn's disease of the colon and ulcerative colitis

Surgery is more often necessary in Crohn's disease than in ulcerative colitis. Eighty per cent of Crohn's colitis patients will require surgery during their lifetimes, while only 25% of ulcerative colitis patients come to operation. Crohn patients with ileocolitis require surgery more often than those with colitis alone. The most common indications for surgery in right-sided Crohn's are obstruction, abscesses, fistulae and generalized weakness, with loss of weight and diarrhoea, which does not respond to medical treatment.

In left-sided disease, the most common indications are perianal sepsis, fistulae and also weight loss and diarrhoea not responding to medical treatment.

In ulcerative colitis, surgery is either performed as an emergency or electively.

Emergency surgery in ulcerative colitis

Indications include:

- *An acute fulminating attack which does not respond to medical treatment, especially if toxic megacolon develops*
- *Colonic perforation*
- *Massive bleeding*

Elective surgery in ulcerative colitis

Elective surgery must be considered if patients have pancolitis which does not respond well to conservative treatment. Such patients are chronically ill, with loss of weight, continual diarrhoea and nutritional imbalances. If the patient is young and has already had the disease for ten years, there is also the fear that carcinoma may develop. Dysplastic changes on histology are an indication for colectomy.

Stenoses, fistulae and perianal sepsis may also be indications for surgery.

Systemic complications, such as skin lesions and eye lesions that do not improve on conservative treatment, are indications for colectomy.

Colectomy does not help for complications such as sclerosing cholangitis and ankylosing spondylitis.

Surgical procedures which can be performed

Crohn's disease

- *Defunctioning ileostomy. This is recommended in very sick patients.*
- *Segmental colectomy or hemicolectomy. This can be used for localized lesions. Unfortunately, there is an approximately 50% recurrence rate after fifteen years.*
- *Total colectomy with ileorectal anastomosis. This can be considered if the rectum is not narrowed and there are no perianal lesions.*

Recurrence occurs in about 15% within fifteen years if a panproctocolectomy and an ileostomy are performed.

In principle, one can say that ideal Crohn should be operated on as conservatively as possible. Crohn colitis patients do better with more radical surgery.

Ulcerative colitis

It must be remembered that, in contrast to Crohn disease, total panproctocolectomy cures the disease. In the emergency setting, the rectum is preserved because patients are very ill and a smaller operation is indicated. In elective operations, it is advisable to perform a total panproctocolectomy. When the rectum is spared too many failures occur, and the risk of malignancy persists.

Two approaches can be considered. These include:

- *Total panproctocolectomy and the creation of a continence reservoir ileostomy (Kock procedure).*
- *Colectomy with removal of the rectal mucosa, with the creation of an ileal reservoir that is anastomosed to the anal canal. In expert hands, this is the operation of choice these days.*

Management of perianal disease

If the lesions are associated with ulcerative colitis, they are relatively easy to treat. They usually improve when the ulcerative colitis has been controlled by conservative treatment. Abscesses must be treated surgically. They usually clear up in ulcerative colitis, but tend to form fistulae in Crohn's disease.

Metronidazole is useful in the treatment of perianal sepsis. Low fistulae are highly resistant to treatment and wide excision with skin grafts and total panproctocolectomy is usually necessary in Crohn's disease. Fistulae which are asymptomatic can sometimes, be left as they are.

Prognosis of ulcerative colitis

The prognosis is largely determined by the extent of the disease. Proctitis and proctosigmoiditis have a very good prognosis on conservative treatment. In total colon involvement, the risk of death is more than 2% per annum. If a total proctocolectomy is performed, the risk of death is the same as that of the general population. Surgery is performed within five years in about one out of fifty patients with proctitis alone, one out of twenty with left colon involvement and one out of three with total colon involvement.

C. ISCHAEMIC LESIONS OF THE INTESTINAL CANAL

Acute mesenteric vascular insufficiency

- **An embolus**

The heart is usually the source, from a mural thrombus, an infarct, or a clot from the atrium of a fibrillating heart.

- **Arterial thrombosis**

This is usually found in patients with underlying atherosclerosis. Rare causes include a dissecting aortic aneurysm and other rare arterial diseases.

• **Venous thrombosis**

This occurs in patients with portal hypertension, abdominal sepsis, trauma or other causes of hypercoagulability.

Mucosal necrosis already commences within three hours of the onset of ischaemia. Bacterial overgrowth takes place, further contributing towards clotting in small vessels, with increased ischaemia. The necrosis later involves the full thickness of the bowel. Timing depends on factors such as the state of collateral vessels.

Toxic substances are absorbed and the patient develops cardiovascular collapse. The bowel can bleed and perforate, with epritonitis.

Clinical presentation

This condition is found mainly in elderly patients. There is constant, severe, poorly localized abdominal pain. In the early stages, there are few clinical signs. Later, abdominal distention and tenderness develop. Eventually the patient develops peritonitis, rigidity of the abdominal wall and shock.

The most important characteristic of this condition is severe, continual pain with few abdominal signs. If there are signs of peritonitis, there is already dead bowel.

Special investigations

• **Laboratory investigations**

Leucocytosis, raised serum amylase and metabolic acidosis can be found. If the bowel is already dead, serum inorganic phosphate levels will be raised.

• **X-rays**

In the early stages, no abnormalities can be seen. Later, there are adynamic air/fluid levels in the small intestine and thickening of the bowel wall. If necrosis has already commenced, there may be gas in the bowel wall and the portal venous system.

• **Special tests**

Certain experimental tests are being investigated. $Xenon^{133}$ is dissolved in saline and injected intraperitoneally. Deal bowel takes up Xe^{133} and this can be observed by means of a gamma camera.

Parasynthesis of the abdominal fluid may reveal dark, haemorrhagic fluid with high inorganic phosphate levels. If this is positive, the bowel is already dead.

Differential diagnosis

In acute abdomen acute pancreatitis must be differentiated from strangulated bowel. Serum amylase levels which are raised tenfold indicate pancreatitis. A swollen pancreas can be seen on CT.

Strangulated bowel must, in any case, be operated on as an emergency procedure.

Management

It is essential to operate on any patient where severe abdominal pain has featured for longer than eight hours, and a diagnosis cannot be made. Examine the bowel mesentery. If there is no mesenteric pulsation, examine the superior mesenteric artery. Sometimes an embolectomy, a thromboendarterectomy or a bypass can be done.

If the diagnosis is acute venous thrombosis, pulsation can often still be observed. The mesentery is thickened by oedema and clots can be squeezed out of veins.

Gangrenous bowel must be resected, provided a short segment of small bowel can be spared. It is sometimes difficult to decide whether retained bowel is really viable or not. Certain experimental methods have been tried. Intraoperative Doppler measurements seem to hold the most promise for the future. If doubtful bowel is left behind, it is wise to reopen the abdomen twelve hours later to reinspect the bowel.

Patients must be resuscitated aggressively, as they will often have lost a lot of fluid. It is also advisable to heparinize them postoperatively, as reclotting often occurs.

Prognosis

The mortality is about 50%. If more than half of the small bowel is resected, the mortality is 75%.

The mortality in venous thrombosis is 30%. If patients do not receive anticoagulants in the postoperative months, 30% will experience further clotting.

Bowel ischaemia without clotting of mesenteric vessels

In about 20% of patients with bowel ischaemia, there is no clotting in larger vessels. Bowel ischaemia arises due to a low flow state. This is caused by cardiac failure, septic shock and drugs, especially digitalis. This condition must be borne in mind when an elderly patient with cardiac failure, on digitalis and a diuretic, develops abdominal pain.

Management involves improvement of the patient's general condition. Arteriography may be performed to confirm the diagnosis and to simultaneously administer vasodilators like papaverine. Segments of dead bowel must be resected and re-exploration may be useful.

The mortality of this condition is higher than 75%.

Ischaemic colitis

This is a disease of the elderly. It is caused by atherosclerotic obstruction of the colonic blood supply. It can also be caused by surgical damage to the blood supply of the colon during resection of aortic aneurysms, or low flow states, as encountered in cardiac failure or abdominal sepsis.

Two clinical types are found:

- **Adequate collateral flow**

The ischaemia is transient. The mucosa undergoes partial necrosis, but the bowel recovers or heals by fibrotic stenosis.

- **Inadequate collateral flow or a low flow state**

The bowel undergoes total necrosis.

Clinical presentation

The disease has a sudden onset. Patients present with abdominal pain, bloody diarrhoea, tachycardia and fever. This is generalized tenderness, more prominent on the left side. Sigmoidoscopy shows blood coming from higher up in the bowel.

Special investigations

Abdominal X-rays are non-specific. Barium enema shows narrowing of the left colon with "thumbprint" filling defects. These are caused by irregular oedema of the mucosa. Colonoscopy shows a haemorrhagic mucosa with ulceration.

Differential diagnosis

The condition must be differentiated from Crohn disease, ulcerative colitis and amoebic colitis. Its sudden onset in elderly patients who have other signs of atherosclerosis, combined with the barium enema findings, distinguishes this condition from the others.

Management

Fluid and electrolyte losses must be supplemented and antibiotics must be administered. If the disease improves, conservative treatment must be continued. Some patients recover completely and others later develop a stenosis.

If the condition does not improve, a bowel resection must be performed. A colectomy and Hartmann closure are usually possible, with later restoration of bowel continuity by means of an ileorectal anastomosis.

Chronic ischaemia of the intestinal canal

The intestinal canal has a rich blood supply, deriving from the coeliac artery, the superior mesenteric artery, the inferior mesenteric artery and collateral flow from the internal iliac artery. Isolated occlusions in these larger arteries do not usually give rise to symptoms. Multiple occlusions at the origins of the large arteries may lead to inadequate blood supply to the intestinal canal which manifests as pain after meals. This condition is also known as visceral angina.

Clinical presentation

Pain in the abdomen lasting fifteen to thirty minutes after meals is an important symptom. The pain usually lasts for at least an hour. Patients lose weight because they are too scared to eat. Some patients develop diarrhoea.

On auscultation, a bruit can be heard in most cases.

Special investigations

Angiography, especially lateral and oblique views, is necessary to show stenosis and anomalies of the main branches of the aorta.

Management

When the diagnosis has been confirmed arteriographically, revascularization must be undertaken. The obstruction and stenosis are usually situated at the origin of the main arteries. Endarterectomy is sometimes possible, but bypasses from the aorta, using dacron prostheses, are often easier.

Prognosis

If the obstruction is not relieved, the patient will eventually develop bowel infarction. The prognosis is good if revascularization can be achieved.

Compression of the coeliac artery

This syndrome is found in young women, where the medial arcuate ligament partially occludes the coeliac artery and causes abdominal pain after meals. If the ligament is transected, the symptoms sometimes improve. The syndrome must not be diagnosed lightly.

D. RADIATION DAMAGE TO THE INTESTINAL CANAL

Irradiation of malignant tumours of the cervix, uterus, bladder, ovaries and prostate often causes radiation damage to the small intestine and/or rectum. There is usually an early transient reaction, followed in some patients by late complications. The incidence of radiation damage following 6 000 Rads is as high as 30%.

If there have been previous operations with small bowel adhesions, the incidence is even higher. The dividing mucosal cells of the intestinal canal are radiosensitive.

In the early stages, patients develop pain, nausea, vomiting and sometimes bloody diarrhoea. Red, oedematous mucosa, which bleeds easily on contract, can be seen on sigmoidoscopy. In most cases, this picture resolves spontaneously.

In some patients, there is damage to the blood vessels of the bowel wall. Fibrosis in the walls of the blood vessels leads to total occlusion, with ischaemic changes. Ulceration occurs, followed by fibrosis, which can lead to stenosis. The mucosa develops telangiectasia, which can bleed recurrently.

The lesions in the rectum must be differentiated from residual malignancy.

Conservative treatment must be attempted initially. Iron supplements are often necessary for iron deficiency anaemia. Hydrocortisone enemas also afford some relief.

If the patient bleeds a lot or develops stenoses or fistulae, it is advisable to do a proximal defunctioning colostomy. If small bowel stenoses develop, affected bowel must be excised and one must make certain that the re-anastomosis is performed on normal bowel. It is not always possible to resect; a short circuit procedure must then be done.

E. TUMOURS OF THE GASTROINTESTINAL CANAL

The small bowel

Polyps and benign tumors of the small bowel

Hamartomatous polyps are found in the small intestine. A hamartoma is an abnormal arrangement of normal tissue. It is not a neoplasm. The hamartomatous polyp may be single or multiple.

Peutz-Jegher syndrome

This is a familial congenital condition which manifests with multiple hamartomatous polyps, especially in the small bowel, and mucocutaneous pigmentation. Patients present with symptoms and signs of small bowel obstruction and sometimes bleeding.

A few cases of malignant transformation have been described, but the condition must not be regarded as being premalignant.

Surgery is indicated only when complications present.

Benign tumours

Leiomyomas, lipomas, neurofibromas and haemangiomas are all found in the small intestine, but are rare.

Malignant small bowel tumours

Adenocarcinoma

This is a very rare tumour. It is mainly found in the jejunum. These tumours are found in patients over forty. The tumour is probably there for a long time before it causes symptoms, since 80% of patients already have metastases at the time of resection.

Patients present with vague complaints of pain and attacks of obstruction with colic. If a patient presents with small bowel obstruction and there is no question of adhesions or hernias, consider carcinoma of the small bowel.

The tumour must be resected, together with its lymphatic drainage. The five year survival rate is lower than 25%.

Lymphoma of the small intestine has already been discussed.

The carcinoid syndrome

These tumours arise in the chromaffin cells of the intestinal canal. Five per cent of these tumours arise in the foregut, 80% in the midgut, which includes the appendix, and 10% in the hindgut, mostly in the rectum.

Most tumours arise in the appendix. The second most common site is the small intestine, especially the ileum. Multiple tumours are found in 30% of patients. Carcinoids are sometimes associated with medullary carcinoma and phaeochromocytoma in familial syndromes. There is also a higher incidence of other tumours such as lung carcinoma, colonic carcinoma and even cancer of the breast in patients with carcinoid tumours.

Carcinoids are small, yellow, solid tumours, situated in the submucus area of the bowel. Argentaffin and argyrophilic reactions can be demonstrated by means of special staining techniques. The size of the tumour is of clinical importance. If the tumour is smaller than 1 cm in diameter, the chance of metastasis is less than 5%. If the tumour is larger than 2 cm in diameter, the chance of metastasis is greater than 75%. In small bowel tumours, 40% of patients already have metastases to lymph nodes by the time the disease is discovered. In tumours of the appendix, metastasis to lymph nodes is very rare, less than 3%. Carcinoid of the colon has often already spread to lymph nodes, as the diagnosis is not usually made while the lesion is smaller than 2 cm in diameter.

Midgut carcinoids secrete serotonin and a variety of other substances such as neurotensin, gastrin, somatostatin, secretin, pancreatic polypeptide and probably other unknown enzymes. Fore- and hindgut carcinoids do not secrete serotonin, but do secrete gastrin, somatostatin and glucagon.

Clinical presentation

Small tumours are usually asymptomatic. Only 30% of patients with this disease will develop symptoms such as pain, obstruction or bleeding. Ten per cent of patients with small bowel carcinoids will develop the carcinoid syndrome.

The carcinoid syndrome

Biologically active substances secreted by the tumours are catabolised to inactive substances in the liver. If there are metastases in the liver, or if the primary tumour is in the bronchus or ovary, these substances go straight into the bloodstream, causing the syndrome. Most cases with the syndrome synthesize large amounts of serotonin. Other peptides also play a rôle. The tumour secretes neuropeptide, histamine, catecholamines, prostaglandins and even calcitonin. Various substances are responsible for various elements of the syndrome. Serotonin is chiefly responsible for diarrhoea. Neuropeptide and histamine are the main cause of facial flushing.

Special investigations

Raised 5-hydroxy-indole-acetic acid levels are usually found in the urine. If there is any doubt, pentagastrin can be given. This elicits the syndrome and serum serotonin levels rise.

Management

The management of the most common tumour found in the ***appendix*** *has already been discussed. It will not normally have spread and the carcinoid syndrome is not usually found.*

If the tumour arises in the ***small bowel****, it must be regarded as a malignant tumour and* *treated as such. A wide resection of the bowel, together with the lymphatic drainage of the region, must be performed, but metastases in the mesentery or liver must be diligently sought. If resectible metastases are found in the liver, they must be removed. Multiple metastases must also be shelled out and removed, even if all tumour tissue cannot be resected. The less tumour tissue there is, the more easily the syndrome can be treated pharmacologically.*

Drugs which may prove helpful include corticosteroids and H1 and H2 histamine receptor antagonists. Somatostatin blocks secretion of some peptides and, if administered intravenously, relieves the symptoms of vasodilatation and vasoconstriction. It also limits diarrhoea, to an extent.

Chemotherapy plays a rôle. Doxorubicine helps somewhat. Interferon reduces symptoms but has no real effect on the tumour.

Carcinoid of the **colon** *is relatively rare and is found mainly in the rectum. If the tumours are smaller than 2 cm in diameter, they have not usually spread and can be excised locally. Larger tumours, or those with visibly enlarged lymph nodes, must be removed by means of standard cancer resections.*

Prognosis

Carcinoid is a slow-growing malignant tumour. The five year survival rate following resection in small bowel carcinoid is higher than 70%. More than 40% of patients with metastases survive five years. It is always advisable to resect carcinoid, even if only partially.

The colon

Colonic polyps

The term polyp is used for a wide variety of masses which bulge into the lumen of the intestinal canal. Polyps can be sessile or pedunculated, benign or malignant, they can arise in the mucosa or in the submucosa, and can be inflammatory, hyperplastic, hamartomatous or neoplastic.

The term polyposis is used to indicate the presence of multiple polyps.

Pathology

Inflammatory polyps

- **Benign lymphoid polyp:** Small polyps are found in the rectosigmoid colon. These polyps consist of normal lymphatic tissue, without sinuses.
- **Inflammatory pseudopolyps:** These usually consist of oedematous shreds of mucosa situated between ulcers and are most commonly found in ulcerative colitis.

Hyperplastic polyps

These are mainly found in the rectosigmoid colon and are smooth, discrete sessile polyps. Microscopically, they have a central fibrous nucleus, surrounded by hyperplastic glandular tissue with cystic dilatation. There is an abnormal increase in goblet cells and round cell infiltration of the *lamina propria.*

Hyperplastic polyps form the majority of polyps found in the rectum and sigmoid colon and have no malignant potential.

Hamartomas

- **Juvenile polyps**

These are found mainly in children. They are round, smooth, pedunculated polyps. On section, small cysts filled with mucus can be seen, and they are therefore also called retention cysts. Epithelial tubules, lined with mucus-secreting cells are found in a fibrous stroma. The *muscularis mucosae* does not form part of the polyp. This is probably why juvenile polyps amputate and bleed spontaneously. This type of polyp is not premalignant.

- **Juvenile polyposis**

Two familial juvenile polyposis syndromes have been described, namely juvenile *polyposis coli* and generalized juvenile gastrointestinal polyposis.

The Cronkhite-Canada syndrome is probably not familial. Although the polyps are also hamartomas, malignancy is more common in patients with the familial juvenile polyposis syndrome.

The Cronkhite-Canada syndrome consists of polyps distributed throughout the gastrointestinal tract, alopecia, atrophy of the nails and hyperpigmentation.

Patients have a severe, watery diarrhoea, streatorrhoea and they lose protein in the stools.

Neoplastic polyps

These are adenomas. Three histological types have been described, namely tubular adenoma, tubulovillous adenoma and villous adenoma.

Tubular adenoma

These are most commonly found in the sigmoid colon, but can occur anywhere in the colon. They vary in size from smaller than 1 cm to more than 4 cm in diameter. They are usually pedunculated, round polyps, with irregular surfaces. In exceptional cases they are sessile.

A fibrous central area, which runs continuously from the submucosa through the stalk to the head of the polyp, can be seen on section. Histologically, the stalk can be seen to be covered by normal colonic mucosa. The polyp itself is covered by adenomatous epithelium, consisting of an accumulation of glands or tubules, with a scanty fibrovascular stroma. There may be areas with a villous growth pattern, but if this comprises less than 20% of the polyp, it remains a tubular adenoma.

These adenomas have a spectrum of differentiation ranging from well-differentiated, orderly epithelium, with relatively uniform hyperchromatic nuclei, to increasing degrees of dysplasia and even anaplasia and increasing numbers of mitotic figures. The atypical epithelium may infiltrate the fibrovascular central part and even the stalk. It then becomes a **tubular adenoma with malignant change**.

Tubulovillous adenoma

If more than 50% of the adenoma has a villous growth pattern, it is called a tubulovillous adenoma. The villous parts are more inclined to have areas of malignant transformation.

Villous adenoma

Villous adenomas are usually larger than tubular adenomas. If the villous adenoma exceeds 2 cm in diameter, there is a 50% chance that there are areas of malignant transformation. These polyps are usually single lesions in the rectum. They can be multiple and arise anywhere in the colon. They are usually sessile and velvety, with a cauliflowerlike appearance. They vary in size from 1 to 10 cm.

On histological examination, fingerlike, branching papilli, with a thin fibrovascular central part covered by epithelium, can be seen. The epithelium varies from well differentiated to a chaotic growth pattern with hyperchromatic anaplastic cells. Carcinoma in situ is found in 50%, and infiltrating carcinoma in 30% of villous adenomas.

Clinical presentation

The clinical presentation of these important neoplastic polyps, with their malignant potential, will be discussed here. The clinical presentation depends on the size, nature and site of origin of the polyps. Small polyps are often asymptomatic. The most important clinical sign is rectal bleeding. The blood can be bright red if the polyp is in the rectum, or dark red and mixed with stools if it is situated higher up in the colon. The bleeding is usually intermittent and not massive.

Changes in bowel habit are uncommon. If they do present, consider carcinoma elsewhere in the colon.

A very large villous adenoma in the rectum can secrete a great deal of mucus, with loss of fluid and electrolytes, especially potassium. Patients can then present with hypokalaemic alkalosis and hypoalbuminaemia. It has been said that **a tubular adenoma bleeds** and **a villous adenoma weeps**.

Usually, there are no signs to be found on examination. A rectal examination must be performed. One must remember that a large villous adenoma in the rectum may be missed because the fingerlike protrusions may be soft and therefore impalpable. If there is a hard area in such a polyp, consider carcinoma.

Polyps are usually discovered on sigmoidoscopy.

Special investigations

- **Barium enema**

Polyps appear as round filling defects on barium enema. A round mass on a stalk is sometimes visible. It is particularly important to study the postevacuation films. A thin layer of barium usually remains on the polyp and can be seen as a positive barium shadow.

Double contrast studies must be done so that the positive shadow of the polyp, which is covered in barium, can be accentuated by the surrounding air.

- **Colonoscopy**

This is a very reliable way of diagnosing polyps. The whole colon is inspected, as polyps tend to be multiple. The rôle of colonoscopy will be more fully discussed in the section on management.

Differential diagnosis

On barium enema, polyps must be distinguished from air bubbles, pieces of faecal matter, diverticula and calcified lymph nodes in the drainage area of the colon. Colonoscopy is important in confirming the diagnosis, to obtain histological material for microscopic diagnosis and to differentiate neoplastic polyps from non-neoplastic polyps.

Management

Polyps must be removed when they cause symptoms, they are premalignant or have already undergone malignant transformation at the time of diagnosis. The majority of polyps are pedunculated and thus lend themselves to simple removal by means of snare coagulation. In the past, rectal polyps were removed using a rigid sigmoidoscope. Since colonoscopy has become available, it has become generally accepted that all patients with polyps, wherever they may be situated, require a complete colonoscopy with snare coagulation and removal of all visible polyps. The polyp must be extracted with the colonoscope and sent for histological examination. If the polyp is simply a tubular adenoma, no further treatment is necessary.

About 3% of polyps removed colonoscopically will show signs of malignant transformation. In such cases, a decision must be made whether to stop at polypectomy or to go on to colon resection. If the carcinoma is confined to the polyp, has not infiltrated through the muscularis mucosae *and has not penetrated into the stalk, then polypectomy is adequate. If these conditions are not met, the lesion must be regarded as an early carcinoma and the appropriate piece of colon must be resected.*

It is far more difficult and dangerous to remove sessile polyps colonoscopically, and this should be left to the experts. Bleeding and perforation occur in 2% of cases.

If malignant transformation is found in a sessile polyp, a partial colectomy must be performed. If the polyps cannot be removed colonoscopically for technical reasons, a limited colon resection must be performed. Large rectal villous adenomas can cause problems. In skilled hands, they can be removed using the colonoscope and coagulation snare. If they are malignant, an anterior resection or an abdominoperitoneal resection must be performed, depending on the situation of the polyp. It is sometimes necessary to approach a large sessile polyp via a posterior approach (York-Mason) through the coccyx and to excise it under direct sight.

Prognosis

Villous adenomas tend to recur after removal with coagulation snare, probably because it is difficult to remove a large sessile polyp completely. Patients are also inclined to develop new polyps. Patients with adenomas have a higher incidence of carcinoma of the colon, even if the adenomas are removed. It is therefore important to follow these patients up colonoscopically in the long term. After removal of all the polyps, colonoscopy must be repeated after a year and then every three years.

Familial polyposis

This is an autosomal dominant congenital condition. Both sexes are affected. Hundreds or even thousands of tubular adenomas in the rectum and colon are characteristic of this disease. The rectum is always affected.

Patients usually present with rectal bleeding. Although the tendency to develop polyps is present at birth, they usually develop after puberty.

All of these patients will develop cancer of the colon before the age of forty unless they are treated. They have so many adenomas that the relatively slight malignant potential of a single adenoma is so much multiplied in a single patient, that they all develop carcinoma.

The disease can be cured by prophylactic panproctocolectomy and ileostomy, but continence is then lost. In the past, some surgeons spared the rectum, did an ileorectal anastomosis and then destroyed the rectal polyps with a coagulation snare. In most series, carcinoma of the rectum still arose in some patients.

Currently, the rectal mucosa is removed and a pouch of small bowel is anastomosed to the anus (Parks procedure or modifications). This operation is difficult and requires special skills, but obviates incontinence and simultaneously removes the danger of potential carcinoma development.

Gardner syndrome

This is also a congenital disease. The syndrome includes polyposis of the colon and, to a lesser extent, of the small bowel, desmoid tumours, osteomas of the skull and jaw and sebaceous cysts.

These patients are equally at risk for colonic carcinoma and also have an increased incidence of gastric carcinoma and periampullary carcinoma.

The treatment is the same as that for familial polyposis.

Turcot syndrome

This is a rare familial polyposis associated with medulloblastoma or glioblastoma of the brain or spinal cord. It differs from the previous two diseases in that there are usually fewer than 100 polyps in the colon. The malignant potential, although strongly present, is less prominent in this syndrome, because the presence of other malignant tumours in the central nervous system dominates the outcome.

Malignant tumours

Carcinoma of the colon

Carcinoma of the colon and rectum will be discussed together. After cancer of the lung, carcinoma of the colon and rectum is the second most common malignant tumour and the second most common cause of carcinoma death. Carcinoma of the rectum is twice as common in men as in women. Carcinoma of the right colon is slightly more common in women than in men.

Aetiology

Because carcinoma of the colon and rectum are common in affluent communities, environmental factors, especially diet, are regarded as important aetiological components. High meat and fat intake and a lack of fibre have been implicated. It has been suggested that animal fats increase the amount of neutral sterols and bile salts in the intestinal canal and this changes the flora, by encouraging the growth of bacteria such as *clostridia* and *bacteroides* species. These bacteria transform the fats and bile salts and convert them to carcinogens and cocarcinogens.

The important rôle of fibre is explained as follows: Fibre speeds up transit of the bowel contents and thus reduces the time of exposure of the fats to the bacteria. It has also been suggested that the large fibre mass dilutes the carcinogens and prevents contact with the mucosa. Genetic predisposition may be another important underlying factor. It has been widely accepted that there are cancerprone families. In such families, colonic carcinoma and other extracolonic adenocarcinomas are found, e g endometrial carcinoma, breast carcinoma and ovarian carcinoma. These patients have been classified according to Lynch type I and Lynch type II syndromes.

Recognized premalignant conditions which are also of a genetic nature, such as familial polyposis and Gardner syndrome, are well known. Granulomatous inflammatory disease such as ulcerative colitis and Crohn disease have already been discussed.

Pathology

Ninety-five per cent of malignant tumours of the colon and rectum are adenocarcinomas. Forty per cent are found in the rectum, 20% in the sigmoid colon, 20% in the caecum and ascending colon and the other 20% scattered throughout the rest of the colon. Multiple carcinomas are found in 5% of patients.

The macroscopic growth pattern of carcinoma of the right colon usually shows polypoid, cauliflowerlike fungating masses. These tumours tend to secrete mucus into the lumen of the glands or even into the interstitium of the bowel wall. These tumours have various degrees of differentiation from relatively well differentiated to anaplastic.

Spread of colonic carcinoma

Colonic carcinoma spreads by means of direct infiltration, lymphatic, haematogenous, intraluminal and transperitoneal spread.

- **Direct infiltration**

Carcinoma, especially of the left colon, tends to infiltrate circumferentially. It takes about two years for the lesion to engulf the bowel and narrow it. It also spreads longitudinally through the intramural lymphatics in the submucosa. It seldom spreads further than 3 cm from the macroscopically visible tumour, but to be absolutely safe, 5 cm is regarded as the maximal possible spread. It spreads through the wall into the serosa and infiltrates the surrounding tissue. It can also infiltrate adjacent organs and the abdominal wall.

- **Lymphatic spread**

About 50% of colonic and rectal carcinomas have already spread to lymph nodes by the time they are diagnosed. Although the adjacent modes are usually the first to be affected, followed by the more distal nodes, there is sometimes spread to the distal nodes without the adjacent nodes being affected. Carcinoma of the rectum spreads, not only to lymph nodes related to blood vessels, but also to the obturator nodes on the pelvic wall.

If the carcinoma is poorly differentiated, lymphatic spread occurs early.

- **Blood spread**

This takes place via the portal system to the liver. Tumour cells also reach the lungs and other organs via the lumbar and vertebral venous drainage and the systemic circulation.

Excessive intraoperative handling of the tumour must be avoided to reduce the risk of tumour embolization.

- **Intraluminal spread**

Residual carcinoma sometimes arises in the suture line after resection of a carcinoma. Some researchers believer that this occurs because of implantation of cells becoming detached in the bowel lumen. They recommend that the bowel should be ligated immediately on either side of the tumour before manipulation is commenced. It has now become more generally accepted that recurrence of tumour at the suture line is more likely to be caused by submucosal spread of carcinomatous cells in the lymphatics.

- **Transperitoneal spread**

If the carcinoma has spread through the wall, cells can disseminate in the peritoneal cavity, giving rise to multiple superficial peritoneal metastases. They can also grow in the Douglas pouch and can be palpated as a hard ridge (Blumer ridge) per rectum.

Clinical presentation

This disease is found in people over forty-five. Symptoms and signs depend on the site of the lesion in the colon.

The right colon has a wide lumen, a thin, elastic wall and liquid contents. Tumours of the right colon have a fungating growth pattern. In the wide caecum, the tumour can become large before symptoms arise.

Patients complain of fatigue and weakness, due to underlying anaemia. They do not often complain of blood in the stools, but occult blood tests are positive and patients develop a hypochromic anaemia. They complain of RIF pain. The symptoms are sometimes ascribed to "chronic appendicitis" or peptic ulceration, because the pain is aggravated after meals. In a small group, the patient himself discovers a RIF mass.

Change in bowel habit is not usually part of the symptom complex.

The left colon has a smaller lumen and semisolid faeces. Tumours in this area tend to infiltrate circumferentially and cause stenosis of the bowel. A change in bowel habit, usually constipation, or sometimes alternating constipation and diarrhoea, is an important symptom. Patients complain of vague pain but somtimes develop partial obstruction with colicky pain. They can also develop total colonic obstruction.

Blood in the stools is common. The blood is usually mixed with the stools, but blood and mucus may also be present simultaneously.

An LIF mass is sometimes palpable.

The rectum has a wide lumen. The carcinoma is usually an ulcer with rolled edges. The most common symptom is blood in the stools. The blood can be either on the outside or mixed with the stools. Patients can also pass blood and mucus. They complain of tenesmus and a feeling that the rectum is not empty after defaecation.

Patients must be thoroughly examined for signs of metastasis, such as enlarged inguinal or supraclavicular nodes. Masses, or an enlarged liver, are sometimes palpable in the abdomen.

A rectal examination must always be done. At least 30% of colorectal tumours are palpable per rectum. More than 50% of colorectal tumours will be found on sigmoidoscopy.

Special investigations

A full blood count must be done to diagnose and treat anaemia. Serum proteins and liver enzymes must be measured. A raised alkaline phosphatase is suggestive of liver metastases. Measurement of carcino-embryonic antigen (CEA) is useful for the following reasons: preoperative CEA levels can be correlated with postoperative levels. If the high preoperative levels have not dropped postoperatively, there are probably metastases. If the level drops and later rises, there is probably residual disease. Remember that CEA is not specific for carcinoma of the colon, but can be found in other carcinomas and a variety of benign conditions.

- **Barium enema**

This was always the investigation of choice. To a large extent, it has now been replaced by colonoscopy. Carcinoma in the left colon shows as a constant stenosis with shoulder formation, a circumferential filling defect and destruction of the normal mucosal pattern (apple core appearance). If there is doubt about a stenosis, glucagon must be given. This will relax a spastic stenosis. If there is still doubt, colonoscopy must be performed.

Carcinoma of the right colon appears as a large polypoid filling defect or a rigid stricture of the bowel, with destruction of the normal mucosal pattern.

Carcinoma of the rectum is not diagnosed on barium enema, but by means of sigmoidoscopy.

- **Endoscopy**

The fibre-optic endoscope, which is 60 cm long, is easy to use and will reach 70% of colorectal carcinomas. Colonoscopy requires special skills, but has become an essential diagnostic tool. If a carcinoma is found, a biopsy must be taken and the rest of the bowel must be examined for a second carcinoma or other adenomas elsewhere in the bowel.

- **Computer tomography**

This is useful to show whether a rectal carcinoma is confined to the abdominal wall and to look for liver metastases.

Differential diagnosis

It is very important to consider carcinoma of the colon and rectum in patients who present with hypochromic anaemia. All cases of rectal bleeding must be investigated for carcinoma, regardless of whether there is a possible benign cause for bleeding, such as haemorrhoids. All filling defects or constant stenoses in the colon must be examined colonoscopically to differentiate conditions such as amoeboma, Crohn disease and ulcerative colitis from carcinoma.

Although spastic colon is the most common cause of abdominal pain and change in bowel habit, carcinoma must always be borne in mind.

Management

- **Colonic carcinoma**

The tumour must be widely excised, including the lymphatic drainage. The lymphatic drainage, lymphatics and lymph nodes are closely related to the arterial blood supply of the bowel. In order to remove the regional lymph drainage together with the primary lesion, bowel resection must be based on the fact that removing the relevant lymph nodes will mean that the blood supply to a relatively well defined area of the colon will have to be sacrificed.

Because the colon is filled with faeces, there is more danger of breakdown of the suture line, with leakage, peritonitis and wound sepsis. The colon must therefore be prepared for elective surgery. Prophylactic antibiotics are also required.

It is sometimes even necessary to create a temporary proximal stoma to protect the suture line until it has healed.

- **Preoperative preparation**

It is very important to explain the nature of the operation carefully to the patient, especially if a temporary or permanent stoma is planned. It may be necessary to allow a patient who already has a stoma to talk to the patient. A stoma sister must see the patient preoperatively and, in con-

sultation with the surgeon, she must mark the most suitable site for the stoma on the skin.

- **Nutritional status**

If the patient is anaemic, a preoperative blood transfusion may be necessary. Protein deficiencies must be supplemented and a short period of hyperalimentation may be necessary.

Bowel preparation

- **Mechanical bowel lavage**

It is extremely important to clean out the bowel. Various methods are available. Patients can be placed on a low-residue diet or even an elemental diet such as Vivonex for three days.

The bowel is emptied mechanically by means of a combination of purgatives and enemas the day before the operation.

A method often used currently is bowel lavage with Golightly, a mixture of sodium sulphate and polyethylene glycol. Patients tolerate it well and it empties the bowel very well. This also obviates the problem of overhydration, which is encountered when 2 to 4 litres of balanced electrolyte solution is used for lavage.

The use of nonabsorbable antibiotics per mouth to reduce the bowel flora has now been replaced by prophylactic systemic antibiotics. Ampicillin, gentamycin and metronidazole form a good combination. Alternatively, a third generation cephalosporin can be used. The first dose is given preoperatively, the second dose intraoperatively and the last does postoperatively.

- **The urinary tract**

A bladder catheter is inserted under sterile circumstances in theatre. It is sometimes necessary to insert ureteric catheters for difficult abdominoperineal resections, so that they can be easily palpated and avoided during the operation.

The operation

The anastomosis is constructed by using an inner layer of absorbable sutures and an outer interrupted layer of nonabsorbable sutures. A corrugated drain must be left at the site of the anastomosis. Leakage, if it takes place, usually occurs five to seven days postoperatively. The drain can be shortened on day seven and removed on day nine.

- **Tumour of the right colon**

Do a right hemicolectomy, including the lymphatic drainage adjacent to the ileocolic and right colic blood vessels. An ileotransverse colonic anastomosis is then made.

- **Tumour of the transverse colon**

Resect the transverse colon, including the hepatic and splenic flexures, because the right colic vessels, the middle colic vessels and the marginal artery must be removed. The ascending colon is then anastomosed to the descending colon.

- **Tumour of the descending colon**

A left hemicolectomy is performed and includes the splenic flexure. The transverse colon is anastomosed to the sigmoid colon.

- **Tumour of the sigmoid colon**

The sigmoid colon and part of the descending colon are resected, because the inferior mesenteric artery and its branches must be removed to eliminate the lymphatic drainage. Mobilize the splenic flexure and suture the descending colon to the rectum.

Management of rectal carcinoma

Two factors play a rôle in the management of rectal carcinoma. The carcinoma must be cured and where possible, the sphincters must be preserved. However, continence must not be maintained at the cost of a curative procedure.

- **Abdominoperineal resection**

This comprises removal of the rectum and anus, with a permanent sigmoid colostomy. The patient's legs are placed in lithotomy and two teams operate simultaneously. The abdominal team begins the operation and determines operability. The perineal team dissects out the anus and its sphincters and the specimen is eventually removed from below.

- **Anterior resection of the rectum**

An abdominal approach is used. The sigmoid colon and the part of the rectum containing the tumour and a free border of 5 cm are excised. The descending colon is sutured to the rectum, either by hand or with the EEA stapler. Continence is thus preserved.

Prerequisites for performance of an anterior resection

The following factors must be taken into account:

1. The height of the lesion above the anal canal

   The principle of transecting the rectum 5 cm distal to the carcinoma to ensure a curative procedure holds. Five cm of rectum must be left behind so that suturing can be done comfortably and rectal continence can be preserved. Bearing these facts in mind, the lesion must be situated at least 10 cm from the anal canal to qualify for an anterior resection. In practice, this means that if the rectal carcinoma can be felt per rectum with a finger, it is situated too low and an abdominoperineal resection will have to be done.

2. The type of carcinoma. *If the tumour is advanced and forms an infiltrating ulcer, especially if it is poorly differentiated, an abdominoperineal resection is preferable.*

3. In men with a small pelvis or very obese patients, *it is more difficult to construct an anastomosis and the surgeon is sometimes forced to do an abdominoperineal resection. The EEA stapler is sometimes helpful when a difficult, low anastomosis must be constructed.*

Other sphincter-preserving procedures

- **Fulguration**

In elderly, unfit patients, electrocoagulation of the tumour can be considered, on condition that it is situated below the peritoneal reflection of the rectum. The tumour is diatherized in sessions and the charred tissue is scraped away with a Volkman spoon.

- **Irradiation**

Certain French researchers use irradiation rather than abdominoperineal resection in operable rectal carcinoma. They claim good results.

Adjuvant irradiation

A common problem in advanced rectal carcinomas that are situated low down is the relatively high incidence of local recurrence. Irradiation is used pre- and postoperatively to try and reduce this incidence. In prospective series, less local recurrence was found after irradiation, but it does not, unfortunately, improve the five year survival rate.

The Hartmann procedure

This is a very useful operation in older, weaker patients with relatively low-lying rectal carcinoma. The carcinoma is excised, but instead of removing the anus, the distal rectum is closed and an end sigmoid colostomy is created.

The rôle of chemotherapy

A combination of 5FU and levamisole has been shown to improve survival in patients with positive lymph nodes.

Complications in colorectal surgery

- **Wound infection**

Wound sepsis is found in more than 5% of cases, despite bowel preparation and antibiotic prophylaxis. It may cause wound dehiscence.

- **Anastomosis leakage**

This is very common in a low anterior resection. There is sometimes only a slight leakage at the corrugated drain. Such patients can be treated conservatively with hyperalimentation and antibiotics. If there are signs of infection, it is advisable to initiate free drainage and to create a temporary proximal colostomy.

- **Urinary complications**

This is a common problem after abdominoperineal resections. The catheter must be left in the bladder for at least five days. If it is removed and the patient develops retention, it can be replaced and left in for longer. Patients can be taught to urinate normally with the help of parasympathomimetic agents.

About a third of men become impotent after excision of the rectum, due to damage to the nervi erigentes.

Prognosis

The results of surgical excision are better in colonic carcinoma than in rectal carcinoma. The prognosis is determined by means of Dukes' staging.

Dukes' A

The lesion is confined to the mucosa – five year survival 90%.

Dukes' B

The lesion infiltrates through the bowel wall – five year survival 70%.

Dukes' C

The lymph nodes are involved – five year survival 30%.

Dukes' D

Distal metastases – five year survival 5%.

The Dukes' staging has recently been altered as follows:

Dukes' A

Confined to the mucosa – five year survival 90%.

Dukes' B1

Infiltration through the muscularis mucosae, but confined to the bowel wall – five year survival 80%.

Dukes' B2

Infiltration through the serosa – five year survival 60%.

Dukes' C1

Fewer than four lymph nodes involved – five year survival 40%.

Dukes' C2

More than four lymph nodes involved – five year survival 20%.

Dukes' D

Distal metastases – five year survival 5%.

The Jass staging

In this staging, the appearance of the tumour edge – whether it is pushing or infiltrating – and the degree of lymphocyte infiltration of the lesion, are factors taken into account. A patient with a pushing, rather than an infiltrating edge and lymphocyte infiltration, has a more favourable prognosis.

At the time of diagnosis, about 10% of patients are completely inoperable. A further 20% have distal metastases. The five year survival of all patients who are operated, is about 40%.

Poorly differentiated tumours have a poorer prognosis than well-differentiated tumours, regardless of the Dukes' staging.

Young patients fare less favourably.

It has been shown that patients who receive blood transfusions intraoperatively fare less favourably than others. The immunosuppressant effect of blood transfusion is a possible explanation. This phenomenon has been observed in renal transplant patients.

Certain researchers suggest that if CEA levels rise in the follow-up period, the patient must be investigated for residual disease. In 30% of such patients, further excision might be possible.

The rôle of screening tests

It has been recommended that the following programme be implemented in all patients older than forty:

- Annual rectal examination.
- Annual occult blood tests on faeces.
- Sigmoidoscopy at fifty and then every three years.
- Colonoscopy must be done if the occult blood is positive.

Although it is not yet proven, such a programme should facilitate early discovery of malignant polyps and early colonic carcinoma.

F. FUNCTIONAL CONDITIONS OF THE COLON

Spastic colon syndrome

This is of great interest to surgeons, as it is the most common cause of abdominal pain and because it mimics so many surgical conditions. It is a disturbance in the normal motility of the intestinal canal, especially the colon. Motility studies have shown differences in the bowel contractions of patients with spastic colon syndrome and those of normal people. The colon patients have increased response to parasympathomimetic agents and cholecystokinin. There is also increased motility in response to emotional stimuli.

Clinical presentation

The syndrome is more common in women and presents between the ages of twenty and sixty. There are two clinical types. In the spastic colon type, abdominal pain and constipation are found. The second type comprises painless diarrhoea and mucus. Both types can be found in the same patient.

The pain is experienced midabdominally or in one or both of the iliac fossae. The pain usually improves on defaecation.

On examination, tenderness can be found over the course of the colon, especially the sigmoid colon. Pain and a gurgling noise can sometimes be elicited over the caecum.

Some patients complain of flatulence and bloating. They pass small, hard, round stools.

Many patients will already have had several operations, such as appendicectomy, cholecystectomy, wedge resections of the ovary and release of adhesions, without relief of symptoms.

Management

It is essential that the condition be borne in mind and that, firstly, unnecessary operations be avoided, and secondly, the condition should not be labelled as psychosomatic. Patients have pain, even if it is of a functional nature. A complete history must be taken and a thorough clinical examination performed. A sigmoidoscopy with biopsy must be done, as well as a barium enema. Only after this a positive diagnosis of spastic colon can be made with confidence and the patient can then be fully informed about her condition. She must be told that there is no question of cancer, as this is often an underlying fear.

Good stooling habits must be encouraged. Patients must be placed on a high fibre diet and must receive antispasmodics during attacks. They must be seen regularly and given support. They must be told that the condition cannot be cured, as it is functional. At the same time, they must be reassured that there is no underlying disease, especially not one requiring surgery.

G. RARE CONDITIONS OF THE INTESTINAL CANAL

Pneumatosis cystoides intestinalis

This is a condition in which gaseous cysts develop in the bowel wall. It is of importance to surgeons, because patients can present with bowel obstruction, blood per rectum and free air under the diaphragm.

The cysts are situated beneath the serosa of the mucosa and contain a mixture of oxygen and nitrogen under pressure. They are lined with endothelial cells and have giant cells and inflammatory cells in their walls.

The cause of this condition is unknown. Some have suggested that the gas is formed by gas-forming bacteria. Pneumatosis of the large bowel is associated with chronic pulmonary disease. it is possible that coughing fits cause alveoli to rupture and that this gas from the mediastinum reaches the retroperitoneal tissues and forms gaseous cysts in the bowel wall. The disease sometimes develops after colon endoscopy and mucosal biopsy.

Patients present with constipation and diarrhoea and pass foamy mucus. The cysts resemble polyps on sigmoidoscopy and rupture on biopsy.

An X-ray abdomen will show small air sacs in the bowel wall. A pneumoperitoneum may be present. The barium enema appearance can be confused with multiple polyps.

The condition must be treated conservatively. Underlying disease, e g peptic ulcer, must be treated. Oxygen administration for a week often resolves the condition. Metronidazole must also be administered.

Rarely, a segment of bowel must be excised if obstruction develops that will not resolve on conservative treatment.

Idiopathic ulcer of the small bowel

The patient presents with an acute abdomen; and a small bowel perforation is found on laparotomy. Usually a local stricture is present, with distended proximal bowel. If the stricture is resected, a solitary ulcer is found.

Histologically, a nonspecific ulcer with underlying fibrosis can be seen.

The aetiology of this condition in unknown. Sometimes there is underlying vascular disease. Ulcers can also be caused by potassium tablets with slow-release coatings. Typhoid and tuberculosis must be excluded. Usually no aetiological factor can be found.

Duplication cysts of the intestinal canal

This is a rare condition that can occur anywhere from the oesophagus down to the rectum. Patients present with bowel obstruction. At laparotomy, inspissation of a segment of bowel is found. This comprises a cyst of the bowel wall, lined by bowel mucosa, which fills with secretions and thus obstructs the bowel.

These cysts probably arise as a result of an embryological developmental fault of defective recanalization.

The affected part of the bowel must be excised, with reanastomosis.

Endometriosis

Endometrial tissue grows in the wall of the sigmoid colon, rectum and other parts of the intestinal canal. The precise pathogenesis of the disease is unknown, but the cells probably reach the peritoneal cavity via the Fallopian tubes.

The tissue responds to the monthly hormonal cycle in the same way as the normal endometrial tissue of the uterus. The patient may bleed rectally during menstruation. Pain and constipation may also occur.

On rectal examination, painful nodules are palpable, but the mucosa is intact on sigmoidoscopy.

The lesions usually respond well to progesterone treatment. If obstruction occurs bowel resection can become necessary.

H. CONDITIONS OF THE RECTUM

Rectal prolapse

There are two types of prolapse: incomplete mucosal prolapse and complete full-thickness bowel prolapse. This condition is particularly common in two age groups. In young children, incomplete mucosal prolapse is especially common, although complete prolapse is found. Complete full-thickness prolapse usually occurs in elderly women. Partial mucosal prolapse, forming part of a grade three haemorrhoid, is also found in this age group in both sexes. Rectal prolapse usually begins at the anterior wall of the rectum as a sliding hernia through the pouch of Douglas, then the whole bowel inverts and forms an intussusception.

Rectouterine

Clinical presentation

Incomplete prolapse

- **Incomplete prolapse in children:**
  In children, the sacral cavity is not fully developed and the rectum and anus thus form a straight line. It usually occurs in malnourished children who have diminished perirectal fat. These children are constipated and sit and strain for a long time and the mucosa comes out as an incomplete prolapse. Later, the condition can become aggravated and form a complete prolapse.
- **Prolapse in the elderly:**
  Ninety per cent of patients who develop prolapse are women over sixty and have often had a number of children. Patients usually begin with a small prolapse which reduces spontaneously, but which, with time, enlarges and must be reduced manually. The anal sphincter stretches and this leads to permanent prolapse with ulceration and discharge of blood and mucus onto the clothing.

On examination, the patient can produce the prolapse easily on straining. Differentiation must be made between complete and incomplete prolapse. A complete prolapse usually has concentric mucosal folds which resemble rings. If the prolapse is palpated between the fingers, a double layer of bowel can be felt.

Incomplete prolapse is distinguished by the fact that the mucosa has radial folds and a sulcus between the various quadrants. It therefore actually consists of advanced prolapsing mucosal folds.

A rectal examination must be performed after the prolapse has been reduced, to test the status of the sphincter tone. The sphincter is often so badly stretched that the patient will remain incontinent even after repair of the prolapse. Sigmoidoscopy and barium enema must be performed to exclude other conditions higher up in the bowel.

Differential diagnosis

Firstly, it is important to distinguish between prolapsing haemorrhoids and complete rectal prolapse, as has already been described. Large polyps and malignant tumours can sometimes be confused with prolapse. Reduction and sigmoidoscopy with biopsy confirms the diagnosis.

Management

Incomplete mucosal prolapse of childhood is treated conservatively. Nutritional status must be corrected. Stool softeners must be given and the perineum anterior to the rectum must be supported by the mother during defaecation. Usually, the condition resolves spontaneously by the age of four.

Incomplete mucosal prolapse in adults is treated with a haemorrhoidectomy.

Complete prolapse is often found in aged, unfit patients. If the patient is not fit for surgery, a circumanal stainless steel wire can be inserted subcutaneously around the anus (Thiersch wire). The anus is closed so that it only admits one finger. The wire tends to erode through the skin. It can be replaced after a few days. This method is useful in old, weak patients.

If the patient is fit for abdominal surgery, the following procedure is recommended (the Wells operation):

- *The rectum is completely mobilized*
- *An Ivalon sponge is sutured to the presacral fascia and folded around the rectum so that 1 cm of bowel remains exposed on the anterior wall.*
- *The sponge is then sutured to the bowel.*
- *The levator ani is sutured anterior to the bowel and the pouch of Douglas is obliterated.*
- *These procedures prevent prolapse by causing adhesion formation between the rectum and the sacral cavity.*

An alternative operation is based on the same principle:

- *A Teflon net is sutured to the rectum and presacral fascia (the Ripstein operation).*

Prognosis

The operation is successful in 80% of cases. A small percentage will continue to prolapse. A more serious problem is that incontinence will persist in aged people whose sphincters have been stretched too much for too long.

Sepsis sometimes develops in the Ivalon sponge and this will not resolve until the foreign body (Ivalon or Teflon) is removed.

Giant solitary rectal ulcer

This condition can develop as a complication of complete rectal prolapse. It sometimes develops without any obvious prolapse being noted.

It is a problem found in young women with constipation. The patient sits on the toilet and strains for long periods. A sliding hernia of the anterior border of the rectum arises and the mucosa prolapses into the anal canal, where it is strangulated by the sphincter mechanism. Because the pelvic floor is intact, a complete prolapse does not occur.

The ulcer has a typical macroscopic appearance. A large, solitary ulcer is found, with surrounding hyperaemic swollen mucosa. It may closely resemble a carcinoma ulcer. The histology may also be confusing. The *muscularis propria* thickens. The crypts branch and become hyperplastic. Glands may be displaced into the submucosa and this can be confused with carcinoma.

Management

This condition must be treated conservatively. Improve stooling habits by education. Use stool softeners.

If there is already a prolapse through the anal canal, the Wells operation should be performed.

The rectal pain syndrome

This syndrome consists of periodic pain and a sensation of fullness and pressure in the rectum. A variant of this condition is known as *proctalgia fugax*. Patients develop a severe pain in the rectum which wakes them at night.

Other causes of severe rectal pain such as fissure-in-ano, perianal abscess and carcinoma must be excluded.

Reassurance is important. Galvanic stimulation of the perianal muscles and hot baths may help.

I. THE ANUS

Haemorrhoids

Haemorrhoids are varices of the normal venous plexus in the anus, which forms the vascular cushions of the anal canal. The venous drainage is divided in the internal haemorrhoidal plexus, which drains to the superior haemorrhoidal veins and thus to the portal system. The venous plexus is situated above the mucocutaneous junction and is thus covered proximally by pink mucosa and distally by dark red mucosa.

The external haemorrhoidal plexus lies distal to the mucocutaneous junction and is therefore covered by skin. This plexus drains back to the systemic venous system, but the two plexi communicate freely with each other.

Haemorrhoids are divided into internal haemorrhoids (origin in the internal haemorrhoidal plexus) and external haemorrhoids (origin in the external haemorrhoidal plexus).

Internal haemorrhoids

These haemorrhoids usually arise at three classical sites – left lateral, right anterior and right posterior, i e at 4, 7 and 11 o'clock. Secondary haemorrhoids may arise between these classical positions.

Haemorrhoids are divided into four grades:

Grade I

Enlarged haemorrhoids in the classical positions, which do not prolapse.

Grade II

Enlarged haemorrhoids which prolapse with defaecation, but reduce spontaneously.

Grade III

Enlarged haemorrhoids which prolapse, but do not reduce spontaneously and must be replaced manually.

Grade IV

Irreducible prolapsed haemorrhoids.

Aetiology

There is a familial tendency. Constipation and straining at stool cause haemorrhoids. The venous return is impaired when the patient sits on the toilet for a long time and strains, the plexus then becomes engorged and the haemorrhoids tend to prolapse. Pregnancy, obesity and a low fibre diet also play a rôle.

Clinical presentation

Patients tend to ascribe any symptoms in the anal area to haemorrhoids. The earliest symptom is usually rectal bleeding. The blood is on the outside of the stool and is bright red. It may spatter the toilet bowel. Sometimes, patients can bleed so severely that they become anaemic. If the haemorrhoids prolapse, the patient complains of something sagging. Patients also complain they they have noticed mucus and even stool on their underwear.

Haemorrhoids are not painful. If there is pain, another diagnosis must be considered, although thrombosed haemorrhoids with inflammation are painful.

On examination there is often nothing visible. The haemorrhoids can only be seen if they prolapse. Internal haemorrhoids cannot be palpated on rectal examination. The diagnosis is usually confirmed by proctoscopy. It is absolutely essential to do a sigmoidoscopy to exclude rectal pathology. This must not be done intraoperatively, as action could then be taken on the findings without the patient's permission. Barium enema must also be done if there are other symptoms such as constipation or blood mixed with the stools.

Differential diagnosis

All the other causes of rectal bleeding must be considered. Polyps, carcinoma, ulcerative colitis and Crohn disease must be excluded on sigmoidoscopy and biopsy.

Prolapsing haemorrhoids must be differentiated from rectal prolapse, which has already been discussed. Anal conditions such as *condylomata acuminata* (anal viral warts), sentinel pile (fissure-in-ano) and carcinoma of the anus, must be considered.

Management

The majority of patients with haemorrhoids can be treated conservatively. This includes dietary adjustment, fluids and a high fibre diet, as well as education about stooling habits.

This treatment is usually successful in Grade I and II haemorrhoids. If the patient bleeds, the haemorrhoids must be sclerosed. No anaesthetic is necessary. Phenol in oil is injected into the base of the haemorrhoid submucously (not into the vein). The injections must be repeated two or three times. Grade I and II haemorrhoids are suitable for sclerosis.

If haemorrhoids prolapse and bleed, excision is necessary. There are more conservative methods, such as placing small elastic bands around the bases of the internal haemorrhoids. Ischaemic necrosis of the haemorrhoids then takes place. Patients sometimes complain of a lot of pain from this method and another complication is haemorrhage when the necrotic haemorrhoid drops off.

Haemorrhoidectomy

The three enlarged haemorrhoids are dissected free until they swing from the pedicle. The venous pedicle is then tied off with a silk suture and transected. The pedicle retracts into the anal canal. One must take care to leave bridges of mucosa between the raw areas at 4, 7 and 11 o'clock to prevent anal stenosis. To minimize postoperative pain, make sure that the pedicles are not caught in the internal sphincter, but have pulled back to a position above the sphincter. Only small tulle gauze swabs must be used to cover the raw areas.

A mild secondary haemorrhage sometimes occurs on the seventh and eighth days. If this is severe, the patient must be put to bed and sedated. If the bleeding persists, a Foley catheter can be inserted into the rectum, the balloon inflated and light traction applied. This may stop the bleeding. It is very seldom necessary to have to ligate the pedicle formally under anaesthetic.

It is advisable to provide patients with an anal dilator, to be used for a few weeks.

Complications of haemorrhoids

Strangulated prolapsed haemorrhoids

If haemorrhoids prolapse and are not reduced, they become oedematous and clot. If haemorrhoids are not reduced, mucosal necrosis will later arise, with secondary infection. Thrombosis may also develop in the external haemorrhoidal plexus, forming a swollen red mass. This may resolve or also undergo necrosis.

Management

If the patients present with prolapsed, oedematous haemorrhoids, it is often possible to reduce the haemorrhoids manually under sedation and then keep the patient in bed. If the haemorrhoids have already undergone thrombosis, the following approaches are possible:

- **Conservative management**

Put the patient to bed and elevate the foot of the bed. Administer analgesics and apply ice-packs on the anus to reduce oedema. Usually the condition resolves spontaneously after a few days. The thrombosed haemorrhoid heals, leaving small skin tags (self-healing).

- **Anal stretching (Lord's procedure)**

If the haemorrhoids prolapse and will not reduce, the anus can be stretched under anaesthetic using the fingers. The patient is then put to bed and the foot of the bed is elevated. After this procedure, the haemorrhoids often reduce spontaneously. The stretch must not be done if necrosis is already present, as this may cause spread of sepsis.

- **Emergency haemorrhoidectomy**

Thrombosed haemorrhoids can be treated by means of a haemorrhoidectomy. This must be performed by only a skilled surgeon, as it is sometimes difficult to leave mucosal bridges between the raw areas, due to the generalized oedema. In order to avoid the possibility of spread of sepsis, or even thrombophlebitis suppurativa, the operation must not be performed if necrosis with secondary infection is already present.

External haemorrhoids

Differentiation must be made between a perianal haematoma and thrombosis of the external haemorrhoidal plexus.

Perianal haematoma

This usually follows a period of longterm straining due to constipation, a coughing fit or strenuous sporting activity. A vein from the external plexus ruptures under the perianal skin and causes a localized haematoma. This is a very painful, round, berry-like swelling. The haematoma can organize and disappear gradually, leaving only a skin tag. It can also undergo pressure necrosis, with formation of an ulcer which can become secondarily infected.

If this is seen in the early painful stages, it can be opened under local anaesthetic and the haematoma evacuated. The skin tags are removed. This usually relieves the symptoms immediately. If they present later, they can be treated conservatively.

Thrombosis of the external plexus

This usually occurs secondary to prolapsed, strangulated internal haemorrhoids. The condition must be treated conservatively with analgesia, icepacks and bedrest.

Fibrous polyps and anal papillae

Fibrous polyps are found in the anal canal and are remnants of previous thrombosed haemorrhoids. They can prolapse through the anus and cause problems with anal hygiene.

Anal papillae are hypertrophied papillae just below the crypts of Morgagni. If they enlarge much, they can prolapse through the anal canal. The polyps and papillae must be excised if they cause symptoms.

Fissure-in-ano

Fissure-in-ano is a very painful ulcer, which is usually found in the midline posteriorly in the anal canal. It is extremely painful because it involves the mucocutaneous junction. It usually runs from the anal papillae, which undergo hypertrophy, to the skin, forming an oedematous, raised tag at the lower end of the fissure (the sentinel pile).

This is usually situated posteriorly, because the mucosa is more fixed. The fissure probably arises when hard stools are passed during constipation and tear the mucosa. The pain causes spasm of the anal sphincters and the pressure on the mucosa causes ischaemia and retards healing.

A fissure can be acute or chronic. Chronic fissures are present for long periods, reach deeply into the fibres of the internal sphincter and have raised oedematous sides.

Clinical presentation

Patients experience severe pain on stooling, with mild bleeding. The pain subsides gradually, but remains vaguely present due to sphicter spasm. Patients develop constipation and a vicious circle develops with severe pain on stooling, sphincter spasm and constipation. On examination, a sentinel pile is often found. The sphincter is in spasm and the patient will not allow any rectal examination.

Management

Apply a local anaesthetic ointment such as lignocaine 2% to the fissure. With lignocaine on the finger insert carefully. When the pain has been anaesthetised, the sphincter will relax and can be examined.

Differential diagnosis

Other causes of ulcers, such as tuberculosis, Crohn disease and ulcerative colitis, must be considered, especially if the ulcer does not present in the midline. Carcinoma of the anus must be excluded. This is hard and has rolled edges. Histology will confirm the diagnosis.

Management of acute anal fissure

Conservative management

The anus is dilated gradually to relieve sphincter spasm, using lignocaine ointment. The patient can continue to use the anal dilator and lignocaine ointment daily. Stool softeners must also be given.

Anal stretching

Under general anaesthetic the anus is stretched to admit four fingers. This breaks the sphincter spasm and leads to healing of acute fissure-in-ano.

Internal sphincterotomy

If the fissure does not heal after stretching only, the lower part of the fibres of the internal sphincter can be transected laterally in the anal canal. Excise the sentinel pile. The fissure then usually heals.

Chronic anal fissure

If the fissure has been present over a protracted period and reaches deep into the muscle fibres, it is necessary to excise the base of the fissure as well as the sentinel pile. The lower part of the internal sphincter is then also transected.

Prognosis

Internal sphincterotomy is a very successful procedure. Unfortunately, some patients complain of incontinence of flatus. Fortunately, this improves in time.

Perianal abscess and fistula-in-ano

The perianal abscess is the precursor of the fistula-in-ano, and they will be discussed together. The structures in the pelvis comprise two funnelshaped tubes. The inner tube consists of the rectum and anal canal and this is surrounded by an outer funnelshaped muscular tube, formed by the *levator ani*, the puborectalis and the external anal sphincter. The intersphincteric plane lies between these two muscular tubes. This plane is comprised of connective tissue joining the two tubes. Abscesses tend to form mainly in the intersphincteric plane in the anal glands of Chiari, which encircle the anal canal and open in the crypts of Morgagni above the valves of Ball. The abscess tends to spread along the intersphincteric space and to present under the skin immediately adjacent to the anus.

If the abscess ruptures, it is often followed by a fistula which runs perianally from the skin through the intersphincteric space, through the lower third of the internal sphincter, opening in the crypts of Morgagni. An intersphincteric abscess can also spread through the external sphincter to the ischiorectal fossa to form an abscess there. This is relatively rare. If it now breaks through to the skin, it forms a transsphincteric fistula with one opening in the skin and one into the crypts of Morgagni.

An intersphincteric abscess can also spread upwards in this plane and break through above the external sphincter, with a high transsphincteric fistula. Because the abscess and fistula are so interdependent, Eisenhammer named this condition fistulous abscess.

Clinical presentation

The disease is more common in women. Patients present with a painful perianal swelling which is red and warm. It can also present more laterally in the ischiorectal fossa. Sometimes patients present with pain and fever without the abscess being visible next to the anus. The abscess can be palpated higher up in the anorectum, in the submucous area or higher up in the intersphincteric space.

A patient with perianal fistula can present with a purulent discharge. If the external opening is found on the skin posterior to the transverse line running from 3 o'clock to 9 o'clock across the anus, the internal opening will be palpable in the midline posteriorly. If it is anterior to this line, the internal opening will be directly opposite the fistula opening (Goodsall's law).

The majority are intersphincteric perianal abscesses and most fistulae are therefore low intersphincteric fistulae.

Differential diagnosis of fistula-in-ano

Other causes that must be borne in mind include Crohn disease, ulcerative colitis and tuberculosis. Conditions with which it can be confused include hydradenitis suppurativa and pilonidal sinus.

Management

Most perianal and ischiorectal abscesses will heal if they are saucerized. Some will go on to form fistulae-in-ano. Eisenhammer recommends that the condition be regarded as a fistulous abscess and treated as such. The abscess must be saucerized and the lower third of the sphincter split down to the crypts of Morgagni to expose the fistula. Both conditions are thus treated simultaneously. If there is doubt about the anatomy, the abscess must only be saucerized. The majority of fistulae can be excised after a sound has been passed from the external opening through the lower third of the internal sphincter to the crypts of Morgagni. The low transsphincteric fistula can in the same way be excised or exposed.

High fistulae must not be transected, as this will cause the patient to become incontinent. The best method is probably extrasphincteric excision of the fistula, via a posterior approach, under direct vision, without splitting the sphincter. This must be attempted by only a skilled surgeon. Fortunately it is rare.

Anal tumours

Malignant tumours of the anal canal are relatively rare and form only 3% of the total of anorectal tumours. Because anal tumours tend to spread upwards to involve the rectum, they are often confused with rectal carcinoma. There are three types of malignant epithelial tumours: Squamous carcinoma of the mucosa in the anal canal above the mucocutaneous junction; squamous carcinoma of the cutaneous epithelium of the anal canal, which reacts like a squamous skin carcinoma at any site; and malignant melanoma of the epithelium above the mucocutaneous junction.

Clinical presentation

Patients present with pain, blood and mucus. They often complain of haemorrhoids. On inspection, a tumour may be seen in the perianal area, but more often than not nothing is visible. The diagnosis is often made on proctoscopy and biopsy.

The anal canal must be examined very thoroughly, under anaesthetic if necessary, to determine whether the tumour is confined to the anal skin or whether it has infiltrated higher into the anal canal and rectum. The inguinal lymph nodes must be examined carefully, as anal canal tumours spread to the inguinal lymph nodes.

Management

Tumours involving the anal canal above the mucocutaneous junction must be irradiated preoperatively and then treated with an abdominoperineal resection. If the inguinal nodes are palpable, a block dissection must be performed a week later. The anus must be excised widely, including sections of the ischiorectal fat, and the defect can then be covered by a skin graft. If lymph nodes are involved, adjuvant chemotherapy can be considered, because squamous carcinoma responds more favourably to chemotherapy than does adenocarcinoma of the rectum.

If the tumour is confined to the skin of the anal canal and it is possible practically, a wide local excision and skin grafts can be done.

Prognosis

The five year survival rate of anal canal tumours which originate above the mucocutaneous junction is 30%. If the tumour arises in the skin of the anal canal, the five year survival is 50%. The prognosis of malignant melanoma is poor, despite radical surgery.

Differential diagnosis

Bowen disease (intraepidermal carcinoma-in-situ), basal cell carcinoma and Paget disease are sometimes found in the anal canal.

Pruritis ani

Pruritis is a common condition found in both sexes at any age. The condition often begins as pruritis and ends up as a raw, painful, bleeding dermatitis around the anus, the result of constant scratching. This condition is exacerbated by the heat in bed and patients often scratch in their sleep. While the patient is distracted by other people or work, the pruritis is bearable, but as soon as he is alone and relaxes, he resumes the scratching. The condition can restrict the patient's normal activities drastically.

It is essential to try to make a definitive diagnosis and treat the underlying cause. The aetiological factors can be divided into five main groups:

- Infections: bacterial, fungi and parasites
- Anorectal conditions
- Skin diseases
- Systemic conditions
- Idiopathic

Infections

Bacterial infections often follow on damage to the surrounding skin caused by scratching and are thus secondary to other causes of pruritis. Sometimes the pruritis arises due to peritoneal fistulae, which excrete pus. Bacterial infections can sometimes arise in the skinfolds of patients who sweat a lot between their buttocks and have problems with hygiene. A syphilitic chancre must be borne in mind.

Fungi such as dermatophytosis and Candida must be considered. Always look for athlete's foot, which can spread to the anus. If the patient has Candidiasis, consider underlying diabetes.

Viruses such as *Condylomata acuminata* may be a cause.

Pruritis also develops secondary to the use of antibiotics, especially the tetracyclines. Look for intestinal parasites, especially worms such as *Enterobius vermicularis*. Scabies is sometimes a cause.

Anorectal conditions

Prolapsing haemorrhoids, polyps and hyperplastic anal papillae lead to excessive secretion of mucus and to pruritis. Skin tags around the anus caused by previous thrombosed haemorrhoids make it difficult to maintain normal hygiene around the anus. Tumours such as Bowen disease, Paget disease and carcinoma must be considered.

Skin diseases

Psoriasis, lichen planus and atopic eczema can cause pruritis. Contact dermatitis, caused by a variety of agents such as local anaesthetic, various ointments, douches and soaps, must be considered.

Systemic conditions

Diabetes with secondary Candidial infection must always be borne in mind. Other systemic diseases which cause pruritis include Hodgkin disease, gout, uraemia and polycythaemia.

Excessive use of alcohol, milk, coffee and fruit juices is sometimes the cause.

Pruritis is also found in mentally disturbed patients.

Idiopathic pruritis

In a small group of patients no obvious cause can be found.

The diagnosis is usually made after a careful history has been taken and followed by a thorough general examination and laboratory tests. Microscopic examination of skin scrapings in the area may reveal mould, fungi or parasites. The stools must be examined carefully to exclude parasites. Serological tests must be done to diagnose venereal disease and urine and blood tests must be done to exclude diabetes and uraemia. A biopsy of any suspicious lesion in the area must be taken for histological examination.

Management

Any underlying aetiological factors must be treated. Patients may not use any soaps or ointments in the area. The anus must be thoroughly washed with warm water after defaecation. Dietary adjustments may be necessary. A water-soluble corticosteroid cream is useful.

Psychiatric treatment is sometimes necessary.

Pilonidal sinus

This name is derived from the Greek words "pilus" = a hair and " nidus" = a nest. The condition consists of an abscess or sinus containing hair in the midline in the cleft between the buttocks. The presence of one or more pits, lined with squamous epithelium, containing granulation tissue and loose hair in their depths, is characteristic of the condition. The origin of the pits is controversial. Some believe that they are congenital remnants of inadequate fusion of neural canal remnants (*canalis reuniens*). It is more likely that the pits are acquired, and caused by hair penetrating the skin in the area. The small pits then become lined by squamous epithelium. The condition also develops between hairdressers' fingers.

Whatever the origin of the pits, they are always found in this condition. Patients present with an abscess or a draining sinus. On examination, the small pits can be seen, especially with the aid of a magnifying glass, and hairs sometimes protrude from their openings.

Management

The key to management of this condition is excision of all the pits and removal of all the hair in the area, until the wound where the pits have been excised has healed completely.

All surrounding hair must be shaved away by the surgeon. The infected sinus must be opened and all hairs in the sinus and tracts removed. Other pits must be carefully sought, using a magnifying glass and they must be excised locally. The wound must be left open to granulate.

The patient must be seen weekly and all hair in the area must be removed, by shaving or by the use of depilatory creams, until the wound has healed completely. The patient must continue to use the depilatory cream to prevent recurrence. These methods give better results than wide excision or excision and immediate suturing.

The recurrence rate is lower than 10%.

J. INTESTINAL FISTULAE

A fistula is an abnormal communication between two epithelial lined surfaces. Intestinal fistulae thus arise between bowel and bowel, between bowel and the urinary tract and between bowel and the skin. The management of external fistulae, fistulae between bowel and skin, is a great challenge, as this condition has a high mortality rate.

Fistulae can arise due to underlying disease such as Crohn disease or carcinoma, from penetrating wounds or as a complication of surgery to the intestinal canal. More than 90% of fistulae are complications of surgery.

Fistulae can be classified as end fistulae, where the two ends of the intestinal canal are no longer continuous; and side fistulae, where the intestinal canal is still continuous, with a fistula occurring from the side wall of the bowel.

A high output fistula of the proximal bowel, which produces more than 500 ml/24 hours, as opposed to a low output fistula of the distal small bowel is another useful classification.

Fistulae following surgery arise as a result of disruption of the suture line due to tension, ischaemia, infection or distal obstruction. They can arise if the bowel is caught up by a suture when the abdominal wall is being closed. Drainage tubes can erode through the bowel. If bowel wall ischaemia arises due to an injury to the blood supply intraoperatively, perforation and fistulae can also arise.

Clinical course

Five to ten days postoperatively, the patient develops fever and abdominal pain. Later a discharge appears from the wound or drainage tube and eventually faecal material drains freely. Fistulae cause dehydration and electrolyte imbalance. The associated sepsis and destruction of skin and tissue by the intestinal and pancreatic juices causes anaemia and hypoalbuminaemia. Because the patient cannot be fed normally, he loses weight rapidly. The patient eventually develops organ failure.

Management

Intestinal fistulae are inclined to close spontaneously if a positive nitrogen balance can be maintained and one of the following factors is not present:

- *If it is an end fistula, it will not close because the two ends of bowel are separated.*
- *If there is obstruction in the bowel distal to the fistula, it cannot close. It acts as an outlet valve for the bowel proximal to the obstruction.*
- *If the fistula drains first into an abscess cavity and then secondarily onto the skin, it will not close until the abscess cavity has been widely drained.*
- *If a specific infection is present, such as tuberculosis or a fungal infection, this must be treated first.*
- *If a foreign body, such as a drainage tube, is present in the fistula, it cannot close.*
- *If there is underlying disease, such as carcinoma or Crohn disease, the fistula will not close.*
- *If the tract has epithelialized, it will not close.*

The treatment must be administered in logical order:

- *Restore the blood volume and fluid and electrolytes.*
- *Drain any abscesses that may be present.*
- *Monitor the fistula. Measure the fluids excreted so that they can be replaced accurately. Protect the surrounding tissue and skin by applying stomahesive. Superficial suctioning of the fistula is also useful.*
- *Insert a central catheter and commence hyperalimentation.*

At this stage it may be necessary to determine the nature and site of the fistula, using radiological investigations. Contrast medium can be given by mouth and through the fistula to determine whether it is an end- or side fistula and whether or not distal obstruction is present. Any abscess cavity can be seen with X-rays and ultrasound.

If it is a side fistula and there is no distal obstruction, the fistula can be expected to close spontaneously within a month if the patient's nutritional status is maintained with hyperalimentation. If the fistula has not closed within six weeks, the studies must be repeated to try and find a reason.

The following operations must be considered:

- *Excision of the fistula, with end-to-end anastomosis. if there is obstruction, or underlying disease like Crohn disease, these must be resected simultaneously.*
- *Bypassing the fistula. Sometimes there is so much sepsis and adhesion formation around the fistula that it is better to locate the bowel proximal to the area and suture it end-to-side to bowel distal to the fistula.*

Prognosis

About 60% of fistulae close spontaneously. The mortality of the disease is still 10%.

K. ABSCESSES OF THE ABDOMINAL CAVITY

Intraperitoneal abscesses

The main causes of intraperitoneal abscesses include: perforations of the gastrointestinal tract, complications following surgery to the gastrointestinal tract, trauma and infection of the female genital system.

An abscess forms either proximal to an inflamed viscus, such as appendicitis, diverticulitis and cholecystitis; or as a result of contamination of the peritoneal cavity when the intestinal canal is opened during surgery or from outside by penetrating trauma.

The anatomy of intraperitoneal abscesses

Abscesses develop in relation to the liver and diaphragm and in the gutters alongside the colon and the pelvis. The subphrenic space, the paracolic gutters and the pelvis communicate freely with each other.

Abscesses can also develop in any place between bowel loops.

The subphrenic spaces

The right and left intraperitoneal spaces can be divided into suprahepatic and infraheptatic spaces. The space between the right lobe of the liver and the diaphragm is divided into an anterior suprahepatic space and a posterior suprahepatic subphrenic space, although these are not anatomical concepts, but clinical concepts which are useful in treatment.

On the left side, there is only one suprahepatic subphrenic space.

There are infrahepatic spaces to the right and left; to the right between the liver and hepatic flexure of the colon and to the left between the left lobe of the liver and the stomach. There is a second space in the lesser sac behind the stomach.

The right paracolic gutter communicates with the right infrahepatic space and is known as Morrison's pouch.

The pelvic space and the fold between the uterus and rectum is known as the pouch of Douglas.

Clinical presentation

One of the possible predisposing factors is usually present. The patient has fever, tachycardia and pain. If the patient is on antibiotics, the symptoms and signs are often masked.

A patient who has undergone an operation and has a persistent ileus, feels ill and has a fever, probably has intraperitoneal sepsis.

If a subphrenic abscess develops, patients complain of chest pain, dysponea and pain which radiates to the shoulder. On examination, there may be pain on compression of the costal margin and there may be an effusion in the pleural cavity.

A patient with pelvic abscess may develop urinary symptoms or diarrhoea.

If a patient who has had major intestinal surgery has a persistent ileus and develops multi-organ failure or bleeding from stress ulceration or disseminated intravascular coagulation, it can be accepted that he has intraperitoneal sepsis.

On examination, a mass is palpable. Pelvic abscesses are usually felt per rectum.

Special investigations

A leucocytosis indicates infection. Pulmonary, renal and liver function abnormalities indicate organ failure and, indirectly, sepsis.

- **X-rays**

An elevated diaphragm, fixation of the diaphragm and fluid levels under the diaphragm can be seen on chest and abdominal X-rays. It is important to take lateral views to determine whether the abscess lies anteriorly or posteriorly in the suprahepatic space.

- **Ultrasound and computer tomography**

This is useful not only for diagnosis of subphrenic abscesses, but also for abscesses elsewhere in the abdominal cavity.

- **Radionuclide scans**

Gallium^{67}- and Indium^{111}-marked leucocytes are sometimes useful in tracking down abscesses.

Management

It is sometimes possible to treat subphrenic inflammation with antibiotics before an abscess has formed, but it is usually necessary to drain an abscess.

If possible, an attempt must be made to drain the abscess without contaminating the rest of the peritoneal cavity. In subphrenic abscesses, this is attempted via an extraperitoneal approach. If the abscess is situated posteriorly suprahepatically on ultrasound, an extraperitoneal approach through the bed of the 12th rib is used. If the abscess is situated anteriorly suprahepatically, it can be reached via an extraperitoneal approach just below the costal margin.

If a pelvic abscess extends up to the anus with mucus secretion per anum, it can be drained into the rectum. All other abscesses are approached and drained via a laparotomy. If multiple intraperitoneal abscesses are found, it is advisable to close the abdomen temporily and to re-explore it after twenty-four hours and then again every forty-eight hours until all abscesses have cleared up.

Subphrenic abscesses must be drained using suction drainage. Drains may not be removed until a sinugram has shown that the abscess cavity has been obliterated, otherwise the abscess will recur.

Percutaneous catheter drainage

Well localized abscesses can be drained with a catheter, percutaneously, under ultrasound guidance.

Prognosis

Multiple intraperitoneal abscesses have a mortality of 50% if multi-organ failure arises. Localized abscesses related to perforated appendix or diverticulitis and pelvic abscesses have a mortality lower than 5%.

Retroperitoneal abscesses

Abscesses in the retroperitoneal space usually arise secondary to acute pancreatitis or pyelonephritis. Penetrating injuries to the duodenum and colon are another important cause.

Primary psoas abscesses are found in young men. They often follow sports injuries and infection is usually caused by *Staph. aureus*, which reaches the haematoma via the bloodstream. Secondary psoas abscesses arise due to spread from adjacent septic organs, e g Crohn disease.

These abscesses must be drained and treated with antibiotics. It must be borne in mind that psoas abscesses can also arise from tuberculosis of the vertebral column. The management of pancreatic abscesses has already been discussed elsewhere.

Skin and soft tissue 6

Skin and soft tissue lesions are among the most common complaints that surgeons have to deal with. The majority are benign, but because benign conditions have to be distinguished from potentially fatal conditions such as malignant melanoma, it must be emphasized that no suspicious lesion should ever be treated by any means precluding a histological diagonsis. Curettage or cauterization of a lesion, particularly a pigmented lesion, which destroys the lesion without allowing for histological diagnosis, is to be condemned.

What does the patient complain of?

Patients usually present with a swelling on the skin surface, in the skin or in the subcutaneous tissue. A patient may also complain of an ulcer.

What must the clinician note?

- Is it a swelling covered with intact empidermis, which looks abnormal?
- Is it a swelling covered with normal epidermis?
- Is it a swelling where the overlying epidermis has been destroyed – an ulcer?

Epidermal swellings which appear to be intact, but abnormal, must be judged according to colour, shape, area, colour and edges.

Pigmentation is extremely important in differentiating between melanoma and other pigmented lesions.

Ulcers must be judged by the types of edge with which they present:

- Punched ulcers: trophic, ischaemic or syphilitic ulcers.
- Undermined edges: tuberculosis or a carbuncle.
- Raised and rolled edges: malignant tumours, squamous carcinoma and basal cell carcinoma.

What must the clinician consider?

Skin cancer is the most common of cancers in South Africa. Basal cancer accounts for 80% of skin cancer, but is the least dangerous. Malignant melanoma is the rarest form, but is also the most dangerous for the patient.

PIGMENTED SKIN LESIONS

Any pigmented skin lesion must be viewed with suspicion; and malignant melanoma must be differentiated from other pigmented lesions.

Malignant melanoma

Malignant melanoma is relatively rare, but its incidence is increasing at the rate of about 6% per annum. This applies particularly to melanomas of the lower limbs in women and of the trunk in men. This can probably be ascribed to a change in clothing fashions, leading to increased sun exposure. There are four main clinical types of malignant melanoma:

Lentigo maligna melanoma

This arises in a Hutchinson freckle. A Hutchinson freckle, or *Lentigo maligna*, is a large brown or black spot with irregular, raised areas, on sun-exposed skin, often on the faces of people over sixty. The edges are serrated; and greyish-white spots, which represent scars or regression, can sometimes be seen.

Histologically, there is proliferation of dysplastic cells at the junction of the epidermis and dermis. This lesion becomes a *Lentigo maligna* melanoma in about 50% of cases. Discrete, black, malignant nodules then arise.

Superficial spreading melanoma

This consists of a dark brown, irregular lesion and small, greyish-pink nodules. The lesion is sometimes ulcerated.

Histologically, all three of the typical cell types containing melanin, namely epithelioid cells, spindleshaped cells and small cells, are present, but epithelioid cells dominate the epidermis. These cells are inclined to spread laterally in the epidermis, but can also break through the epidermal basal membrane and spread to the papillary dermis and deeper layer.

Nodular maliganant melanoma

This is the most malignant of the three types of malignant melanoma. They consist of dark blue or black nodules.

Histologically, the lesion mainly comprises spindle-shaped and epithelioid cells containing melanin. These cells tend to infiltrate to the deeper parts of the skin and even to the subcutaneous tissues. Anaplasia and mitotic figures are more prominent than in the two aforementioned lesions.

Lentigo maligna acrale

This is found on the feet and soles of black people. It consists of black, raised lesions with ulceration. It has a poor prognosis.

Clinical presentation

A malignant melanoma can arise in an existing nevus, or *de novo*. A pigmented lesion which is enlarging, changing colour, itching or ulcerating and bleeding should arouse suspicion of malignant melanoma.

An irregular surface with loss of skin folds and hair, especially when associated with satellite pigmentation and enlarged palpable lymph nodes in the drainage area, is very suspicious.

This also applies to pigmented lesions on the palms or soles of the feet.

The diagnosis must be confirmed histologically, by taking a punch biopsy through the thickest area of the lesion, or by excision of the lesion for complete histology and staging.

Histological staging

Clarke's levels

Level I: Lesion confined to the epidermis. Mortality 0%.

Level II: Lesion infiltrates the papillary dermis. Mortality 8%.

Level III: Lesion infiltrates through the papillary dermis down to the reticular dermis. Mortality 35%.

Level IV: Lesion infiltrates through the reticular dermis. Mortality 46%.

Level V: Lesion infiltrates the subcutaneous tissues. Mortality exceeds 50%.

Breslow's infiltration depths

- Less than 0,76 mm: No deaths.
- 0,76 to 1,5 mm: 25% mortality within five years.
- 1,5 to 3,0 mm: More than 50% mortality within five years.
- Deeper than 3,0 mm: Mortality higher than 75% within five years.

Clinical staging

Stage I: Any primary lesion without lymph nodes or distal metastases.

Stage II: Lymph nodes involved.

Stage III: Distal metastases.

Factors determining prognosis

- Tumour depth
- Ulceration
- Site of lesion – trunk worse than head, and neck worse than limbs

- Metastasis to lymph nodes

If lymph nodes are involved, depth of infiltration no longer plays an independent rôle in the prognosis.

Management

The concept that microscopic spread to lymph nodes can be predicted by depth of infiltration of the primary lesion, has attractive implications for the treatment of this disease. In retrospective analysis of series it was found that if the lesion infiltrates deeper than 1,5 mm but shallower than 4 mm, elective excision of lymph nodes in the drainage area will be advantageous.

When this hypothesis was tested in random prospective trials, no advantage could be shown. Because of inadequacies in those trials, further prospective trials are now being done. The practice of wide excision of the primary lesion, leaving a 5 cm free border, has recently been questioned. Current findings indicate that in a superficial lesion (less than 1,5 mm penetration) a 1 cm free border is adequate. In deeper lesions, a 2 cm free border is adequate. Wounds must be closed primarily where possible. The rôle played by the width of the excision is also being tested in a prospective trial.

Current approach

Stage I malignant melanoma

- *Biopsy of the primary lesion to determine diagnosis and Breslow depth of infiltration.*
- *Beslow infiltration less than 1 mm – excision of lesion with 1 cm border and wound closure.*
- *Regular follow-up of the patient, with emphasis on lymph node examination.*
- *Breslow depth of infiltration greater than 1 mm – excision of the primary lesion, with a 2 cm free border.*
- *Primary closure where possible, otherwise skin transplant.*
- *Depth of excision – up to deep fascia.*
- *If the melanoma has spread to the subcutaneous tissues (Clarke level V), take the deep fascia as well.*

Stage II malignant melanoma

- *Excise the primary lesion, leaving a 2 cm border and close primarily.*
- *Immediate block dissection of the draining lymph nodes must be performed.*

Block dissection of the neck

- *Spare the sternocleidomastoid muscle.*

Block dissection of the groin

- *Restrict the dissection to the groin. There is no proof that dissection of the iliac nodes improves prognosis.*
- *Inguinal dissection has a high morbidity, with wound breakdown and skin necrosis, lymphocoele with infection and oedematous leg in about 20% of cases.*
- *Suitable adjuvant chemotherapy is not available.*

Stage III malignant melanoma

- *Melanomas spread to the liver, lungs and brain. They also tend to involve unusual organs such as the intestinal canal, spleen, heart and kidneys. There is not really any effective chemotherapy available.*
- *Radiotherapy is not very effective, except in combination with nitrose-ureas in brain metastases.*
- *Immunotherapy has sometimes achieved surprisingly good results in isolated cases, but was disappointing in prospective trials.*
- *Injection of metastases with BCG sometimes causes the lesions to disappear, but results of prospective trials were equally disappointing for this method.*
- *Isolated limb perfusions are done in some centres. The best approach is to refer patients with advanced disease to centres where multidisciplinary treatment, including excision, irradiation and chemotherapy, is available.*

Differential diagnosis

Moles

These are very common, and malignant melanoma is rare. Malignant melanoma can develop *de novo*, but about 50% arise in moles. The melanocytes lie in the basal layer of the epidermis, where it joins the dermis.

In children, proliferation of these cells takes place. This is also known as junctional activity, characterized by mitosis, pleomorphic cells and intradermal infiltration. If it arises before puberty, it is known as a juvenile melanoma and is not an indication of malignant transformation. If junctional activity is found in adults, it is regarded as a premalignant phenomenon.

Junctional nevi are flat and hairless. The majority of moles are intradermal nevi. The melanocytes are found deep to the basal layer of the epidermis in the dermis. The moles are raised and hairy. They are not premalignant.

Compound nevi have melanocytes at the junction and deep in the dermal layer. Because of the junctional activity, they are also premalignant.

A blue nevus is an intradermal nevus with deeply situated melanocytes which shine through as blue colouring. They are not premalignant.

Because melanomas are rare and moles are very common, all moles cannot be removed. Remove moles which change colour, itch or bleed. Remove moles if a patient requests removal. All moles which are removed must be sent for histology.

Basal cell papilloma (seborrhoeic keratosis)

This is a benign overgrowth of the basal cells of the epidermis. It is found in the elderly, often in blacks. It is pigmented, raised, rough, greasy and usually multiple. It scratches off easily. If there is doubt about the diagnosis, excise and send for histology.

Pigmented basal cell carcinoma

This is the most common malignant skin tumour and is found on the face, neck and trunk. It is a pearl-like nodule with small blood vessels. It can form a small central ulcer, sometimes with pigmentation. A biopsy must be taken for histology.

Histiocytoma (sclerosing haemangioma)

Small, raised tumour, usually on the lower leg. Discrete, does not ulcerate. It contains haemosiderin, which resembles pigment.

Histology will confirm the diagnosis. It is benign.

Cafe-au-lait spots

These are small, flat, pigmented spots on the skin. They are often associated with neurofibromatosis, sometimes with phaeochromocytoma and, if found around the mouth, with Peutz-Jeghers syndorme. They do not undergo maligant transformation.

Haematomas

Small subcutaneous haemotomas, especially on the soles and palms, can be confused with melanomas. If there is any doubt they must be examined histologically. Subungual haematomas can also cause confusion.

Squamous cell carcinoma

These comprise 30% of skin carcinomas. They usually arise in the parts of the skin which are exposed to the sun. They are often preceded by solar keratosis, a form of epidermal dysplasia. Sometimes these lesions arise in old sinuses, venous ulcers or old burns (Marjolin ulcer).

The lesions arise as small, raised plaques, which gradually enlarge and ulcerate, with a necrotic base and raised edges. Later, the tumour infiltrates deeply and spreads to lymph nodes. Luckily, spread usually occurs late and seldom occurs at all in lesions smaller than 1,5 cm. If the lesion is confined to the epidermis, it is called carcinoma in situ or Bowen disease. The tumour infiltrates the dermis and even the subcutaneous tissue.

The majority are well differentiated, with keratin pearls, but can also be anaplastic, with a virtual abscence of keratinization and with giant cells and many mitoses.

The diagnosis is made on biopsy, which must include part of the raised edge.

Management

The majority of lesions do not spread. The primary lesion must be excised with a 1 cm free border. Affected lymph nodes must be treated by block dissection. If there is distant metastasis, chemotherapy can be considered. Primary lesions not suitable for excision can be irradiated.

Basal cell carcinoma

This tumour is twice as common as squamous cell carcinoma (60% of skin cancers). The tumour seldom metastasizes, but tends to infiltrate locally. These tumours are sometimes found in the skin at the corner of the eye, where they can infiltrate deeply, and are therefore difficult to excise fully. They are found, as are squamous cell carcinomas, on areas of the skin exposed to the sun and are especially common in fair-skinned people.

The tumour arises in the basal cell layer of the epidermis of the skin or the sebaceous glands of the skin. The lesion consists of a raised nodule with small superficial blood vessels and a waxy, pearly surface. Pigmentation is sometimes present.

Later, the lesion ulcerates and the ulcer takes on a typical rolled, pearl-like edge, in contrast to the rolled edges of the squamous cell carcinoma.

Histologically, the lesion comprises bundles of dark, spindle-shaped cells from the deeper layers of the epidermis, which infiltrate the upper dermis. The cells form nests of basal cells which surround the spindle-shaped cells. Giant cells and mitoses are absent. Various patterns are found. Some are solid cell masses, others take on a cystic pattern, with microcysts lined with keratin. They are then known as basosquamous cell carcinomas. This phenomenon does not mean that the tumour will adopt the behaviour pattern of squamous call carcinoma. They are not more malignant and do not metastasize. The diagnosis is confirmed on biopsy.

Management

The lesions can usually be excised with a 5 mm margin; and the skin is then closed primarily. If the lesion is unsuitable for excision, it can be irradiated. Lesions in the area of the ocular canthus must be excised and monitored histologically to make sure that the lesion has been excised completely. If this lesion infiltrates the sinuses and base of the skull, it becomes very difficult to remove totally. There can sometimes be widespread tissue loss due to the destructive local infiltration of these lesions.

DIFFERENTIAL DIAGNOSIS

Keratoacanthoma

This is a benign overgrowth of a sebaceous gland which becomes necrotic in its centre and collapses, leaving a deep skin lesion. It is benign.

Clinical presentation

It is found in adults, usually on the face, but can arise at any site where there are sebaceous glands. There is a raised area with a central keratinlike plug, which undergoes necrosis and then loosens and falls out, causing scarring. It takes two to three weeks to develop and heals within two to three months.

Management

Because it causes an unsightly scar anyway and looks so malignant, it must be excised and the skin closed. This confirms the diagnosis and yields a better scar.

Pyogenic granuloma

All wounds heal by formation of granulation tissue. At times chronic infections stimulate an overgrowth of granulation tissue, covered by epithelium. This well-vascularized nodule tends to bleed and secrete purulent fluid. Later, the lesion stabilizes as the overlying epithelium becomes better established. This lesion does not disappear spontaneously and, because it can be confused with squamous cell carcinoma, it must be excised and sent for histological examination.

Keratosis

Solar keratosis is a raised plaque of hyperkeratotic skin, found especially on the hands, face and ears. It is a premalignant condition, and if the lesion is already hard and immobile, malignant transformation to squamous cell carcinoma must be considered. The lesion must be excised and sent for histology. Multiple keratotic lesions can be treated with 5-Fluoro-uracil ointment.

Senile keratosis is a term used for solar keratosis or seborrhoeic keratosis (basal cell papilloma).

Keloid

As a wound heals, the granulation tissue is replaced by collagen and fibrous tissue. A good wound usually has scant fibrous tissue and results in a small scar.

If there is infection or traction on the wound edges, more fibrous tissue forms and the wound becomes thicker and wider. This is known as a hypertrophic scar. In some people, this overgrowth of fibrous tissue, beyond the line of the wound, occurs spontaneously. This phenomenon is especially common in blacks. The scar gradually deteriorates and may be very tender and itch. The keloid scar tends to recur if excised and resutured. If the wound is irradiated after suturing, keloid formation can be prevented.

Malignant melanoma

Although this is usually a raised, pigmented lesion, it can sometimes be amelanotic and present as an ulcer, which is difficult to differentiate from squamous cell carcinoma. Histology will confirm the diagnosis.

Kaposi sarcoma

This is found mainly on the lower limbs of middle-aged black men. It starts as small, reddish, painless nodules. If it enlarges at a later stage, it ulcerates and becomes secondarily infected.

This disease can run a long, slow course in aged black patients, but is sometimes more aggressive, involving lymph nodes and viscera, with hepatosplenomegaly.

It sometimes responds well to irradiation.

Glomous tumour

This is a rare tumour, very painful when pressure is applied to it. It is commonly found under the fingernails and arises in the glomus bodies. The tumour cells are glomous cells.

The treatment is excision.

SUBCUTANEOUS CYSTS

Sebaceous cysts

They arise in the sebaceous glands and are thus found more commonly on the neck, behind the ears and on the scalp. A sebaceous cyst comprises a round mass which is fixed to the skin and has a punctum. There is often more than one cyst to be found. It sometimes becomes infected and a thick, creamy discharge oozes from the punctum.

The cyst must be opened and its lining removed completely. If the cyst is infected, it is first simply drained and removed later.

Implantation dermoid

These are often confused with sebaceous cysts. They arise as a result of implantation of the dermis, which continues to grow, forming a cyst filled with keratin. An implantation dermoid is also a round skin mass, but does not have a punctum. These must be excised.

Dermoid cysts

These arise at the embryological junctional folds of the face and neck, especially at the eyebrows. They are lined with squamous epithelium and contain keratin. They are not fixed to the skin.

These cysts must be excised.

OTHER SKIN CONDITIONS

Haemangiomas

Capillary haemangiomas

These are usually present either at birth or shortly thereafter. They consist of red, raised flat skin lesions which blanch on pressure. Common types include the port wine stain and strawberry nevus.

Campbell de Morgan spots and spider nevi are seen in older people.

Haemangiomas sometimes ulcerate and become secondarily infected, after which the lesions disappear. Some angiomas disappear spontaneously in time. Port wine stains are difficult to treat and should preferably be covered by cosmetics.

Cavernous haemangiomas

These dark blue lesions are found in the skin and subcutaneous tissues. They usually disappear spontaneously before the age of eight. If they do not disappear, they can be excised, if this is practically possible. Irradiation is sometimes used, with success, if the tumour is at a life-threatening site, e g the throat.

Tumours of the sweat glands

These rare tumours present as solid, round, smooth, well-defined nodules and are found especially on the scalp. The hidradenomata have a cylindromic appearance on histological section. Multiple tumours can cover the scalp and are then known as a turban tumour. Tumours of the apocrine glands of the axillae, perineum or vulva are known as siringomas. Sweat gland tumours sometimes undergo malignant transformation. The treatment is excision.

Infections

Hidradenitis suppurativa

This is a rare condition, but when it presents it is chronic, difficult to treat and causes great pain and discomfort. It is characterized by multiple sinuses which drain pus and are typically found where apocrine glands are common, namely the axillae, groins and perineum.

The lesions sometimes resolve on antibiotic treatment, but must usually be resected. If they occur in a limited area, the raw areas can be allowed to granulate. When excision does become necessary, such a large area usually requires excision, that a skin graft becomes necessary.

Carbuncle

These usually arise in hair follicles and are more common in the nape of the neck. They are caused by Staphylococcus, which causes necrosis due to the coagulase it secretes. A hard indurate, with multiple sinuses, is present. Carbuncles are more common in diabetics.

The pus must be cultured, so that the appropriate antibiotics can be prescribed. If the carbuncle does not improve rapidly, a cruciate incision must be made and the necrotic tissue excised. The skin must not be closed.

Hyperhydrosis

These patients sweat excessively. It can affect the hands, feet and axillae. If the hands are involved, it can prevent the patient from performing his normal daily tasks. The hands can sweat so much that it becomes impossible to write or type.

If the feet sweat excessively, the shoes and socks will always be wet, causing an unpleasant odour and rotting of the shoes.

Conservative treatment with aluminium chloride applications must be attempted. Deodorants are available. Conservative treatment often fails, making surgery essential.

A cervical sympathectomy is performed for the hands and a lumbar sympathectomy for the feet. If the problem is confined to the axillae, the axillary skin, with its sweat glands, can be removed and replaced by a skin graft. If the area is relatively limited, a subcutaneous excision of sweat glands can sometimes be done. The size of the problem area can be determined by painting the axilla with iodine and then sprinkling starch onto this area. In the area where the skin sweats, the iodine will turn blue as it moistens.

THE NAILS

Haematoma

This is usually extremely painful and, depending on the degree of the force causing the haemotoma, an underlying fracture must be excluded on X-ray, because osteomyelitis can arise if it becomes secondarily infected. The treatment of a painful haemotoma is to bore through the nail with a warm needle and allow the blood to drain. In the differential diagnosis, a malignant melanoma and a glomus tumour, which are also very painful, must be borne in mind.

Paronichia

This is an infection which arises in the nailfold of the fingers. The cause is always Staphylococcus. If the condition is not treated promptly, the infection can spread further under the nail and can even involve the pulp space. In the early stages, the condition can be resolved by antibiotics. If pus has already accumulated, it must be drained. Early on, only a small part of the nail can be removed, but later the whole nail must be removed.

Ingrown toenails

The big toe is usually affected. The distal free edge of the nail causes pressure necrosis in the nailfold, which ulcerates and becomes secondarily infected. There is sometimes overgrowth of granulation tissue. The majority of patients can be treated conservatively with success.

Immerse the feet in water as warm as the patient can endure, to soften the nail. Lift the sides of the nail out of the nailfold and place a small cotton plug dipped in tinc.-Benzoin Co under the nail in the nailfold to prevent pressure. Teach the patient to perform this procedure himself. This simple maneouvre solves the problem in most cases. It sometimes becomes necessary to operate on the nails.

SOFT TISSUE TUMOURS

How does the patient present?

Patients present with a solid mass in the subcutaneous tissue or in a muscle compartment, most often in the region of the thighs. At times the mass is situated in the shoulder/scapular region. The nodule can also be found near a joint.

Patients can also complain of loin pain and a retroperitoneal mass may be palpable.

What must the clinician consider?

Any solid mass found deep in muscle compartments, or in the retroperitoneal area, must arouse suspicion of a soft tissue tumour. Solid masses related to joints elicit suspicion of a synovioma.

Soft tissue sarcomas arise from the primitive germ cells. the ectoderm gives rise to the malignant neurilemmomas; and the mesoderm gives rise to the other sarcomas. Most sarcomas also have a benign variant, arising from the same cells.

Some sarcomas are difficult to classify according to cell origin. Poorly differentiated tumours are difficult to classify, even with the help of an electron microscope.

Lipocyte tumours

Benign lipoma: This is soft, grows slowly and has a capsule. Clinically, it is cooler than the surrounding tissues and has slipping edges. Deeply situated lipomas are suggestive of liposarcoma. Histologically, they consist of normal lipocytes.

Liposarcoma: This is a relatively common sarcoma, found most often in men. It is most often situated in the thigh-gluteal region in the deep muscle compartment and is also the most common type of retroperitoneal sarcoma.

It has a pseudocapsule and shells out easily. It is divided into three histological types:

- **Well-differentiated liposarcoma (20%):** Histologically, these are difficult to distinguish from lipomas and have a good prognosis.
- **Myxoid liposarcoma (46%):** These can have different degrees of differentiation. The well-differentiated myxoid liposarcoma has a good prognosis. If a lipoma has a mucoid appearance on removal, a myxoid liposarcoma must be suspected.
- **Pleomorphic liposarcoma (34%):** This is the most malignant type of lipoma. The cells are anaplastic, with pleomorphic cells and mutiple nuclei which stain darkly hyperchromatically. These tumours spread to the lungs, and other organs.

Muscle cell tumours

Benign rhabdomyomas

These are rare tumours, found in the head and neck area. A rhabdomyoma of the tongue muscles is a typical example.

Rhabdomyosarcoma

These are three histological types, namely embryonic, alveolar and pleomorphic rhabdomyosarcoma.

- **Embryonic rhabdomyosarcoma**

  This is a tumour of childhood and is most frequently found in the head and neck, bladder, and vagina. It tends to resemble a bunch of grapes (botryoid growth).

- **Alveolar rhabdomyosarcoma**

  This is a tumour of young people and is found chiefly on the limbs. It is more aggressive than the embryonic type, and spreads via the bloodstream and also lymphatically. Histologically, it resembles a vague glandular structure.

- **Pleomorpic rhabdomyosarcoma**

  This is a tumour found in adults, usually over fifty. It is found mainly in the muscle compartments of the thigh. The tumour is poorly differentiated, with hyperchromatic nuclei. It can be so poorly differentiated as to make histological recognition very difficult. It spreads through the bloodsteam, especially to the lungs.

Leiomyoma

This is a benign tumour of smooth muscle which is found particularly in the gastrointestinal canal. Clinically it presents as an obstruction or bleed due to ulceration on the surface of the tumour. It can be found retroperitoneally.

Leiomyosarcoma

These are found mainly in the gastrointestinal canal. They present as obstruction or bleeding and spread through the bloodstream to the liver. These sarcomas, which are found retroperitoneally, have a poor prognosis. At times the tumours occur in the skin and subcutaneous tissues, where they have a better prognosis.

Tumours of the fibroblasts

Benign fibrous histiocytoma is a common tumour which presents as a nodule in the skin, often on the lower limbs. Malignant fibrous histiocytoma is the most common soft tissue sarcoma. It arises from histiocytes and fibroblasts. It spreads haematogenously and to lymph nodes. This is the sarcoma which most often spreads to lymph nodes.

Superficial sarcomas have a better prognosis than deep-lying tumours. Retroperitoneal tumours have a poor prognosis.

Fibrosarcoma is a malignant tumour which, when found, is usually on the extremities of patients over fifty. Differentiation varies from well-differentiated to totally anaplastic tumours with a poor prognosis.

A variant, the dermatofibrosarcoma protuberans, is a rare skin tumour which tends to recur locally, but very seldom spreads. It presents as a pink or blue mobile nodule in the skin and grows very slowly.

Tumours of the neural sheaths

Most neural sheath tumours are benign and are particularly common in patients with neurofibromatosis, or Von Recklinghausen disease. Benign tumours are called neurilemmomas. Malignant neural sheath tumours are called Schwannomas. These are usually found on the limbs. They either arise *de novo* from the sheaths which envelope small nerves, or in patients with neurofibromatosis.

Patients with malignant Schwannomas arising in neurofibromatoses often have tumours with a poor prognosis, situated on the trunk. These tumours seldom metastasize to lymph nodes and most often spread via the bloodstream.

Tumours of the synovial tissues

These tumours are almost always malignant. They do not generally arise from the synovium of large joints, but more often from tendon sheaths, synovial bursae and aponeuroses. They are found distally on the limbs.

Two histological types have been described:

- The monophasic type, with mainly spindle-shaped cells.
- The biphasic type, consisting of spindle-shaped cells and epithelioid cells, giving a glandular appearance to the tumour. The monophasic tumour has a poorer prognosis.

These tumours tend to recur locally and spread through the bloodstream to the lungs and to lymph nodes.

Tumours of the vascular endothelium

Benign tumours are especially common in children. Haemangiomas and haemangio-endotheliomas are the most common types. The malignant haemangio-endotheliomas are usually found on the scalp, face, chest and extremities. They spread through the bloodstream and the lymph nodes and have a poor prognosis.

Haemangio-pericytomas arise in the pericytes of Zimmerman, which are found on the capillaries. About half these tumours follow a malignant course and tend to recur locally.

Kaposi sarcoma is a variant of angiosarcoma. Lymphangio-sarcomas arise in limbs with chronic oedema. If they arise in the swollen arm that follows radical mastectomy, they are known as the Stewart-Treves syndrome.

Other soft tissue tumours

- Epithelioid-sarcomas are found on the limbs and may be synovial in origin.
- Alveolar soft tissue tumours are found on the limbs of young patients and may arise in Schwann cells.

Management of soft tissue tumours

Factors influencing prognosis and management

The site at which the tumour presents

Tumours which present more distally on the limbs have a more favourable prognosis, probably because they are diagnosed earlier due to their superficial situation. They can also be treated without sacrificing essential anatomical structures and thus without loss of function. Retroperitoneal tumours have a poorer prognosis. They are discovered later and are more difficult to excise widely.

In the thigh region, it is very important that the site of the tumour is determined precisely, in relation to the muscle compartments.

Size of the tumour

The larger the tumour, the poorer the prognosis. Larger tumours will more often already have invaded muscle compartments and important structures such as large nerves and blood vessels, and metastasized. It is difficult to excise them widely without destroying important structures, resulting in loss of function.

Histological appearance and differentiation

The most important prognostic factor is the differentiation of the tumour. Although certain tumours such as synoviomas and rhabdomyosarcomas generally have a poorer prognosis, the differentiation is the overriding consideration. **Two tumours with the same degree of differentiation have the same prognosis, regardless of the histological type.** Poorly differentiated tumours spread more often and are more likely to recur locally after excision.

Age

Rhabdomyosarcomas have a better prognosis in children than in adults.

Practical approach

The primary lesion must be removed surgically, with histologically proven tumourfree edges. The removal of the tumour must be planned so that the limb is spared. To plan the extent of surgery, size, localization and differentiation of the tumour must be determined.

Size and localization are initially determined by means of clinical examination, computer tomography and, where necessary, arteriography. One must determine whether the lesion is confined to a particular muscle, muscle group or muscle compartment. One must also determine whether important structures, such as blood vessels, nerve or bone, are involved. When the size and localization of the tumour have been determined, tissue must be obtained for histological examination.

Biopsy technique

Excision biopsy must not be performed. It opens tissue planes and contaminates tissues with malignant cells.

Incision biopsy

This must be done by the surgeon who is to perform the operation. The incision must be planned so that it can be removed later, along with the specimen.

- The incision must be made directly over the tumour, and, without opening tissue planes, deepened down to the tumour.
- A wedge of tumour must be removed, including surrounding tissue, the outer border and the deeper parts of the tumour.
- Absolute haemostasis must be achieved and the wound must be closed firmly, layer for layer, without drainage.
- The specimen must be handed over to the pathologist personally.
- A frozen section must be made before the wound is closed to ensure that representative tissue has been removed. After this, the pathologist can do histological examinations, including electron microscopy.
- The management is planned after the degree of differentiation has been determined.
- Some researchers believe that a needle biopsy, done by an experienced surgeon, is adequate.

Staging

This is based on histological grading – G, localization – T, and metastasis – M.

Histological grading

G0 – Benign. Cells fully differentiated.

G1 – Low grade malignancy. Moderate differentiation, few mitotic figures. The matrix is well developed.

G2 – High grade maliganancy. Poor differentiation. Cells show pleomorphism and hyperchromatic nuclei. There are many mitotic figures and the matrix is poorly developed.

Localization

T0 – The tumour is well encapsulated and confined to a compartment.

T1 – It infiltrates beyond the pseudocapsule, but is still confined to the compartment.

T2 – It infiltrates through the capsule and has spread out of the compartment.

Metastasis

M0 – No metastasis.

M1 – Metastasis to lymph nodes or via the bloodstream or both.

Management according to staging

G0 T0 M0 – Local excision.

G1 T1 M0 – Excision of the compartment containing the tumour.

G2 T1 M0 – Excision of the compartment containing the tumour, followed by local irradiation and chemotherapy.

Every attempt must be made to spare the limbs. In well-differentiated, small tumours, confined to the compartment, surgery, with excision of the compartment, is probably adequate.

Multimodal treatment can be given for all other tumours, namely a combination of compartment excision, followed by irradiation and chemotherapy. In most series, limbs are spared in 95% of cases and the five year survival rate is higher than 60%.

THE FEMALE BREAST

How does the patient present?

- With a lump in the breast
- With a change in the appearance of the breast
- With deformity
  - The skin is retracted
  - The nipple is retracted
  - The breast is situated higher than usual
  - There is eczema around the nipples
- With pain
- With a discharge from the nipple

What must the clinician consider?

A lump

Common conditions

- Carcinoma
- Fibroadenoma
- Fibroadenosis

Rarer conditions

- Cystosarcoma phylloides
- Fat necrosis
- Gynaecomastia in men

Deformity

Retracted skin:

- Carcinoma
- Fat necrosis

Retracted nipple:

- Carcinoma
- Duct ectasia
- Congenital

Eczema around the nipple:

- Paget carcinoma

Pain

- Acute – inflammation
- Dull (cyclical, menstrual)
- Cysts (fibroadenosis)
- Continuous
  - fibroadenosis
  - carcinoma

Nipple discharge

Not bloody:

- Lactation
- Duct ectasia
- Fibroadenosis

Blood:
- Intraductal papilloma
- Carcinoma

What does the clinician wish to ascertain from the history?

- Is the patient pregnant – painful swollen breasts?
- Has she given birth recently? Abscesses can arise at this stage.
- Is there a family history of carcinoma of the breast – mother, grandmothers, sisters?
- Is the patient on any drugs? – Digitalis and oestrogen cause gynaecomastia.

What is found on examination?

On inspection

Expose both breasts. Have the patient sit and stand in front of her. Note:

- The size – one breast may be larger than the other.
- The position – one breast may be situated higher.
- The nipples and areola – is the nipple retracted or is there eczema around the areola?

Raise the arms

This elicits differences in position or accentuates changes which have already been noted on inspection.

Allow the patient to lean forward and note the skin and the nipples. There is now traction on Cooper's ligaments and skin or nipple retraction is accentuated. The above signs are indicative of carcinoma.

Wrinkling of the skin or skin ulceration may be visible. Skin oedema (peau d'orange) indicates carcinoma.

A swollen, red, shiny breast suggests a breast abscess.

On palpation

Is there evidence of a mass or perhaps several?

- A single rubberlike, hard, irregular, poorly defined, immobile mass indicates carcinoma.
- A mass fixed to deep-lying tissues or skin confirms carcinoma.
- A single, rubberlike, hard, regular, well-defined, mobile mass indicates fibroadenoma.
- Multiple masses indicate fibroadenosis.
- Multiple masses with a prominent, well-defined, dominant mass indicate a cyst.
- Multiple masses with a dominant, hard, poorly defined mass are suggestive of carcinoma.
- Also examine the mobility of the mass.
- Can nipple discharge be produced?

Regardless of the nature of the discharge, if a mass is present in the breast, assess it on its own merits. The nipple discharge only serves to draw attention to the mass.

If there is no associated mass – is the discharge bloody? Does it come from one duct? A bloody discharge which comes from one duct, indicates an intraductal papilloma. A bloody discharge issuing from multiple ducts, is suggestive of carcinoma, but may also be the result of duct ectasia with infection.

A nonbloody discharge is more commonly due to fibroadenosis or ductal ectasia.

The axilla

Allow the patient to rest her hand on your shoulder and palpate the axilla from the front. Feel carefully for the pectoral, apical and lateral or humeral groups.

Also palpate the axilla from behind, with the patient seated on a chair. This makes it easire to feel the posterior group of axillary lymph nodes.

- Are the lymph nodes enlarged?
- Are the lymph nodes matted?
- Are the lymph nodes still mobile?
- Are there nodes in the opposite axilla or the supraclavicular region?

Also examine:

- The opposite breast
- The bone skeleton: skull, clavicles, ribs and spinal column
- Is there a prominent spine which indicates collapse of a vertebral body?

Examine the lungs

- Is there an effusion?

Examine the abdomen

- Is the liver enlarged?
- Is there ascites?
- Do a rectal examination. + PV

Special investigations

Mammography

X-rays of the soft tissues of the breast and axillae.

Indications

- Nodular breasts with a dominant nodule.
- Pain in the breast, particularly if it is unilateral and no lump is palpable.
- Large breasts, which are difficult to examine, where there is doubt about the presence of a lump.
- Bloody discharge from the nipple, especially from multiple ducts, if no lump is palpable.
- The opposite breast in a women who already has carcinoma of the ipsilateral breast.
- To remove an impalpable lesion under mammographic guidance with a hooked needle, which is placed in the breast.

Screening tests

Mammography, when used as a general screening test in large populations, is not cost-effective. It is a useful investigation for checking high risk patients annually. These risk factors include:

- Previous carcinoma in one breast, where mammography is performed on the opposite breast.
- A history of carcinoma which presented at a young age in family members.
- Mammography is useless in young women under thirty-five, because the breast tissue is too dense.
- Mammography is not useful where there is a lump. The decision whether to operate on a single lump does not depend on mammography. If the result for malignancy is negative, the lump must be removed in any case. Mammography yields false negative results in 5% of cases.

Aspiration cytology

A 20 cc syringe and an ordinary needle are used. Penetrate the mass with the needle, applying slight suction to the syringe. Move the needle and make a few stabbing movements. Place the contents of the needle on a slide and seal it with sealing material. Carcinoma can be diagnosed in 95% of cases.

A negative result must be ignored in a clinically suspicious lesion and material must be obtained for histology. If the lesion is cystic, it must be aspirated until empty and the fluid must be sent for cytology.

The mass must disappear completely after aspiration and if any residual mass is palpable, a biopsy must be taken for histological diagnosis.

Needle biopsy

This is performed on a mass with clinical stigmata of carcinoma in order to confirm the diagnosis histologically.

Carcinoma of the breast

This is the most common malignant tumour found in women. One out of fourteen will contract the disease. It causes 20% of cancer deaths in women and twenty-two out of a hundred thousand die anually of breast cancer.

- **Older women:** There is a steady increase in incidence until the menopause, whereupon the incidence remains constant for five years and then slowly rises again.
- Women with **fibroadenosis** – particularly with epithelial hyperplasia.
- **Childless women**, or those who had their first child after thirty.
- A positive **family history of breast cancer.**
- A history of **early menarche and late menopause.**
- Women who have already had **cancer of the opposite breast**, or endometrial-, ovarian- or colonic carcinoma.

Aetiology

Three factors play a role:

- Viral
- Hormonal
- Genetic

Viruses

It is well known that viruses transported by milk cause cancer in mice. Thus far no concrete proof has been found that this applies to humans.

Hormones

Hormones play a rôle at different stages of the natural course of carcinoma of the breast. The disease is more common in women who have had long, uninterrupted cyclical ovarian function. On the other hand, removal of the ovaries before puberty protects the patient against cancer. Hormonal manipulation plays a rôle in the treatment of the disease. Seventy per cent of breast cancer cells have oestrogen receptors which influence the prognosis. Use of the "pill" does not increase the incidence of breast cancer.

Genes

The risk of developing breast cancer is two to three times greater in families where a close family member has had breast cancer.

Pathological classification

Originating in the ducts

Non-infiltrating

- *Intraductal carcinoma (comedocarcinoma)*

Infiltrating

- *Infiltrating ductal carcinoma (scirrhous carcinoma)*
- *Medullary carcinoma*
- *Colloid carcinoma*
- *Tubular carcinoma*
- *Paget disease*

Originating in the lobules

Non-infiltrating

- *Lobular carcinoma in situ*

Infiltrating

- *Lobular carcinoma*

Intraductal carcinoma (comedocarcinoma: 5% of breast cancers)

This is so named because it proliferates until the ducts are packed full of anaplastic cells, which can be expressed from the nipple. The carcinoma eventually infiltrates through the basal membrane.

Infiltrating ductal carcinoma (75% of breast cancers)

This is a hard lesion and is sometimes known as scirrhous carcinoma. Histologically, it consists of a dense stroma of connective tissue, with nests or cords of cancer cells.

Medullary carcinoma (5% of breast cancers)

This is a large, soft, fleshy tumour. Histologically, it has very little fibrous stroma, with strings of carcinoma cells and well-developed lymphocyte infiltration.

Colloid carcinoma

This is a soft carcinoma, characterized by a lot of mucin, with islands of cells in the mucin. Sometimes the cells contain a lot of mucin in their cytoplasm and have a signet ring appearance.

Paget disease

This starts as an intraductal carcinoma which grows up into the lactiferous duct and involves the skin of the areola. Paget cells, which infiltrate the epidermis, are characteristic of the disease. Paget cells are large, hyperchromatic cells surrounded by a clear ring, caused by intracellular accumulation of mucopolysaccharides.

Tubular carcinoma

This is difficult to differentiate from sclerosing adenitis. It forms glandular structures in the fibrous stroma. Only the anaplastic appearance of the cells distinguishes them from sclerosing adenosis.

Lobular carcinoma

This arises in the acini or terminal ductules of the lobules. Clinically it does not present as a mass, but is usually found coincidentally on histological sections of biopsies done for other reasons, e g fibroadenosis.

Histologically, we find acini filled with neoplastic cells. It is often found bilaterally in mirrorimage biopsy of the opposite breast (20%).

The importance of this condition is that it becomes infiltrating in about 20% of cases.

Infiltrating lobular carcinoma

This presents as a poorly defined, rubberlike, hard mass. Histologically, it often comprises single rows of malignant cells or cells which are loosely spread in the connective tissue stroma. Sometimes they are arranged around acini in a typical "bull's eye" pattern. The tumour is rare (5%), but important because it often occurs bilaterally.

Staging

Before a decision is taken on management of breast cancer, it must be staged.

The most commonly used staging method is the TNM staging.

Tumour – T

TIS – Carcinoma in *situ*
– Non-infiltrating intraductal carcinoma or Paget disease without a palpable mass
T1 – Tumour smaller than 2 cm
T2 – Tumour 2–5 cm
T3 – Tumour larger than 5 cm
T4 – Tumour infiltrates skin, chest wall: peau d'orange or ulceration

Lymph nodes – N

N0 – No palpable lymph nodes
N1 – Loose, mobile lymph nodes
N2 – Lymph nodes fixed to each other or to underlying structures
N3 – Supraclavicular lymph nodes or swollen arm

Metastases – M

M0 – None
M1 – Metastases present
MX – Suspected metastases

Modified Manchester staging is useful when the clinician needs to assess operability.

Operable

Stage I

- Mass confined to the breast
- No nodes
- No metastasis

Stage II

- Mass confined to the breast
- No skin or chest wall infiltration
- Mobile nodes in the axilla

Inoperable

Stage III

- Mass infiltrates skin or chest wall
- Lymph nodes larger than 5 cm in diameter and/or fixed.
- Inoperable, due to advanced local disease

Stage IV

- Any local lesion
- Any node involvement with distal metastasis
- Inoperable for distal reasons (metastases)

Management of a breast lump in which malignancy is suspected

- *Needle biopsy. If positive, clinical staging*
- *If* **Stage I**, *X-rays of the lungs and alkaline phosphatase*
- *If negative, surgery recommended*

Standard operation

Modified radical mastectomy, comprising total removal of the breast tissue and a complete dissection of the axilla, without removal of the pectoral muscles.

- **Alternative**

Removal of the mass, together with a 2 cm border of normal breast tissue. The nipple and areola must be spared. Complete dissection of the axilla, via a separate incision. Irradiation of the remaining breast tissue.

In both cases, adjuvant chemotherapy is recommended if the lymph nodes are found to be histologically positive.

Stage II

The lymph nodes are clinically palpable, but mobile. The implication is that there is a much greater chance that distal metastasis has already taken place. Staging must therefore include chest X-rays, alkaline phosphatase, a radio-isotope scan of the liver and a bone scan.

Modified radical mastectomy, with detachment and insertion of the pectoralis minor muscle tendon on the coracoid process, so that a more thorough axillary block dissection can be achieved. If lymph node involvement has been confirmed histologically, adjuvant chemotherapy is administered.

Stage III

The cancer is inoperable because of an advanced local lesion, infiltration of the skin or chest wall, or matted or fixed lymph nodes. The local lesion is usually irradiated and the patient receives chemotherapy after the lesion has been diagnosed histologically and the oestrogen receptors have been measured.

If the local lesion can be removed without cutting through tumour, surgery can be attempted.

Stage IV

The cancer is inoperable due to distal metastasis. The histology and oestrogen receptors must be determined and the patient treated with chemotherapy and/or hormonal treatment. The local lesion can be irradiated or removed surgically.

The management of exceptional cases of breast cancer

Minimal breast cancer

It is described as minimal if no mass is palpable. It is usually discovered on a mammogram. Screening mammograms should be done annually in women over forty who have a close relative with breast cancer. Microcalcification, or a mass with surrounding oedema and outgrowths, are the signs to note. A histological specimen must be taken of such masses with the help of needle localisation. The needle has a small hook at its end to prevent shifting. Mammography must be done to ensure that the point of the needle is in the correct position. After removal of the needle, mammography must be repeated to ensure that the correct tissue has been removed.

If infiltrating duct carcinoma is confirmed on histology, a modified radical mastectomy must be performed.

• The alternative

Excision of the mass and block dissection of the axilla, followed by irradiation of the remaining breast tissue. If the lymph nodes are positive, adjuvant chemotherapy must be given.

Inflammatory breast cancer

This usually presents with a mass larger than 5 cm, with inflammatory skin signs, namely warmth, erythema and thickening of the skin.

Biopsy is required for confirmation of the diagnosis. The management is chemotherapy, with adjuvant irradiation of the breast, or, if possible, surgical removal once the inflammatory tumour has stabilized.

Lobular carcinoma in situ

If only an excision biopsy is done, 20% develop infiltrating lobular carcinoma, 10% in the same breast and an equal percentage in the opposite breast. In larger lesions, an ipsilateral mastectomy must be done, in conjunction with permanent follow-up of the opposite breast.

• Alternative

In the case of small lesions, an excision of the lesion must be done, with annual mammographic follow-up to identify further tumours at an early stage.

Bilateral breast carcinoma

Women with breast cancer have a 5% chance of developing cancer in the other breast. If it is discovered within eighteen months of the first cancer, it is probably due to metastasis from the first tumour. If later, it is more likely to be a second primary.

Carcinoma which recurs locally

If it arises in the skin flaps, it is usually an indication of systemic disease. Confirm the diagnosis and treat with chemotherapy or hormonal therapy.

If the lesion arises in the scar itself, it may be due to cell implantation. Excise and stage completely. If systemic disease is found, treat with chemotherapy or hormonal therapy.

Breast cancer in men

This is usually found in men over sixty-five. Only 1% of breast cancers are found in men.

If the mass is larger than 2 cm, a radical mastectomy must be done. Muscle must be removed, so that one can excise widely around the tumour. In masses smaller than 2 cm, a modified radical mastectomy must be done. Results are poorer than in women.

Breast cancer in pregnancy

This diagnosis is sometimes difficult, because of intumescence of the breast. This can delay the diagnosis. Apart from this factor, there is no difference in prognosis. If the diagnosis has been made, treat breast carcinoma in pregnancy on merit. If it was an early carcinoma, with no nodes, the patient can become pregnant again. If nodes were positive, discourage further pregnancies, as the disease has a poor prognosis.

What influences the prognosis?

Histological grading

It is usually graded from Grades I to III. The more anaplastic the lesion, the poorer the prognosis.

Histological type of tumour

After twenty years of follow-up, the following survival figures are found after treatment:

- Comedocarcinoma 75%
- Papillary carcinoma 65%
- Medullary carcinoma 60%
- Infiltrating lobular carcinoma 35%
- Infiltrating duct carcinoma 30%

Staging

If the lesion is smaller than 2 cm and no lymph nodes are affected, the survival after five years is 85%.

In contrast, if the lesion is larger than 5 cm and the lymph nodes are involved, the five year survival is 40%. Where all cases with positive nodes are followed up, the ten year survival is 25%, while those with negative nodes have a ten year survival of 65%.

From the above facts it is clear that the smaller primary lesion, with negative nodes, has a better prognosis. It is also clear that if lymph nodes are involved, this is strongly indicative of systemic disease. Factors which may further influence the prognosis are early diagnosis and adjuvant treatment of systemic micrometastases if lymph nodes were positive.

Screening tests to make an early diagnosis

Self-examination of the breasts

Published studies show that monthly self-examination of the breasts by women is more effective for early discovery of breast cancer than annual examination by a doctor, or tumours discovered by chance. These patients have a 20% better chance of survival.

Screening mammography

This does not apply to women under the age of thirty-five. Breast tissue is too dense and the incidence of carcinoma in this group is so low that it is not cost-effective. Furthermore, there is a small risk of increased incidence of breast cancer due to the irradiation that the patient will receive over a long period of time.

It has now been recommended that screening mammography should be performed only on women over the age of forty with known risk factors, such as close family members with the disease or a history of carcinoma in the other breast.

Adjuvant therapy to treat possible microscopic systemic disease

Chemotherapy

Adjuvant chemotherapy, namely low doses of chemotherapy in cases where no metastasis is clinically demonstrable but where there have been positive lymph nodes, improves the five year survival in premenopausal patients. Various combinations are used:

The main groups comprise the following:

- *Antimetabolites:*
  5-Fluorouracil
  Methotrexate

- *Alkylating drugs:*
  Cyclophosphamide
  Melfalan
- *Cytotoxic antibiotics:*
  Adriamycin
  Mitoxantrone
- *Spindle toxins*
  Vincristine
  Vinblastine

A common combination is cyclophosphamide + methotrexate + 5-Fluorouracil.

Adjuvant chemotherapy is being studied in prospective series for use when the nodes are negative, but other risk factors such as a large mass (2 – 5 cm), poor differentiation and ER negative, are present; but is not standard practice at present.

Hormonal therapy

Surgical endocrine intervention, such as oöphorectomy and adrenalectomy, have now been replaced by the use of antioestrogen agents such as Tomoxifen and the adrenal steroid aromatic inhibitor, aminoglutethamide.

Before hormonal drugs are used, it is important to determine the oestrogen and progesterone receptor status. About 66% of carcinomas are ER positive and about 66% of these respond to hormonal therapy. Patients with positive ER have a better prognosis.

It is safer to treat older women with Tomoxifen. They react adversely to the side effects of the cytotoxics.

The primary operation

It has become clear from several prospective series that there is no significant difference between the results obtained in operable breast cancers by radical mastectomy (Halstead, with removal of the pectoral muscle), modified radical mastectomy (with retention of the pectoral muscle); and excision of the mass with block dissection of the axillary nodes, all followed by irradiation of the breast tissue.

Breast reconstruction following mastectomy

For the patient's morale it is very important for her to know that plastic reconstruction of the breast can be considered after mastectomy. It is usually advisable to wait eighteen months before considering reconstruction. Two methods are used:

- *Placement of a prosthesis deep to the pectoralis major muscle to restore the contour of the breast.*
- *The use of tissue flaps of muscle, subcutaneous fat and skin, with reconstruction of the nipple. After eighteen months, most women have accepted the situation and do not desire reconstruction.*

Benign conditions

Most breast lumps are benign. It is useful to divide the most likely diagnosis into groups according to age:

Under thirty-five

- Fibroadenosis
- Fibroadenoma
- Mastitis – usually related to lactation
- Carcinoma – rare in this group
- Fat necrosis – very rare

Thirty to fifty

- Fibroadenosis
- Carcinoma
- Fibroadenoma
- Mastitis – sometimes due to duct ectasia
- Fat necrosis – rare
- Intraductal papilloma – rare

Older than fifty

- Carcinoma
- Fibroadenosis
- Fat necrosis
- Mastitis – associated with duct ectasia

Fibroadenosis

It is clear that fibroadenosis is the most common condition found in the female breast. It is found in 50% of women. It is synonymous with fibrocystic disease of the breast, chronic cystic mastitis. The aetiology is not completely clear, but is is a reaction by the breast to the hormonal changes of the normal menstrual cycle, with hypertrophy and regression of the breast tissue. The hyperplastic changes can be initiated by oestrogen. The use of oral hormonal contraceptive preparations reduces the incidence of these changes.

Pathological types

Fibrosis of the breast

This is found to a larger or lesser extent in all forms of fibroadenosis. It is sometimes decidedly marked, with only mild epithelial hyperplasia and virtually no cyst formation, especially in younger women.

Cysts

These are found in the older age group, often just before the menopause. There is stromal and epithelial hyperplasia, with cyst formation of the lobules. These cysts are usually multiple and bilateral and can be microscopic or up to 5 cm in diameter. They sometimes contain a transparent fluid, which gives the breast a bluish tinge. The cysts are sometimes lined by large cells with acidophilic cytoplasm, so-called apocrine metaplasia. The epithelium can also be completely atrophic.

Sclerosing adenosis

This is characterized by reduplication of glands or terminal ducts, with a marked stromal fibrosis, which can compress the ducts to such a degree that they resemble a string of cells in a fibrous stroma and can be confused with carcinoma.

Epithelial hyperplasia

This is characterized by intraductal epithelial hyperplasia with multiple cell layers. The ducts are sometimes filled with cuboid cells. This form of fibroadenosis is associated with an increased incidence of breast carcinoma.

Importance of fibroadenosis

It must be differentiated from carcinoma of the breast. Usually this is easy. Pain just before the menses, mastodinia, is common. Multiple nodules are found, usually in both breasts. Cysts can form discrete nodules and can be painful or painless. There is often a yellow, green or brown discharge from the nipples. Histologically, it is sometimes difficult to distinguish epithelial hyperplasia from carcinoma. The important difference is that there is no infiltration of the basal membrane in fibroadenosis. Although it has never been proven that fibroadenosis is a direct precursor of carcinoma, the incidence of carcinoma is increased fourfold in patients with epithelial hyperplasia.

Diagnosis and symptoms

Cysts

- Aspirate the cysts
- If the fluid contains no blood and the mass disappears completely and does not refill rapidly, nothing further need be done.
- If a cytologist is available, the cells in the fluid can be examined.
- If the mass does not disappear, or if the fluid contains blood and the cyst refills rapidly, remove the mass for histology.

Mastodinia

Pain in the breast, uni- or bilateral, without any obvious cause, is called mastodinia. The pain can be cyclical or persistent.

Cyclical pain

This is usually found just before the menses. It is often associated with fibroadenosis. Other factors are methylxanthine-containing diets (with ingredients such as coffee, tea and chocolate) and the nicotine in cigarettes. If the pain is very severe, the androgen analogue, Danazol, can be tried, but it has many side effects. The prolactin inhibitor bromocriptine helps some patients. Another cause of pain is an inadequate bra, which is either too small or too large. Breast pain can also be caused by jogging for long distances, without an adequate bra.

Persistent pain

If continuous pain presents in a breast and no cause can be found, it is essential to do mammography to exclude an underlying lesion. Carcinoma is seldom the cause of the pain.

Fibroadenoma

This is usually found between the ages of twenty-five and forty. It is a simple, well-defined, mobile tumour. There may be more than one tumour and the condition may even present bilaterally. The harder pericanalicular type is found in younger women. This consists of dilated glands in a fibrous stroma. The softer intracanalicular fibroadenoma is found in older women. In this tumour, the ducts are compressed in a stellate pattern in a fibrous stroma.

There is often a mixture of the two histological types. If the tumour becomes very large, a giant fibroadenoma, it can cause pressure necrosis of the tissues.

Cystosarcoma phylloides

The phylloides tumour is a large fibroadenoma with an active stroma. It is a benign tumour. The stroma sometimes undergoes malignant transformation and can then spread through the bloodstream and sometimes also to the lymph nodes. A small tumour can be excised, leaving a free border of normal tissue. If the tumour is large, a mastectomy must be performed, otherwise local recurrence is a common problem.

Intraductal papilloma

This manifests as a single neoplasm in a single duct, or as generalized papillosis in multiple ducts. The lesion is usually too small to present as a palpable mass and it then presents as a bloody discharge from the nipple, usually from one duct. This neoplasm is benign, but it sometimes infiltrates and becomes a papillary carcinoma.

Discharge from the nipple

If a nipple discharge focuses attention on breast pathology, the most important thing is to make sure that there is no underlying mass. If there is a mass, the further management entails treatment of the mass or masses in the breast, as has already been discussed. If no mass is palpable, attention must be focused on the discharge.

The following questions are relevant:

- What is the nature of the discharge?
- Is it bloody?
- Does it come from one or many ducts?

Blood exuding from one duct is an intraductal papilloma. Pass a sound into the duct and excise – this operation is known as a microdochectomy. The papilloma can be found in the duct and must be examined histologically to confirm the diagnosis.

Blood from multiple ducts – do mammography. If there is a suspicious lesion, excise the segment and make a histological diagnosis. Send the discharge for cytological examination for malignant cells.

A nonbloody discharge from multiple ducts is usually a sign of fibroadenosis. Carcinoma very seldom presents with a bloody discharge from the nipple, but if the blood exudes from multiple ducts, do mammography and cytology to exclude malignancy.

Inflammatory conditions of the breast

Breast abscess

lactating

This is usually associated with the puerperium. *Staphylococcus aureus* causes cellulitis in the tissue around the ducts. The breast is red, very painful and tender. There are often systemic signs of infection, fever and listlessness. The breast is engorged.

Administer antibiotics and empty the breast by careful manual expression of the milk. The baby can suckle on the opposite side in the early stages. It is seldom necessary to suppress lactation with bromocriptine.

One must be wary of treating the patient for too long on antibiotics, as a destructive, smouldering infection may be present, which should preferably be drained. Radial incision and insertion of a finger to break down lobulations, followed by insertion of a corrugated drain, is the treatment of choice. If possible, make the incision in an inferior position without cutting through normal breast tissue, in order to effect drainage.

Periareolar abscess

Abscesses which arise in the breasts of nonlactating women, usually recur repeatedly after drainage. A lactiferous duct fistula arises due to obstruction by keratin plugs in lactiferous ducts, where squamous metaplasia of the lining of the duct has arisen. The abscess resolves when the fistula is formally excised. A sound must be inserted from the opening at the edge of the areola to the nipple. A keratin plug is usually squeezed out. The fistula must then be excised and left to granulate.

Chronic inflammation of the breast

Duct ectasia

Intraductal debris and keratin accumulate in multiple dilated lactiferous ducts. A duct can rupture into the surrounding tissue, with an auto-immune inflammatory response of plasma cells and giant cells. Usually, culture is negative after drainage of such an inflammatory swelling. Plasma cell mastitis is an alternative name for this condition. After recurrent secondary infection, multiple abscesses can be found in the subareolar region, with nipple retraction, which can mimic carcinoma.

If the condition is confined to a segment, it can be excised. Sometimes so many ducts are involved that a cone excision becomes necessary. A halfmoon circular incision must be made around the areola, the areola and the nipple lifted and the ducts excised. The skin is then closed, and a corrugated drain left in position.

Tuberculosis

This can affect the breast itself, or arise as a result of a retromammary abscess from the thoracic cavity. The axillary lymph nodes may be involved by systemic tuberculosis, with secondary lymphoedema of the breast skin, which mimics the peau d'orange seen in breast cancer. The diagnosis can be made on biopsy and treated with antitubercular drugs.

Fat necrosis

This can be caused by trauma, but about half these cases have no history of trauma. A tender, well-defined mass can sometimes present, with skin retraction which can make it look like carcinoma. The lesion consists of a central focus on necrotic fat cells, surrounded by neutrophils and macrophages, which is later infiltrated by mononuclear leucocytes. The macrophages eventually remove the necrotic tissue, which is then replaced by fibrosis, which will retract the skin.

The importance of this lesion is to differentiate it from carcinoma by means of biopsy.

Gynaecomastia

This condition is found in young boys at puberty, or in older men, around the age of sixty. It can be uni- or bilateral, painful or painless. The cause is physiological (hormonal) at puberty. It must be treated conservatively and usually disappears within a year.

In older men, hormonal causes must be considered. Increased secretion of oestrogen, e g by testicular or adrenal tumours, is a very rare cause. Reduced breakdown of endogenous oestrogen due to liver cirrhosis is sometimes the cause. It can also be caused by oestrogen administration in prostatic carcinoma. The most common cause in older men is drugs. Digitalis, cimetidine and spironolactone are common culprits. The condition must be differentiated from carcinoma by means of biopsy and the treatment is simple excision.

The inguinal area and scrotum 7

What does the patient complain of?

- A lump in the groin region
- A dull pain in the groin region
- A severe pain in the groin region

What else does the clinician wish to ascertain?

- **About the lump**

Is it always present, or does it come and go? Does it appear when the patient stands and disappear when he lies down? Does it move downwards into the scrotum?

- **About the pain**

Is the pain there constantly, or does it disappear when the patient lies down? Is the pain associated with nausea?

- **Other information**

Is it the only lump, or are there similar lumps, eg in the opposite groin, axillae, or the neck? Are there any lesions on the lower limb?

What must the clinician consider?

- **Inguinal hernia**

In the early stages, a hernia can present with only a dull pain, without the patient having noticed any lump.

A lump which appears when the patient stands, and disappears when he lies down, is usually an uncomplicated inguinal hernia.

Do not ignore the possibility of a saphenous varix. This also protrudes when the patient stands, and disappears when he lies down. It is found in the femoral triangle.

- **Femoral hernia**

This presents with a lump in the inguinal area, which may disappear when the patient lies down, but is more inclined to persist even in the supine position.

- **Enlarged inguinal lymph nodes**

Painful, tender, palpable lymph nodes are usually secondary to an inflammatory nidus in the drainage area – in the lower leg, perineum, scrotal skin, penis and abdominal wall.

Painless enlarged lymph nodes may form part of the generalized lymphadenopathy of lymphoma and Hodgkin disease. Usually other nodes are also palpable. Painless enlarged lymph nodes may contain metastases from skin tumours, melanoma or squamous cell carcinoma of the drainage area.

- **Lipoma**

A lipoma, or other rarer benign tumours of the inguinal canal, presents as a solid, painless mass.

- **Ectopic testis**

A testis may be palpable in the inguinal region. The scrotum may be empty or have only one testis in its normal position.

- **Cystic masses**

A hydrocele of the cord, a cyst of the canal of Nuck, a saphenous varix and an aneurysm of the femoral artery must be considered.

THE SCROTUM

What does the patient complain of?

- A painless mass
- A mass with vague pain
- A very painful mass
- Absence of the testis

What else does the clinician wish to ascertain?

- Did the mass appear suddenly?
- Did it arise following physical activity?
- Does the urine burn and is there a urethral discharge?
- Does the mass disappear when the patient lies down?

What must the clinician consider?

- A solid painless mass in the scrotum – consider testicular tumours, seminoma and teratoma.
- A cystic, painless mass – consider a hydrocele.
- A mass with vague pain – consider testicular tumours, or chronic infections such as tuberculosis or syphilis.
- A very painful mass – consider torsion of the testis and epididymo-orchitis or a strangulated indirect inguinal hernia.

INGUINAL HERNIAS

A hernia arises when the lining and contents of a body cavity protrude abnormally, through a weak point or hiatus, into other body cavities or tissue planes.

The components of such a hernia are a sac, the contents of the sac and the hernial neck or ring (the weak point or hiatus).

- **An uncomplicated hernia** usually reduces spontaneously or can be manually reduced. It appears when the pressure in the body cavity is raised, e g by coughing.
- **An irreducible hernia:** The hernia does not reduce spontaneously and cannot be reduced manually, but there is no complication such as obstruction or strangulation present.
- **An incarcerated hernia:** The hernia is not only irreducible, but the contents of the hernia (bowel) are incarcerated and there is usually obstruction.
- **A strangulated hernia:** This is a serious complication, where the blood supply of the contents of an incarcerated hernia (bowel) is compromised, causing ischaemia and eventual bowel necrosis.
- **A Richter hernia:** In this type of hernia, part of the bowel wall becomes incarcerated, with strangulation. Total obstruction does not occur and the main blood supply of the bowel is not compromised. This usually occurs when there is partial protrusion of the small bowel into a femoral hernia.
- **A sliding hernia:** This is a hernia where the hernial contents form part of the hernial sac. In the inguinal region, this will consist of caecum on the right and sigmoid colon on the left. It can also contain bladder.

Comparison between indirect and direct inguinal hernia

Indirect inguinal hernia

This hernia can arise due to imcomplete closure of the *processus vaginalis*, or it can force a new sac open, adjacent to the cord in the obliterated *processus*, which projects into the scrotum. The sac comes through the internal opening and lies in the inguinal canal. It can run through the external opening into the scrotum.

Direct inguinal hernia

The sac bulges out directly through the posterior wall of the canal, through Hesselbach's triangle. It stretches the transverse fascia or splits the fibres. Hesselbach's triangle is formed by the inferior epigastric artery laterally, the edge of the rectus sheath medially and the inguinal ligament inferiorly.

Clinical differentiation between the two hernia types

- Reduce the hernia.
- Use a finger to close the internal opening, situated between the anterior iliac spine and the pubic tubercle.

- Raise the intra-abdominal pressure by asking the patient to cough.
- If the hernia still appears medial to one's finger, it is a direct hernia, which protrudes directly through Hesselbach's triangle.
- If the hernia can be controlled by closing the internal opening and appears when the finger is removed, it is an indirect hernia.

At operation, the hernia is classified by noting the relationship of the hernial neck to the inferior epigastric artery. An indirect hernia lies lateral to the artery and a direct hernia lies medial.

Complications of inguinal hernia

The most important complication is strangulation. A strangulated hernia is hard, painful and irreducible.

Management of inguinal hernias

Hernias found in children and young men are usually indirect, with a patent processus vaginalis. If an older patient presents with a hernia, underlying causes of raised intra-abdominal pressure must be considered. The usual causes include chronic cough and constipation. Always consider carcinoma of the colon in older patients. There is controversy as to whether prostatism plays a rôle in hernia formation. It is probably advisable to treat prostatism before performing a hernia repair.

Conservative management

A truss can be applied to indirect hernias in totally unfit patients. It works by closing the inguinal canal. It is not suitable for femoral or direct inguinal hernias. A truss should seldom be considered.

Surgical repair of hernias

The principles of hernia repair are as follows: Reduce the contents of the sac, remove the sac and repair the defect.

Indirect hernia

- *Reduce the bowel.*
- *Dissect the sac away from the cord, ligate its neck at the internal ring and remove the sac.*
- *Plicate the transverse fascia.*
- *Suture the conjoint tendon to the inguinal ligament in order to strengthen the posterior wall.*
- *Reduce the internal ring.*
- *Close the external oblique muscle over the inguinal canal.*
- *In women, the inguinal canal can be obliterated completely after the sac and round ligament have been ligated.*

Direct inguinal hernias

The principles remain constant, except that the sac bulging through Hesselbach's triangle cannot be removed. It must be invaginated into the opening and the transverse fascia sutured over it. Apart from this, the repair is identical.

Femoral hernias

Femoral hernias are more commonly found in women than in men. However, inguinal hernias are still more common, even in women, than femoral hernias. The sac of a femoral hernia bulges out through the femoral canal. The boundaries of this canal are:

- The pubis and reflected inguinal ligament, known as the lacunar ligament, medially
- The femoral vein laterally
- The inguinal ligament anteriorly
- The pectineal section of the pubis posteriorly. The neck is narrow and a femoral hernia can therefore easily become strangulated.

Management

Surgery

The principles of hernia repair are applied. Reduce the contents, remove the sac and repair the defect. The hernia can be approached from the inguinal side, or from the abdominal side. After the sac has been removed, the femoral canal is closed by suturing the inguinal ligament, the lacunar ligament and the fascia, to the pectineus muscle. A femoral hernia can also be approached via the inguinal canal. The conjoint tendon is sutured to Cooper's ligament to close the defect.

If the hernia is operated on from above, the inguinal ligament must be sutured to the pectineal fascia.

Incarcerated hernias

If a patient presents with a irreducible hernia, an attempt can be made to reduce the hernia if the condition has been present for only a few hours and the signs of strangulation, namely hardness and pain, are absent. It must be remembered that a hernial sac can sometimes be reduced without allowing the bowel to escape from the sac (reduction *en masse*). Bowel obstruction can then persist.

It is highly unlikely that bowel which has already strangulated will be able to be pushed back with careful reduction.

Lay the patient on a bed and give IV morphine (0,15 mg/kg). The hernia sometimes reduces spontaneously when the patient relaxes. If this does not occur, do not persist, rather operate.

The operation

Take care that the strangulated bowel is not allowed to slip back into the abdominal cavity. Extend the neck of the internal opening laterally. Remember that the artery lies medially. Pull out the bowel, cover it with warm swabs and wait for half an hour. Often the bowel recovers and it can then be replaced. If not, resect the dead bowel and repair the hernia. Unfortunately, wound sepsis is relatively common and broad spectrum antibiotics should be given.

When a femoral hernia is irreducible, it is better to approach it from above so that one can transect the lacunar ligament under direct vision. If this is done from below, an abnormal obturator artery can be accidentally severed.

Strangulated Richter hernia of the femoral canal

This is one of the pitfalls in surgery. An elderly, obese female patient presents with acute abdomen and the inguinal region is not examined thoroughly, or even if it is, the small hard mass is missed because of the obesity. Surgery is delayed and a strangulated Richter hernia is found on laparotomy.

Other rare hernias

Epigastric hernia

This is a small hernia through the *linea alba* between the xiphisternum and the umbilicus. It contains fat and does not normally have a sac.

Para-umbilical hernia

This is commonly found in obese, middle-aged women. It is a hernia just above the umbilicus through the *linea alba*. It has a sac and is inclined to become strangulated. The hernia must be repaired after weight loss.

Spigelian hernia

This is a hernia through the *linea semilunaris* in the rectus sheath. The patient presents with a mass in the lower abdomen just lateral to the midline. The mass disappears when he lies down. This hernia must be differentiated from a haematoma of the rectus sheath. This is a condition which can arise after slight trauma in patients with bleeding tendencies or degenerative arterial disease. A very tender mass is found in the rectus sheath in the lower abdomen. Skin discolouration and ecchymosis can sometimes be seen. Ultrasound is useful in differentiating between a tumour and a haematoma.

A Spigelian hernia has a tendency to cause obstruction and must be repaired.

Obturator hernia

This is found mainly in older women. The small bowel herniates through the obturator foramen. Pressure on the obturator nerve can cause pain in the anteromedial aspect of the thigh. Patients must undergo emergency surgery.

Lumbar hernia

This is a hernia through the Lumbar triangle. The superior triangle is larger and more commonly involved than the smaller, more inferior Petit triangle. These hernias tend to enlarge and must be repaired.

Littre hernia

This is an inguinal or femoral hernia containing a Meckel diverticulum.

THE ACUTE SCROTUM

The patient presents with a painful mass in the scrotum. If there is a history of trauma, a haematoma must be considered. Haematomas usually resolve spontaneously and it is very rarely necessary to drain them or to ligate bleeders.

Three conditions must usually be differentiated from one another:

- Torsion of the testis or of the appendix of the testis
- Epididymo-orchitis
- Strangulated indirect inguinal hernia

Torsion of the testis

This can occur at any age, but is more commonly found in patients between the ages of fifteen and twenty. A sudden, severe pain arises in the scrotum. The boy is nauseous and may vomit. The testis is swollen, hard and very tender. The testis rides high in the scrotum. The pain does not improve when the testis is lifted.

The patient must undergo emergency surgery. The testis is untwisted and fixed. The opposite testis must also be fixed, to prevent bilateral torsion. If the testis is necrotic, it must be removed.

Epididimyo-orchitis

Orchitis sometimes follows mumps. Epididymo-orchitis is usually due to gonococcal infection, but *E. coli* infection is more common in aged men.

There is a sudden onset of pain. The patient feels ill, is feverish and may develop rigor. The testis is swollen, hard and very tender. The pain improves if the testis is lifted. Gonorrhoea or a urinary tract infection may be present. The prostate is usually tender on rectal examination.

The condition is treated with bedrest, elevation of the scrotum and antibiotics. If this condition cannot be distinguished from torsion, an emergency operation should preferably be performed. No damage will be incurred and the scrotum can simply be drained if there is epididymo-orchitis.

Strangulated indirect inguinal hernia

The patient is usually aware of the fact that he has an inguinal hernia. The hernia is irreducible and becomes hard, tender and acutely painful. Nausea and vomiting are associated. On examination, the abdomen is distended, with increased bowel sounds. The thickened cord containing bowel, can be palpated at the neck of the scrotum.

X-rays show intestinal obstruction (distended bowel loops and air/fluid levels) and distended bowel loops can usually be seen in the scrotum.

The patient must undergo emergency surgery.

Endocrine surgery 8

Endocrine surgery is not directed at the removal of a mass or at the correction of an anatomical defect, but rather at restoring normal hormonal balance and thus physiological function. The surgeon is often called on to recognize subtle abnormalities of normal physiological function. These abnormalities are often a disturbance in normal metabolism in the target organ.

The anatomical abnormalities are often subtle or even so well hidden that the management of such cases is largely aimed at methods of localizing the source of hormonal hyper- or hypofunction.

HYPERPARATHYROIDISM

In this condition, the main physiological abnormality is hypercalcaemia. The patient's complaints will thus arise from metabolic abnormalities associated with hypercalcaemia. The diagnosis will be aimed at differentiating between the various causes of hypercalcaemia, and the treatment, at removing the source of hyperstimulation of calcium homeostasis.

What does the patient complain of?

Patients may be asymptomatic and hypercalcaemia may be a chance finding on blood tests. Calcium homeostasis is so important that it is governed by two hormones, parathyroid hormone (PTH) and calcitonin, and also by vitamin D. The functions of calcium are important and disturbance will usually cause symptoms and signs.

- Calcium is one of the main building blocks of the skeleton and teeth.
- In conjunction with other building blocks, it maintains the structural and functional integrity of the cell membrane.
- It facilitates a large variety of reactions, including
  - release of neurotransmitters at synapses and at neuromuscular junctions
  - gluconeogenesis, glucose transport across the cell membrane and many others.

If there is a disturbance in homeostasis, patients complain of fatigue and muscle weakness, nausea and vomiting, constipation, polydipsia and polyuria, psychiatric symptoms, renal colic and bone- and joint pains.

What does the clinician find on examination?

Clinical examination

Usually very few signs can be found. Hypertension, kyphosis and clubbed fingers may be observed.

Special investigations

Serum calcium is raised and serum phosphate is lowered, but urinary phosphate is raised. PTH levels are raised.

X-rays may show subperiosteal resorption of the phalanges, demineralization of bone, bone cysts and nephrocalcinosis or renal calculi.

What else must the clinician consider?

Hypercalcaemia due to hyperparathyroidism must be differentiated from that caused by metastases. Breast cancer is the most important cause. The primary disease and perhaps the metastases have usually already been diagnosed. PTH is suppressed.

Myeloma and other malignancies can also be identified as causes. PTH is also inhibited.

Vitamin D overdose, milk-alkali syndrome, thiazide diuretics and sarcoidosis must also be considered. **Low PTH levels are the most important distinguishing sign.**

An ectopic source of PTH is a rare cause of hypercalcaemia. The malignant tumour elsewhere has usually already been diagnosed. It is now also known that malignant tumours can produce PTH-like substances which can cause hypercalcaemia.

Primary parathyroidism is treated surgically.

THE ADRENALS

Cushing syndrome

This syndrome is caused by excessive secretion of cortisol. Cortisol has multiple and varied functions. It controls carbohydrate, protein, fat and electrolyte metabolism. It therefore strongly influences the cardiovascular, renal, musculoskeletal and central nervous systems, as well as other organs. It plays such an important rôle in the body's metabolism that one cannot live if both adrenals are removed.

Cortisol plays an important rôle in carbohydrate and protein metabolism. It mobilizes protein (catabolism) and stimulates gluconeogenesis. The blood glucose is raised and glycogen is deposited. Cortisol speeds up the turnover of body proteins in muscle, bone and skin. A cortisol excess therefore causes loss of skin-, muscle- and bone tissue and bone protein. This leads to attenuation of the skin and loss of muscle fibre and bone protein (osteoporosis). Cortisol speeds up the turnover of body fat, including mobilization of fatty acids from fat deposits, oxidation of fatty acids and synthesis of fats.

Longterm stimulation by excessive cortisol causes redistribution of body fat, leading to the buffalo hump and moonface characteristic of the syndrome.

Electrolyte metabolism is also influenced. Excessive cortisol causes sodium and water retention and potassium loss.

Cortisol causes psychological disturbances, because it influences the electrical activity of the brain.

Its anti-inflammatory effect inhibits the lymphocyte and eosinophil response and suppresses immune reactions.

What does the patient complain of?

Patients complain of weakness and depression. They and their families notice a gradual change in their appearance. They complain of loss of libido and amenorrhoea, as well as weight gain, acne and hirsutism.

What does the clinician find on examination?

One finds the typical Cushingoid appearance – moonface, buffalo hump, acne, hirsutism and purple skin striae. One must differentiate between the various causes of hypercortisolism. Twenty per cent are caused by functional adrenal tumours and 80% by adrenocortical hyperplasia, due to overstimulation by excessive adrenocorticotropic hormone (ACTH). The ACTH originates from the pituitary or an ectopic source (e g carcinoma of the bronchus).

Special investigations

- **ACTH and cortisol measurements:** If both ACTH and cortisol are raised, the cause is cortical hyperplasia, secondary to a microadenoma of the hypophysis and, rarely, an ectopic source of ACTH. If ACTH is suppressed and cortisol is raised, the cause is an autonomically functioning tumour of the adrenal cortex.
- **Localization of the tumour:** Computer tomography (CT) is the most useful investigation.

Management

Microadenoma with hyperplasia

Operate on the hypophysis. If this is unsuccessful, or if specialist skills are not available, do a bilateral adrenalectomy and administer replacement therapy.

Functional adrenocortical tumour

Do an adrenalectomy.

Hyperaldosteronism (Conn syndrome)

Primary hyperaldosteronism is a renin-independent hypersecretion of aldosterone. Adenoma is the cause in 85%, bilateral nodular hyperplasia in 15% and, rarely, carcinoma of the adrenal cortex.

Excessive aldosterone causes sodium retention, leading to water retention and an increase in plasma volume, with secondary hypertension. This causes potassium loss, leading to hypokalemic alkalosis.

What does the patient complain of?

Patients complain of headaches, muscle weakness, polydipsia and nocturia. As a result of the hypokalaemic alkalosis, carpopedal spasm and paraesthesia are also found.

What does the clinician find?

Patients have hypertension without retinopathy or oedema.

What must the clinician consider?

Primary hyperaldosteronism must be differentiated from secondary hyperaldosteronism. Loss of total body sodium, gain in total body potassium, major blood losses, dehydration, and constriction of a renal artery stimulate the kidneys to secrete more renin, resulting in increased angiotensin secretion, which stimulates the adrenals to secrete more aldosterone. This causes secondary hyperaldosteronism.

Special investigations

Increased aldosterone and absent renin indicate primary aldosteronism, caused by a functioning adenoma or hyperplasia. Raised aldosterone and raised renin indicate secondary hyperaldosteronism, usually secondary to cardiovascular or renal disease.

Localization

CT is the most useful investigation.

Management

Adenoma

Adrenalectomy.

Hyperplasia

Conservative diuretics which will avoid excessive potassium secretion and spironolactone.

Phaeochromocytoma

The adrenal medulla produces catecholamine, in a ratio of 80% adrenalin and 20% noradrenalin. It also secretes the noradrenalin precursor, dopamine.

Adrenalin interacts with both alpha- and beta receptors to redistribute blood flow by constricting skin and splanchnic vessels and dilating the vessels of the heart, skeletal muscles and brain. This causes tachycardia and anxiety. The metabolic effects are transformation of glycogen into glucose and an increase in the circulating free fatty acids.

Noradrenalin acts on the alpha receptors to cause constriction of all the blood vessels and thus raises both the systolic and the diastolic blood pressure. It has little effect on the central nervous system or metabolism.

A phaeochromocytoma, which is found in the adrenal medulla, secretes excessive adrenalin and noradrenalin. A phaeochromocytoma in the extra-adrenal paraganglionic tissues, usually secretes only noradrenalin.

What does the patient complain of?

Patients complain of episodic headaches, visual disturbances, attacks of excessive sweating, pallor and tachycardia.

What does the clinician find?

Patients are hypertensive. This may be episodic or persistent. It can be precipitated by palpation of the abdomen.

Special investigations

Increased secretion of catecholamine metabolites in the urine during an attack is the best screening test. VMA and metadrenaline are measured.

Localization studies

CT is the best noninvasive localization test. MIBG I^{133} scanning is also a reliable test. Selective venous catheterization, with direct measurement of catecholamine levels in blood samples thus collected, is useful in localizing an extra-adrenal phaeochromocytoma.

Management

Adrenalectomy or excision of an extra-adrenal tumour are indicated. Malignant tumours and their metastases can sometimes be treated with MIBG I^{133}.

The adrenogenital syndrome

A genetically determined enzyme defect gives rise to inadequate cortisol secretion. The feedback mechanism is activated and ACTH secretion is stimulated. This causes adrenal hyperplasia and increased androgen secretion.

How does the patient present?

Patients present with virilism, growth anomalies, renal sodium losses and hypertension.

THE ENDOCRINE PANCREAS

Various endocrine tumours arise in the islets of Langerhans. The most common type is a B cell adenoma with excessive insulin production, resulting in hypoglycaemia.

How does the patient present?

Patients present with symptoms and signs of hypoglycaemia. Hypoglycaemia, in turn, stimulates increased adrenalin secretion. Symptoms associated with raised adrenalin levels include fatigue, weakness, anxiety, excessive sweating and tachycardia. The hypoglycaemia causes irritability, anxiety, sleepiness, confusion, disorientation, speech defects, diplopia, delirium, mania, stupor and eventually coma.

What must the clinician consider?

All the causes of hypoglycaemia must be considered. The two main groups to be differentiated are hypoglycaemia following food intake (postprandial hypoglycaemia) and hypoglycaemia following fasting (fasting hypoglycaemia).

Postprandial hypoglycaemia

This follows on a high carbohydrate meal in patients who have undergone a gastrectomy or gastrojejunostomy. The stomach empties rapidly, glucose is absorbed and this causes an increase in insulin secretion.

Fasting hypoglycaemia

Following a fast, patients develop hypoglycaemia, with the symptoms and signs which have already been described.

Special investigations

The important findings are high circulating serum insulin levels and hypoglycaemia in patients during an attack.

Localizing tests

The tumours in the pancreas are too small to be traced on CT. Arteriography and selective transhepatic venous catheterization, with measurement of insulin levels in the blood samples so obtained, is the most reliable method.

Management

Excision of the insulinoma.

Classification of surgical endocrine conditions

A. THE PARATHYROIDS

Primary hyperparathyroidism

- Adenoma
- Diffuse hyperplasia
- Carcinoma of the parathyroids

Secondary and tertiary hyperparathyroidism

- Parathyroid carcinoma

Hypoparathyroidism

B. The Adrenals

Cushing syndrome

- Cushing disease
- Pituitary adenomas
- Adenoma
- Bilateral hyperplasia

Carcinoma of the adrenal cortex

Eutopic ACTH-producing tumours

Incidentaloma

Hyperaldosteronism

Phaeochromocytoma

Virilizing and feminizing syndromes

C. The pancreas

Insulinoma

- Adenoma
- Carcinoma
- Hyperplasia
- Nesidioblastosis

Glucagonoma

- Adenoma
- Carcinoma

Vipoma

- Adenoma
- Carcinoma

Somatostatinoma

- Adenoma
- Carcinoma

Gastrinoma

- Adenoma
- Carcinoma

D. Multiple endocrine neoplasias

- MEN I-syndrome
- MEN II-syndrome
- MEN IIa-syndrome
- MEN IIb-syndrome

These conditions will now be discussed in more detail.

A. HYPERPARATHYROIDISM

Primary hyperparathyroidism

Primary hyperparathyroidism is caused by excessive production of PTH by a parathyroid adenoma or -adenomas, hyperplasia of one or more, but usually all parathyroids, or very rarely, parathyroid carcinoma.

In large series, it has been found that a single adenoma causes the disease in 80% of cases, multiple adenomas in 5%, hyperplasia of the parathyroids in 13% and carcinoma in 2%. The disease is more common than was initially thought, and, if routine calcium measurements are taken of the general population, two out of 1000 people will have the disease. It is twice as common in women and is found between the ages of thirty and sixty.

Overproduction of PTH mobilizes calcium from bone and inhibits resorption of phosphate by the kidneys, resulting in hypercalcaemia and hypophosphataemia. This leads to calcium and phosphate loss and osteoporosis. The increased secretion of calcium by the kidneys leads to nephrolithiasis and nephrocalcinosis, with renal failure.

Pathology

Adenoma

Single or multiple adenomas are found. There will always be one or more normal or hypoplastic parathyroid glands with the adenoma. Adenomas involve the inferior parathyroid glands in about 75% of cases. The adenoma is a yellow-brown, soft, lobular mass, with fine blood vessels visible on its surface. Adenomas usually weigh between 100 mg and 5 g. Adenomas as large as 30 g have been described.

These adenomas can also be found in aberrant positions in the neck or thorax.

Histologically, all three cell types are found, but one cell type dominates. The most common type of adenoma comprises mainly chief cells. The second most common adenoma comprises mainly clear cells. Oxyphil cell-dominant adenomas are rare.

It is sometimes difficult to distinguish adenomas from hyperplasia on histological grounds. Often the adenoma is enclosed in a thin capsule and normal residual parathyroid gland tissue is visible on the one side.

Diffuse hyperplasia

Hyperplasia of all the parathyroids usually occurs secondary to hypocalcaemia, with the development of secondary hyperparathyroidism. It may sometimes develop as a primary condition. The cause of primary hyperplasia is uncertain. One possible cause is idiopathic hypercalcuria, which supplies a constant chronic stimulus for PTH secretion and eventually leads to hyperplasia and inappropriate function of the gland. The degree of hyperplasia in different glands varies considerably. One gland can weigh as little as 100 mg, while another can weight as much as 15 g. **Under these circumstances, one must be wary of not regarding it as an adenoma.**

The majority of glands show chief cell hyperplasia. Cells form cords and have a follicular pattern. It is characteristic that the fat cells disappear. Clear cell hyperplasia is less common but causes very large glands when it does occur.

Hyperplasia is also found as part of the MEA syndrome.

Carcinoma of the parathyroids

This is a rare tumour. It is difficult to distinguish between a carcinoma and an adenoma. The tumours are usually relatively small. They are harder than adenomas and tend to adhere to surrounding tissues. Hyperchromatism, pleomorphism and variety in nuclear size are present, but not necessarily to a more marked degree than in adenomas.

To confirm a diagnosis of carcinoma, at least one of the following findings must be present:

- Metastases
- Infiltration of the capsule
- Residue following previous removal

Metastases are usually found in lymph nodes and distal blood spread is extremely rare.

Clinical presentation of hyperparathyroidism

The way in which patients present has changed in the last few years. Thirty years ago, patients presented with advanced disease, mainly with bone pain and deformity due to osteitis fibrosa cystica, or Van Recklinghausen disease. This involves osteoclastic resorption of bone and replacement with fibrous tissue, and is typically found in the mandible.

Later, patients often presented with renal calculi, nephrocalcinosis and sometimes renal failure. Currently more than half these cases are discovered by chance on routine calcium measurements. Sometimes patients are completely asymptomatic, but often realize retrospectively that they feel much better following successful treatment, and that they had been aware of fatigue, weakness, psychiatric symptoms such as depression, polydipsia, polyuria, constipation and bone and joint pain.

If the above symptom complex presents, consider hyperparathyroidism, especially if renal calculi, hypertension, peptic ulcer and pancreatitis are associated. **Always look for hypercalcaemia.**

Special investigations

Calcium homeostasis

The diagnosis of hyperparathyroidism is actually the differential diagnosis of hypercalcaemia. About a third of hypercalcaemia cases are caused by hyperparathyroidism, a third by malignant conditions, mainly bone metastases of breast carcinoma, myeloma, leukaemia and other bone metastases, and a third by a variety of conditions, including laboratory errors and a tight tourniquet when drawing blood. Thiazide diuretics, sarcoidosis, hyperthyroidism, Vitamin D overdosage and the milk-alkali syndrome are sometimes responsible.

Firstly, the diagnosis of hypercalcaemia must be confirmed. The blood sample must be taken from a fasting patient, without applying a tourniquet to the arm. The test must be repeated three times. A calcium level higher than 2,6 mmol/ℓ must be investigated further. A low serum phosphate and raised serum chloride support the diagnosis of primary hyperparathyroidism. The next important measurement is the serum PTH level. If PTH is normal or raised, the diagnosis of primary hyperparathyroidism is usually confirmed. This may naturally also be due to ectopic PTH, but then the malignant tumour or tertiary hyperparathyroidism has usually already been diagnosed, or the underlying longstanding renal disease is well known. In all the other causes of hypercalcaemia, the PTH levels are completely suppressed by the high serum calcium. In a few cases there may be uncertainty as to the diagnosis, and then certain additional special investigations can be useful.

- **Hypercalcaemia which is not consistently present**

  The clinical presentation suggests hyperparathyroidism, but the serum calcium is either at the upper limit of normal, or only sporadically slightly raised. The calcium levels must be tested repeatedly. The laboratory measurement must be done on the same day, since calcium levels drop if blood is stored and frozen.

Serum calcium comprises ionized calcium (48%), protein-bound calcium (46%) and calcium bound to organic anions (6%). Total serum calcium thus varies with the plasma protein levels. If protein levels are low, the total serum calcium will be artificially low. Ionized calcium levels are independent of protein levels. Raised ionized calcium levels and recordable or raised PTH levels confirm the diagnosis of normocalcaemic hyperparathyroidism.

- **Hypercalcuria, with or without renal calculi**

There are three causes:

- *Increased calcium uptake in the gastrointestinal tract* (absorption hypercalcuria). These patients have suppressed PTH levels.
- *Tubular leakage of calcium* (renal hypercalcuria). Owing to renal leakage of calcium, these patients have raised PTH levels. The tubular leakage of calcium can be blocked by chlorthiazide. The PTH levels drop to normal. In cases of normocalcuric hyperparathyroidism, the calcium will probably rise and PTH levels will remain unchanged.
- *Primary hyperparathyroidism*. Hypercalcuria is associated with raised urinary levels of cyclic AMP, hyperphosphaturia and reduced tubular resorption of phosphate. The use of other special investigations to differentiate other types of hypercalcaemia will be discussed in the section dealing with differential diagnosis.

X-rays

The classic X-ray bone signs are rarely seen these days in patients with primary hyperparathyroidism, but are still often seen in secondary hyperparathyroidism. The pronounced bone changes of osteitis fibrosa cystica have become extremely rare. If they do occur, alkaline phosphatase is also raised. The usual bone signs, if they do occur, include: subperiosteal bone resorption of the phalanges, with bone cysts, matt glass appearance of the skull, resorption of the ends of the clavicles (rotted stump appearance), loss of the *lamina dura* of tooth sockets (after tooth extraction).

Differential diagnosis

Distinguishing between primary hyperparathyroidism caused by parathyroid disease and that caused by ectopic PTH, can be difficult. If the calcium levels are very high, even as high as 3,0 mmol/ℓ, the erythrocyte sedimentation rate is raised and alkaline phosphatase levels are raised, and there are no bone cysts, consider an ectopic source. Specific radioimmuno assays for tumour PTH can be done, but are not generally available. Usually the presence of a malignant tumour, such as lung carcinoma, hypernephroma or hepatoma, has already been established.

Other causes of hypercalcaemia

Chlorthiazide diuretics can cause a slight rise in serum calcium. Discontinue the drug and measure PTH levels – these will be normal. Hyperthyroidism, especially in the elderly, is a cause of hypercalcaemia. It drops to normal after successful treatment of the hyperthyroidism. People who ingest large quantities of dairy products or calcium-containing antacids can develop hypercalcaemia (the milk-alkali syndrome). Levels drop if intake is limited.

Malignancy and hypercalcaemia

The most important finding is hypercalcaemia and suppressed PTH levels. Serum protein electrophoresis helps in the diagnosis of myeloma and sarcoidosis. X-rays will show metastases of breast carcinoma and the lesions of the skull found in myeloma. Bone marrow studies are helpful in diagnosing myeloma. A chest X-ray may show pulmonary metastases or the diffuse nodular infiltrate of sarcoidosis.

The hydrocortisone suppression test (4,0 mg cortisone eight-hourly for ten days) reduces serum calcium levels in all the abovementioned causes, but only very exceptionally in cases of primary hyperparathyroidism. Malignant tumours are also known to secrete

PTH-like substances which can cause hypercalcaemia.

Management of primary hyperparathyroidism

If a diagnosis of primary hyperparathyroidism has been firmly established, an operation must be performed. It is not necessary to try and locate the precise location of the tumour before exploration in these cases. Localizing investigations are only necessary in re-explorations for recurrent hyperparathyroidism. The thyroid is exposed and the superior vessels and middle vein are ligated so that the thyroid lobes can be mobilized medically. The important landmark, the site where the recurrent laryngeal nerve crosses the inferior thyroid artery, must be located. The inferior parathyroid glands are usually found within 1 cm of this point and the superior glands within 2 cm. Haemostasis must be maintained, because the colour differences between a parathyroid adenoma and a lymph node or thyroid nodule are important in recognition of the adenoma.

Every attempt must be made to locate all four parathyroids. If one enlarged gland is found, it must be removed and sent for frozen section. If an adenoma is found, with compressed parathyroid tissue, nothing further is necessary. If there is doubt about normal glands, a small biopsy can be taken with fine scissors to confirm that the parathyroid gland is normal on frozen section. Such single adenomas are the cause of hypercalcaemia in 85% of cases.

If two adenomas are found and two normal glands, remove both adenomas. If three glands are enlarged, hyperplasia is a more likely diagnosis.

If no adenoma is found, explore the neck thoroughly, including the tracheo-oesophageal grove, the carotid sheath and the superior mediastinum. If an adenoma is still not found, do a thyroid lobectomy on the side on which only one normal gland was found. Remove the thymus and send the tissue for frozen section histology. If an adenoma is still not found and the other glands are normal, close the neck.

Primary hyperplasia of the glands

If all the glands are enlarged, the three largest glands are removed in toto *and half of the smallest gland is removed, to leave a gland of approximately normal size.*

Postoperative course

After the operation, serum calcium levels usually return to normal within forty-eight hours. Sometimes, after longstanding disease and very high preoperative serum calcium levels, patients develop carpopedal spasm and even fitting (the hungry bone syndrome). It may be necessary to administer intravenous calcium supplements for a few weeks.

Longterm prospects

The chances of cure are 95% if a single adenoma is removed. If three and a half glands are removed, there is an 85% chance of cure.

Management of recurrent hyperparathyroidism

The diagnosis of hyperparathyroidism must be reconfirmed. Repeat the tests, and make especially certain that there are no other causes present. Think of familial hypocalciuric hypercalcaemia. Hypocalciuria and a family history of hypercalcaemia are usually found in these cases.

• No adenoma found at the first operation

Usually an adenoma is still present in the neck. An adenoma will be found in the mediastinum in only 2% of cases. Every attempt must now be made to localize the adenoma. Ultrasound, computer tomography and Thallium ^{201}, Technesium ^{99} and subtraction scans must be employed. Selective venous catheterization, with PTH level measurements may be necessary. Digital subtraction angiography must be attempted. The tumour will usually be located in the neck. If these tests do not help, the neck must be explored by an experienced surgeon, with partial thyroidectomy forming part of the exploration.

If nothing is found in the neck, the mediastinum must be explored via a sternotomy approach.

• Hyperplasia has been treated by removal of three and a half glands

Explore the neck. Remove all parathyroid tissue and transplant it into the muscles of the arm. Less than 50 mg tissue must be transplanted in small fragments.

Asymptomatic hypercalcaemia

If there is no contraindication to surgery and the diagnosis has been confirmed, asymptomatic patients must be operated on. If the diagnosis is uncertain, the patient must be followed up and the tests repeated until a definitive diagnosis is made. The patient must then be operated on. Most such cases will develop later complications, of which renal failure and hypertension are the most important. Once these complications have been confirmed, they are already irreversible.

Hypercalcaemic crisis

Hypercalcaemic crisis is caused by disseminated carcinoma with metastases, an ectopic PTH-producing tumour, a large parathyroid adenoma, or hyperplasia. The most common cause is metastatic breast carcinoma.

The serum calcium is usually higher than 3,75 mmol/ℓ. Patients are usually dehydrated, due to vomiting and polyuria. They complain of headache, weakness and severe thirst. They have tachycardia and a low blood pressure and may lapse into a coma. These patients must be rehydrated urgently and hypokalaemia and hyponatraemia must be corrected. Saline must be given, with potassium supplementation, while the central venous pressure is carefully monitored. Furosemide is given as soon as the fluid balance has been restored, to facilitate calcium secretion.

It is particularly important to administer corticosteroids, especially where disseminated carcinoma is the cause. Intravenous phosphate can be given, but hydration must first be restored, otherwise renal failure can develop. Calcitonin, if available, can be useful. Meanwhile, the diagnosis must be confirmed. If PTH levels are high and there is no sign of an ectopic source, the neck must be explored as soon as the patient has been rehydrated.

Secondary and tertiary hyperparathyroidism

In secondary hyperparathyroidism, there is increased PTH secretion secondary to low ionized calcium levels, due to renal failure and malabsorption. Serum phosphate levels are high.

This condition is commonly found in patients on dialysis. They present with osteoporosis, bone pain and metastatic calcification. They sometimes develop skin necrosis and vascular occlusion due to metastatic calcification.

Most patients can be treated medically with 1-hydroxy-vitamin D_3, which enhances calcium absorption and inhibits PTH secretion via a negative feedback effect. If conservative treatment is unsuccessful, a total parathyroidectomy is performed, with auto-transplantation of 50 mg of tissue to the arm. Conservative treatment must also be continued. If patients do not recover after renal transplantation, medical treatment must be continued. If hypercalcaemia persists and especially if metastatic calcification causes problems, it must be accepted that the hyperplastic parathyroid has begun to function autonomically (tertiary hyperparathyroidism). Total parathyroidectomy, with autotransplantation to the arm, is indicated.

Parathyroid carcinoma

This is responsible for approximately 2% of cases of hyperparathyroidism. This carcinoma tends to spread to lymph nodes and only later via the bloodstream. If the condition is recognized at operation, a wide excision, including the ipsilateral thyroid lobe, must be performed. Affected lymph nodes must be removed. If there are already signs of metastasis, the patient has a poor prognosis. These patients usually die of the complications of hypercalcaemia.

Hypoparathyroidism

This is a rare condition. It is sometimes found after thyroidectomy, especially if the operation was performed for carcinoma. Idiopathic hypoparathyroidism is an auto-immune disease and is found in association with adrenal insufficiency.

Clinical presentation

The symptoms are caused by hypocalcaemia. Patients present with paraesthesia, a numb feeling round the mouth, muscle cramps, carpopedal spasm and even convulsions. A dry skin, brittle nails and hair loss can also be found. Tetany is typical in the immediate postoperative period. Latent tetany can be elicited by Chvostek or Trousseau signs.

Chvostek sign

Contraction of the facial muscles if the facial nerve just anterior to the ear is tapped.

Trousseau sign

Occlusion of the circulation to the arm elicits carpopedal spasm.

Special investigations

Hypocalcaemia and hyperphosphataemia are present. Urinary phosphate and calcium levels are low.

Differential diagnosis

Malabsorption and renal disease can cause hypocalcaemic tetany. PTH levels are raised in these patients.

Management

Acute tetany is common in the immediate postoperative period and requires emergency treatment. Administer 20 ml of a 10% calcium chloride solution slowly intravenously, until the tetany subsides. Then add 50 mg of 10% calcium chloride to 1000 ml of saline in 5% dextrose and administer it slowly. Adjust the flow rate to maintain normal serum calcium levels. Administer 1,25 dihydroxy-vitamin D. It may sometimes be necessary to supplement magnesium sulphate in a dosage of 6 g/day intramuscularly. When the tetanus is under control, calcium gluconate can be given orally. The dose of vitamin D required to prevent hypocalcaemia may vary from 25 000 to 200 000 IU/day. Calcium levels must be measured regularly and vitamin D doses adjusted. Dietary phosphates must be reduced and dairy products must be avoided. If the problem persists, administer albumin hydroxide gel to bind phosphates and excrete them into the faeces.

B. THE ADRENALS

Cushing syndrome

This condition is caused by excessive cortisol secretion by the adrenal cortex. This excessive secretion is caused by a functioning tumour in 20% of cases and by overstimulation of a normal cortex by ACTH in 80%. Almost all patients have an ACTH-producing tumour in the pituitary gland. It may be a basophilic or chromophobic adenoma. The majority are micro-adenomas, but sometimes the tumour is large with obvious erosion of the *sella turcica* (Cushing disease).

Tumours outside the pituitary gland which excrete ectopic ACTH-like peptides, stimulating the cortex, are a rare cause. The most common types of tumour are bronchus carcinoma and carcinoid and less commonly, malignant tumours of the pancreas, thymus, thyroid, prostate, oesophagus and colon.

Clinical presentation

This disease is ten times more common in young women than in men. Centripetal obesity, buffalo hump and moonface are classical signs. Acne, hirsutism and purple skin striae are also typical. Patients complain of fatigue, weakness, loss of libido and amenorrhoea. On examination, hypertension and diabetes are usually found.

Special investigations

The aim of special investigations is to determine whether a patient with the stigmata of Cushing disease is really secreting excessive cortisol, and whether this is due to an adrenal adenoma or hyperplasia of both adrenals due to ACTH overstimulation and, if so, what the source is of the ACTH.

Plasma cortisol

Morning plasma cortisol levels will be raised. If there is any doubt, the following confirming tests are done:

- The diurnal rhythm of cortisol: Cortisol levels taken at 08h00 should be two or three times higher than cortisol levels taken at midnight. If these two values coincide, there is strong support for a diagnosis of Cushing syndrome.
- Overnight dexamethasone suppression test (low dose tests): At 23h00, the patient is given 1 mg dexamethasone and 100 mg phenobarbitone per os, after a basal plasma cortisol level has been taken. In normal people, cortisol is then suppressed to below

5 mg/dl. In Cushing syndrome, no suppression will take place.

Measurement of ACTH levels

Direct immuno-assays of ACTH in the blood can be done. If ACTH levels are raised, the syndrome is caused by a pituitary adenoma, or an ectopic source of ACTH is present. If the ACTH is suppressed, the patient has an autonomically functioning adenoma or carcinoma of the adrenal cortex.

The high dose dexamethasone test

Eight mg of dexamethasone is given in divided doses over twenty-four hours. The urine is collected for the next twenty-four hours to measure the 17 hydroxycorticosteroids in the urine for that period. In normal people, excretion will be suppressed to less than 4 mg per twenty-four hours. In patients with an adenoma, no suppression will take place. In patients with Cushing disease, suppression will take place, but to a lesser degree than in normal people.

Computer tomography

This is the most useful investigation for localizing an adenoma or demonstrating bilateral hyperplasia. It is also useful in the diagnosis of pituitary adenomas.

Selective venous catheterization

Collection of venous blood directly from the veins draining the adrenals is sometimes used to localize an adenoma, by determining selective cortisol levels.

Differential diagnosis

Obesity

The fat distribution of obesity usually differs from that of Cushing syndrome. Patients with Cushing syndrome seldom weigh more than 190 kg. The diurnal cortisol rhythm is normal and cortisol is suppressed by dexamethasone.

Diabetes mellitus and hypertension

This may sometimes cause confusion, but the same tests will exclude the diagnosis of Cushing syndrome.

Alcoholism

Alcoholics often have a very similar build with centripetal fat distribution. Tests will differentiate Cushing syndrome.

Management

Cortical adenoma

The treatment of an adenoma is removal of the gland. It is better to do an adrenalectomy via a twelfth rib approach, as these patients fare better postoperatively than those who have had a transperitoneal operation. Ileus does not usually occur and there are fewer pulmonary complications.

During the immediate postoperative period, it will be necessary to supplement cortisone temporarily, as the opposite cortex is suppressed.

Bilateral hyperplasia

The majority of patients have a microadenoma of the pituitary gland. There are techniques to remove these microadenomas surgically. If the skill and experience are available, this is the treatment of choice. If they are not, a bilateral adrenalectomy must be done and the patient must be put onto permanent replacement therapy. Other disadvantages include the fact that the pituitary adenoma secretes large amounts of ACTH and melanotropic hormone, causing excessive skin pigmentation. The pituitary adenoma can enlarge, causing headaches, exophthalmos and even blindness (Nelson syndrome). The pituitary adenoma can be irradiated, but recurrence is common. Following bilateral adrenalectomy, it is essential that replacement therapy be very carefully monitored. A general approach is the following: 300 mg hydrocortisone is given intraoperatively, as soon as the adrenals have been removed. On the first day, 100 mg of hydrocortisone is given eight-hourly. After this, the dosage is halved daily, until 25 mg is given twice daily. In the longterm, patients will need between 20 and 30 mg of hydrocortisone daily and 0,1 to 0,2 mg fluorocortisone daily.

Carcinoma of the adrenal cortex

Fortunately, this is rare. If it does occur, the tumour is large and the syndrome pronounced. This is more common in young people and children. These tumours tend to infiltrate blood vessels and spread. It is difficult to make the diagnosis on histological criteria, as pleomorphism does not necessarily indicate malignancy. If possible, the tumour must be excised widely. Recurrence often occurs rapidly and then one must rely on medical management.

Metyrapone and aminoglutethimide inhibit steroid biosynthesis and may be helpful. Op-DDD may help, but it has severe side effects and may be toxic.

Ectopic ACTH-producing tumours

They are usually malignant and resection is seldom possible. Although the prognosis is poor, a bilateral adrenalectomy is indicated in some patients for symptomatic reasons. Metyrapone and aminoglutethimide are also useful.

Incidentaloma

Since computer tomography has come into general use, incidental masses have been discovered in the adrenals. If no endocrine abnormalities can be demonstrated, and if the mass is smaller than 6 cm and does not enlarge in the follow-up period, no operation is necessary. Such lesions are usually non-functioning adenomas or cysts.

Hyperaldosteronism

Hyperaldosteronism most frequently arises as a secondary phenomenon in chronic liver- and renal disease and cardiac failure. The juxtaglomerular apparatus is stimulated by excessive use of diuretics and reduced plasma volume and renal ischaemia to secrete excessive renin, which stimulates the zona glomerulosa of the cortex, via the angiotensin mechanism, to secrete excessive aldosterone.

Primary aldosteronism is caused either by an adenoma (85%), bilateral micronodular hyperplasia (15%), or, very rarely, carcinoma.

Pathology of primary hyperaldosteronism

Adenoma

Non-functioning adenomas of the adrenal cortex are found in 2% of autopsies. Only a minority of adenomas are actually functional. These adenomas are usually unilateral and smaller than 2 cm in diameter. They are bright yellow and well circumscribed. The yellow colour is ascribed to cells which are overloaded with fat. Cellular pleomorphism is often present. The tumour arises from the zona glomerulosa.

Hyperplasia

Hyperplasia of the zona glomerulosa may be very subtle and difficult to recognise. Micronodular hyperplasia is more commonly found.

Clinical presentation

The patient is usually a young middle-aged women, who complains of headaches, weakness, polydipsia and nocturia. Carpopedal spasm and tetany may be found if there is hypokalaemic alkalosis.

On examination, pronounced hypertension is found, without retinopathy. Oedema is usually absent if renal function is good.

Special investigations

Special investigations are aimed at confirming the diagnosis of hyperaldosteronism; to differentiate primary hyperaldosteronism from secondary hyperaldosteronism and to distinguish adenomas from hyperplasia as the cause of primary aldosteronism.

Electrolyte measurements

A low serum potassium and high serum sodium are found. Eventually, the patient develops hypokalaemic alkalosis. If these changes are not pronounced, hypokalaemia can be elicited by introducing 1 g of table salt daily to the diet.

Aldosterone

Plasma aldosterone is raised.

Renin levels

High renin levels are characteristic of secondary hyperaldosteronism. A low renin level suggests primary hyperaldosteronism, but is not absolutely diagnostic. If the hyperaldosteronism is caused by hyperplasia, renin is not suppressed to the same extent.

The postural test

Normal people have a diurnal rhythm of plasma aldosterone. It is high at 08h00 and lower in the afternoon. Renin secretion is stimulated if a patient assumes an upright position. In normal people, the diurnal position will be maintained when they are constantly recumbent. If such people then rise between 08h00 and 10h00, aldosterone levels will rise, due to stimulation by raised renin levels. An adenoma is autonomic and will not be influenced by postural hyperreninaemia. Patients with hyperplasia respond well.

Suppression tests

Adenomas which produce aldosterone are autonomic and aldosterone production is not suppressed by fluorocortisone or desoxicorticosterone acetate (DOCA).

Localization of the adenoma

An adenoma is localised in 80% of cases, by means of computer tomography. If everything points to an adenoma, but nothing is found on CT, selective venous specimens can be taken to demonstrate unilateral raised aldosterone levels.

Differential diagnosis

Primary hyperaldosteronism must be differentiated from secondary aldosteronism as has been described. Other conditions to consider include the effects of oestrogen-containing contraceptives and alcohol. Plasma renin is also raised in pregnancy and diabetes.

Management

Spironolactone, an aldosterone antagonist and amiloride, a potassium-sparing diuretic, must be used preoperatively to normalize hypokalaemia and hypertension. If hypertension cannot be controlled, methyldopa must be used.

Adenoma

Adenomas are usually unilateral and can therefore be removed via a twelfth rib approach.

Hyperplasia

If a diagnosis of hyperplasia is made preoperatively, patients must be treated conservatively, since only a minority recover completely even after bilateral adrenalectomy. Patients must be given a diet of low sodium content, with a potassium supplement. Potassium-sparing diuretics such as amiloride and triamterine must also be used.

If hyperplasia is found at operation, it is advisable to go ahead with a bilateral adrenalectomy. A group of patients will recover and others will be easily controlled on conservative treatment. These patients must, of course, be given replacement therapy.

Prognosis

After removal of an adenoma, 70% of patients are cured. The remaining 30% are more easily controlled on medical treatment. Patients with hyperplasia have a poorer prognosis and their hypertension is sometimes difficult to control with medical treatment.

Phaeochromocytoma

A phaeochromocytoma is usually a benign tumour found in the adrenal medulla. It secretes large quantities of adrenaline and noradrenalin. It also secretes dopamine and vasoactive peptides. The tumour is often larger than 5 cm in diameter, with a rich blood supply, and is reddish-brown in colour. Although 80% of these tumours are found in the adrenal medulla, about 10% are found in extra-adrenal paraganglionic tissues, especially adjacent to the aorta and in the organ of Zuckerkandl. They can also occur in the neck, mediastinum, pelvis and bladder. They occur bilaterally in the adrenal medulla in 10%, and 10% of them are malignant. Ninety-nine per cent of all tumours are found in the abdominal cavity.

Pathology

Necrosis and bleeding are visible on cross-section. Fibrous adhesions from the capsule give the tumour a lobular appearance. On microscopic examination, the tumour consists of pleomorphic cells with central single, or sometimes double, nuclei. The basophilic cytoplasm contains fine granules which can be demonstrated on colouring with chrome salts. Giant and bizarre cells are also visible, but do not necessarily mean that the tumour is malignant. Malignancy can only be diagnosed with certainty if metastases are present.

Clinical presentation

The classical presentation is one of periodic hypertension with pallor, followed by a glowing facial blush, palpitations, headache, excessive sweating, nervousness and anxiety. A minority of patients present with constant hypertension, tachycardia, retinopathy and signs of hypermetabolism such as weight loss. They may also mimic diabetes, with raised blood sugar levels.

If a young patient presents with a triad of palpitations, headache and excessive sweating and has hypertension, one must look for a phaeochromocytoma.

Phaeochromocytoma is a rare tumour and is found in less than 0,5% of patients with hypertension.

Special investigations

The most important metabolites of adrenaline: metradrenalin, 3-methoxy-4-hydroxy-mandelic acid, metnoradrenalin and VMA and of dopamine: homovanillic acid (HVA) are measured in the urine. If they are raised, the catecholamines adrenaline and noradrenalin can be measured directly in the plasma, using chromatography. Although the normal range values of catecholamines is reasonably wide, levels twice the upper limit of normal should be found.

Provocation tests

All provocation tests are dangerous and they are seldom done any more. If they do become necessary, glucagon is the safest substance to use. The serum levels of catecholamines double after glucagon stimulation. Phentolamine (Regitine) must be kept in readiness in case of a dramatic rise in blood pressure.

Localization tests

Normal X-rays can sometimes show a soft tissue tumour or displacement of the upper pole of the kidney. CT is a very reliable method of localizing the tumour. If there is any doubt, especially with tumours outside the adrenal medulla, metaiodobenzylguanidine-I^{131} (I^{131}-MIBG) (hot guano) can be administered and the body can be scanned. Phaeochromocytoma will show up as a warm area in 90% of cases.

Selective collection of blood specimens in the *vena cava*, the renal and adrenal veins, with measurement of catecholamine levels, can also be used to localize the tumour.

Differential diagnosis

All patients who have recently developed hypertension must be considered. Phaeochromocytoma can sometimes be confused with hyperthyroidism. All the symptoms and signs, such a tremor, tachycardia, excessive sweating and even exophthalmos, can be present. The carcinoid syndrome, with its glowing facial blushing, tachycardia, excessive sweating and even hypertension, must be differentiated. Hypertension in pregnancy is a well known pitfall. Pre-eclampsia and eclampsia can be confused with a phaeochromocytoma which presents in pregnancy.

Management

The management of phaeochromocytoma is surgical removal. Because there are serious complications related to the disease, patients must be thoroughly prepared for surgery beforehand. Patients with phaeochromocytoma may develop cardiac failure, renal failure or stroke. Such patients usually have a relative hypovolaemia, because the peripheral circulatory bed has shrunk due to vasoconstriction. When this vasoconstriction is relieved, hypovolaemic shock sets in. Patients must thus be prepared as follows:

- *Alpha-adrenergic blockade is achieved, using phenoxybenzamine. The initial dosage is 10 mg eight-hourly. The dose can be slowly increased until the blood pressure is controlled. As the blood vessel bed gradually enlarges, the blood volume will adjust and be restored.*
- *As soon as the patient is on alpha blockade, propanalol must be added to achieve beta adrenergic blockade, which controls the tachycardia and arrhythmias in particular. Commence with a dose of 40 mg eight-hourly.*
- *As soon as the hypertension is under control, the myocardiopathy has recovered and the blood volume has been supplemented, the patient can undergo surgery.*

Because tumours are sometimes situated bilaterally or extra-adrenally, a bilateral subcostal transperitoneal approach is preferable.

- *The anaesthetist must have an arterial catheter and a pulmonary artery wedge pressure catheter in position. Phentolamine and nitroprusside must be available to control sudden blood pressure crises.*

- *There is a dramatic rise in catecholamines when the tumour is handled and a drop when it is removed.*
- *The venous drainage must always be ligated first.*
- *Large volumes of fluid may be needed to maintain the blood pressure.*
- *If the patient has been well prepared, these crises are rare.*
- *Propanalol must also be available to control arrhythmias.*

Prognosis

Untreated phaeochromocytoma is a fatal disease. With good preparation, the operative mortality is less than 5%. A small number of patients still have hypertension postoperatively, but this can normally be well controlled on medication. If the syndrome is caused by a malignant phaeochromocytoma, the prognosis is poor. Metastases can be treated with I^{131}-MIBG, but the results are not satisfactory.

Virilizing and feminizing syndromes

The adrenogenital syndrome

The adrenogenital syndrome arises due to a congenital deficiency of the enzyme which controls synthesis of certain adrenocortical hormones. As a result, too few of these hormones are synthesized and the adrenal cortex undergoes hyperplasia, under the influence of increased ACTH stimulation. The hyperplastic cortex then produces excessive androgens. Three main types of virilism are described:

- **Simple virilism**

The cause is a partial deficiency of 21-beta-hydroxylase, resulting in decreased cortisol production. This deficiency causes the hypophysis to secrete too much ACTH causing adrenocortical hyperplasia. The hyperplastic cortex secretes too many androgens.

- **Virilism plus salt loss**

The cause is an almost total deficiency of 21-beta-hydroxylase. The cortisol deficiency is more severe and is associated with an aldosterone deficiency. Virilism is associated with salt- and water losses.

- **Virilism plus hypertension**

This is caused by an 11-beta-hydroxylase deficiency. Deoxycorticosterone is produced in excess, and salt is retained. Patients thus develop virilism and hypertension.

Virilization caused by tumours is found in older patients. No increase in deoxycorticosterone or the breakdown products of 17-hydroxyprogesterone can be found. Treatment with hydrocortisone or ACTH has no effect on androgen secretion.

Feminization is almost always caused by adrenal tumours and most of these are malignant.

Clinical presentation

There is excessive muscle development, obesity, hirsutism and acne. In boys, the penis and scrotum develop rapidly. Libido, pubic-, axillary- and beard hair develop early.

In girls, the clitoris is enlarged, with atrophy of the secondary feminine sexual characteristics, lowered libido and no menarche at puberty.

Special investigations

- **Corticotropin stimulation test**

17-Ketosteroids are raised and 17-hydroxyketosteroids are lowered in this syndrome. If the patient is stimulated with corticotropin (ACTH), the 17-ketosteroids rise further, while the 17-hydroxyketosteroids remain unchanged.

- **Dexamethasone suppression test**

Baseline measurements of 17-ketosteroids and 17-hydroxy-ketosteroids must be taken. The patient is then given 2 mg of dexamethasone six-hourly for two days. If the syndrome is caused by carcinoma, the 17-KS and 17-HKS will not be suppressed.

Differential diagnosis

Testicular and ovarian tumours must be kept in mind. Cushing syndrome and administration of exogenous hormones can mimic the presentation.

Management

- *Congenital enzyme anomalies, with hyperplasia of the cortex, are treated by administration of small doses of hydrocortisone.*
- *Tumours must be removed surgically.*

Prognosis

- Virilizing tumours are usually benign.
- Feminizing tumours are usually malignant, with a poor prognosis.

C. THE PANCREAS

So far, five cell types have been described in the islets of Langerhans. It is highly probable that there are more, which have not yet been recognized.

- The alpha cells secrete glucagon and can form tumours (glucagonoma).
- Beta cells secrete insulin. Beta cell tumours or insulinomas are the most common type of islet cell tumour.
- The D-cells secrete somatostatin. Somatostatinomas have been described. Although some doubt still exists, it has been postulated that gastrinomas also arise from D-cells, or from the very closely related A_2 cells.
- D^1 cells secrete vaso-active intestinal polypeptide (VIP). The Werner-Morrison syndrome (watery diarrhoea) is caused by tumours which develop from these cells.
- PP-cells secrete pancreatic polypeptides. This causes diarrhoea and intestinal hypermobility. Tumours of the islet cells secrete ACTH, vasopressin, catecholamine, serotonin and chorionic gonadotrophin.

Insulinoma

This tumour is the most common type of islet cell tumour. It arises in the B-cells and produces excessive insulin leading to hypoglycaemia.

Clinical presentation

The symptoms and signs are caused by hypoglycaemia and a secondary increase in catecholamine secretion.

The early presentation includes fatigue, weakness, anxiety, insatiable hunger, tremors, sweating and tachycardia. Later insomnia, excitability, confusion and disorientation develop. Even later, delirium, mania, stupor and coma occur.

There is often a delay in diagnosis and fewer than a third of patients are diagnosed within the first year. These patients sometimes end up in mental institutions. Usually the diagnosis is only made when the patient lapses into coma.

In the past the Whipple triad was always used to make the diagnosis. It consists of:

- Symptoms and signs provoked by exercise or fasting.
- While symptoms are present, the blood sugar drops to below 2,2 mmol/ℓ.
- Symptoms resolve immediately on oral or intravenous glucose administration.

Special investigations

Insulin- and blood glucose measurements after a fasting period

Both glucose and insulin drop after a period of fasting in normal people. In patients with insulinoma, the blood glucose drops, but insulin levels remain high because the tumour reacts autonomically. During a spontaneous attack of the disease, the blood glucose will be low and the insulin high.

Measurement of pro-insulin and C-peptide

Pro-insulin is formed in the rough endoplasmic reticulum of the beta cells. Pro-insulin is split proteolytically into insulin and C-peptide. C-peptide is the binding peptide between the A- and B-chains of insulin.

Insulin and C-peptide are released in equivalent concentrations by the beta cells. Patients with insulinomas have raised pro-insulin and C-peptide levels. If patients receive exogenous (self-administered) insulin, insulin will be high, but C-peptide will be low. If both insulin and C-peptide levels are high, they come from an endogenous source (insulinoma).

Stimulation tests

Tolbutamide- and glucagon stimulation were used in the past. The calcium infusion test is a safer and more reliable stimulation test. Pro-insulin and C-peptide levels rise after calcium infusion and glucose levels drop. This does not happen in normal patients or patients with reactive hyperglycaemia.

Preoperative localization

Insulinomas are usual small tumours and are seldom found on ultrasound and CT. ERCP is also not really useful, as the tumour is not of ductal origin.

Angiography

These tumours are relatively vascular and often show as a blush on angiography. Various methods are used to make the angiogram more useful. Selective canulization of blood vessels and subtraction angiography make the investigations more accurate.

Selective catheterization of veins with insulin measurement

Catheters can be placed in the portal venous system via the liver and blood can be collected from the veins draining the pancreas. A type of map is thus created. The area with the highest insulin levels is thus identified as the suspicious area.

Pathology

These tumours are equally common in the head, body and tail of the pancreas. Forty per cent of the tumours are smaller than 1 cm in diameter. Multiple tumours are found in only 10% of patients. If tumours are multiple, 5% of patients will have more than four. MEA I syndrome must be considered in such cases. About 10% of these tumours are malignant.

Remember that nesidioblastosis and islet cell hyperplasia are also found in adults.

Management

The patient must be protected against attacks of hypoglycaemia in the preoperative period. This is done by feeding the patient often. He must be given a glucose infusion the evening before the operation.

Some surgeons recommend that patients be treated with diazoxide to control the hypoglycaemia. They contend that if patients react well to diazoxide preoperatively, "blind" pancreatectomy is not necessary if the tumour cannot be found. Others say that the drug has many side-effects, such as nausea, cardiac arrhythmias, leucopaenia, hypertrichosis and postural hypotension. Another reason for not using it is that it impedes intraoperative blood glucose measurement.

The operation

A bilateral subcostal approach is the best. The pancreas must be clearly exposed so that it can be properly inspected and palpated. A Kocher manoeuvre allows the surgeon to palpate the head between his fingers. The retroperitoneum must be split via the lesser sac to expose the pancreas. It may be necessary to mobilize the spleen and the tail of the pancreas to the medial side. All superficial tumours can be excised locally. Deep-seated tumours of the body and tail must be removed together with a distal resection of the body and tail of the pancreas. Tumours of the head can be excised locally.

Malignant tumours are treated by means of a distal pancreatectomy, if they are situated in the body or tail. If they are in the head, a pancreaticoduodenectomy is performed.

If the tumour cannot be found, there are various possible approaches:

- *Intraoperative selective venous collections, with insulin measurements to determine the area of high insulin secretion.*
- *To do nothing and rely on diazoxide if the patient has responded well to it. To perform further localization studies, using transhepatic venous blood collection.*

• Blind pancreatectomy

Proponents of this method suggest that a distal pancreatectomy from the neck to the tail of the pancreas be done (80% of the pancreatic tissue). A pathologist must then look for the tumour serially and insulin levels are measured half-hourly. There is an 80% chance that the tumour will be situated in the sample. If the insulin levels drop sharply, the tumour has probably been removed. The pathologist may also make a diagnosis of hyperplasia or nesidioblastosis.

If the tumour has not been located and the insulin level has not dropped, all the pancreatic tissue is removed. A thin layer is left round the bile duct which is left to safeguard the blood supply in the duodenum.

This is also the correct treatment for hyperplasia and nesidioblastosis. The chances are 90% that the tumour will be found. If it is not removed, the patient must be treated with diazoxide. If this does not control the disease, or if the side-effects of the drug become unbearable, a total pancreatectomy must be performed.

Glucagonomas

These tumours arise from the alpha cells and secrete excessive glucagon. The syndrome is mainly found in middle-aged women. Patients present with dermatitis, glossitis, stomatitis, constipation and loss of weight.

They are diabetic and anaemic. Hypocholesterolaemia, hypoproteinaemia and a decrease in serum amino acids is often found. The majority of tumours (70%) are malignant.

The treatment is excision of the tumour. All symptoms and signs of the syndrome resolve if the tumour was benign. Malignant tumours recur and chemotherapy (DTIC) must be given.

Vipoma (Werner-Morrison syndrome)

This condition is more common in middle-aged women. Ninety per cent of these tumours are found in the pancreas and the rest in the retroperitoneal sympathetic nerves and the adrenal medulla. About 40% are malignant.

Patients present with watery diarrhoea – up to 10 litres per day, with an average of 5 litres per day.

They develop hypokalaemia, hypercalcaemia, hyperglycaemia, hyperchlorhydria and even achlorhydria.

In about 15% of cases, patients develop hot flushes during diarrhoea attacks. Forty per cent of these tumours are malignant.

The diagnosis is confirmed by measuring raised fasting plasma vasoactive intestinal polypeptide (VIP). The levels of pancreatic polypeptide (PP) and prostaglandin E_2 (PGE_2) must also be measured. Sometimes the VIP is normal, but PP and PGE_2 are raised.

Preoperatively, dehydration and hypokalaemia must be corrected. Steroids and somatostatin are useful. The tumour must be excised. If total excision is not possible, a partial resection (debulking) procedure must be done, followed by streptosotazin and 5-fluorouracil. The patient must be treated symptomatically with steroids and somatostatin.

Somatostatinoma

Somatostatin is a polypeptide secreted by the D-cells of the islets. These cells are also found in the stomach, duodenum, small intestine and colon.

Somatostatin inhibits all gastrointestinal tract hormones. Drainage of the gall bladder and the stomach are inhibited, as is bowel motility. Somatostatin also inhibits secretion of gastric and pancreatic juices.

The majority of these tumours are found in the pancreas, but a few have been found in the wall of the duodenum. The condition is most frequently found in women. Patients present with diarrhoea, loss of weight and hypertension. Gall stones and diabetes are common. Most tumours are associated with liver metastases.

Gastrinoma

This tumour has already been discussed in the chapter dealing with gastrointestinal haemorrhage.

D. MULTIPLE ENDOCRINE NEOPLASIA (MEN) SYNDROME

Cells which secrete amines and polypeptides have several characteristics in common. They store amine (such as catecholamines) A, they absorb amine precursors (such as dopamine) and PU (precursor uptake); and they contain a decarboxylase which is necessary for amine synthesis D. These cells are therefore known as APUD cells.

Although there is controversy on this issue at the moment, most researchers believe that these cells originate from the neuroectoderm and migrate to the different sites at which they are found.

The APUD cells in the pituitary gland secrete ACTH. In the gastrointestinal canal, they secrete 5-hydroxytryptamine, histamine and various polypeptides such as secretin, cholecystokinin, gastrin, glucagon, somatostatin and VIP.

Tumours of the APUD system are responsible for the majority of the endocrine syndromes discussed in previous chapters. Because these syndromes can be caused either by adenomas or malignant tumours, it is more accurate to refer to multiple endocrine neoplasia, rather than multiple endocrine adenomatosis (MEA).

The MEN-syndrome has an autosomal dominant inheritance pattern.

MEN I

This consists of hyperplasia and/or tumours of the parathyroid, pancreatic islets and anterior pituitary gland. A variety of other non-hormone-producing tumours have been described with this.

Ninety per cent of patients have hyperparathyroidism. Forty per cent have an increase in gastrin secretion and 10% an increase in insulin secretion. Acromegaly is rare, but chromophobe tumours are relatively common.

Patients present more often with peptic ulcer. Management is mainly aimed at the parathyroid hyperplasia. All the glands are removed and a small amount of tissue transplanted.

MEN II

This syndrome consists of medullary carcinoma of the thyroid, phaeochromocytoma and parathyroid hyperplasia.

MEN IIa

All have medullary carcinoma. A third also have phaeochromocytoma and parathyroid hyperplasia.

MEN IIb

Medullary carcinoma is always present. Patients also have neuromas of the conjunctiva, lips and oral mucosa, as well as ganglioneuromas in the intestinal canal. They have a Marfanoid appearance, with long limbs, high foot arches and kyphoscoliosis. They sometimes also have phaeochromocytoma, but never parathyroid hyperplasia. Medullary carcinoma is more aggressive in the MEN IIb than in the MEN IIa syndrome.

Medullary carcinoma and phaeochromocytoma are often bilateral in the MEN II syndrome. Family members of patients with MEN syndrome must be examined for raised calcitonin levels which will suggest hyperfunction of the occult lesions in the thyroid.

The treatment is aimed mainly at the medullary tumour, if phaeochromocytoma has been excluded on screening tests. Otherwise, the phaeochromocytoma must be operated on before the medullary carcinoma.

The blood vessels 9

THE ARTERIAL SYSTEM

Arterial obstruction

The blood supply to a limb consists of a main artery and its branches. The branches, which supply the muscles with blood, also serve as collateral vessels via the arterioles, which can return blood to the main vessel after bypassing an obstruction.

The flow in the artery is dependent on blood pressure, the diameter of the blood vessel and the viscosity of the blood.

The flow in the collateral vessels is dependent on the same factors, except that the development of existing potential collateral vessels depends on a pressure gradient. If an obstruction occurs in a large vessel, the pressure distal to the obstruction will immediately fall to very low levels. A difference in pressure between the proximal blood vessels and the vessels distal to the obstruction thus arises (a pressure gradient). This immediately stimulates dilatation of the potential collateral vessels, which enlarge gradually to transport more blood around the obstruction. As the collaterals enlarge, the pressure distal to the obstruction rises. If and when the pressure returns to normal, the gradient will disappear and the stimulus for collateral dilatation will no longer be present. Pressures distal to the obstruction do not usually rise higher than the diastolic pressure proximal to the obstruction, so that the stimulus for collateral dilatation is maintained.

Other factors influencing collateral dilatation include underlying disease of the vascular wall such as atherosclerosis, spasm of the wall due to autonomic nervous control, vascoconstriction caused by catecholamines and the dilating effect of the metabolites which arise in the tissues due to anoxia.

Other consequences of arterial obstruction

Static blood clots. The clot at the obstruction thus tends to extend proximally until it reaches the next large branch of the artery. The clot also tends to extend distally and can even block the openings of the small branches which form collaterals. The success of blood flow through collaterals depends largely on an open inflow tract, with optimal blood pressure, and an adequate outflow tract distal to the blockage. If these factors are not present, there is a tendency towards stasis and further thrombosis.

How does the patient with arterial obstruction present?

The presentation is totally dependent on the adequacy of the collateral flow. If the collaterals are inadequate, there will be symptoms and signs of arterial insufficiency, even when the limb is at rest – acute arterial insufficiency.

If the collateral flow is adequate at rest but insufficient with exercise, chronic arterial insufficiency is present.

Acute arterial insufficiency

This follows a sudden occlusion of a large vessel to a limb, with inadequate collateral flow.

Causes of arterial occlusion

- **Thrombosis**

Thrombosis takes place on an underlying atherosclerotic lesion of the blood vessel wall. Local haemodynamic factors, such as movement of the arteries at joints (knee join), turbulence at bifurcations and the openings to branches and trauma, play a role. Systemic factors include obesity, hypercholesterolaemia, diet, cigarette smoking and diabetes mellitus.

Thrombosis occurs if the atheromatous plaque ulcerates. Underlying narrowing or irregular widening of the vessels will also predispose. If the collateral vessels and their openings are also affected by the disease, the collateral flow will be inadequate.

- **Embolus**

Part of a thrombus on an atherosclerotic plaque may break off and cause obstruction more distally at a bifurcation. The most common source of embolus is the heart. Large thrombi can form in the heart chambers of patients with mitral stenosis who are fibrillating, those with coronary thrombosis with infarction and those with vegetations on their valves due to subacute bacterial endocarditis. Aortic aneurysm is also a source of emboli.

- **Injuries**

Joint dislocations, particularly posterior subluxation of the knee joint and fractures, can cause avulsion of the artery, or only the intima, with thrombosis.

Direct arterial injury by missile or stab wounds can also cause acute arterial insufficiency.

What does the patient complain of?

Pain

There is sudden onset of severe pain at the site of the obstruction overlying the artery, followed by pain in the remainder of the limb. This is followed by continuous, nagging pain, which is worst in the toes and feet; and is known as rest pain. The patient finds that if he exposes the leg and lets it hang over the edge of the bed, the pain subsides slightly.

Paraesthesia

Patients complain of pins-and-needles and hyperaesthesia of the skin of the toes and soles. Gradual hypoaesthesia sets in, with total loss of sensation in the toes and feet.

What does the clinician find?

The limb is pale and cold, due to spasm in the skin arterioles. Later this spasm relaxes and blood flows slowly back into the skin. Because excessive oxygen is withdrawn by the ischaemic tissues, the limb becomes blue. No pulses are palpable distal to the obstruction. The calf muscles are tender and swollen due to oedema. The muscles later harden and paralysis sets in. The patient can no longer move his toes.

The skin develops areas of oedema and blisters arise. This is an indication that the endothelium of the capillaries has been so severely damaged by ischaemia that it has become extremely permeable to fluid.

This complex of symptoms and signs is known as an acute threatened limb. The next step is gangrene of the tissue.

Remember that nerves are more vulnerable to ischaemia than muscle, and muscle is more vulnerable than skin. By the time gangrene of the skin develops, the muscle has usually already been irreversibly damaged.

Natural course of arterial insufficiency

If collateral flow is inadequate, the limb will become gangrenous, with resultant loss of the limb. If collateral flow is sufficiently adequate to prevent gangrene, but the patient has continuous rest pain, peripheral gangrene of the tips of the toes or ischaemic ulceration, the limb is chronically threatened. Such a limb will be lost if the blood supply cannot be improved considerably. If the collateral flow improves to such an extent that the flow is adequate at rest and the patient only develops pain on exercising (claudication), it is known as chronic arterial insufficiency.

What causes must the clinician consider?

Thrombosis with underlying artherosclerotic vascular insufficiency

This is the most common cause. Patients give a history of previous claudication. There are signs of chronic arterial insufficiency in the limb. There is no source of emboli (fibrillation).

Embolus

A source of embolism is present (fibrillation). There is no history of chronic arterial insufficiency (no claudication). There are no signs of arterial insufficiency.

Management of acute arterial insufficiency

The aim is to increase the circulation to the limbs by improving collateral blood supply or by restoring flow through the main artery by relieving or bypassing the obstruction.

If the most probable diagnosis is an embolic obstruction, the embolus must be removed as an emergency procedure. If the most probable diagnosis is thrombosis, the patient must initially be treated conservatively.

Conservative management

- *Put the patient to bed and administer analgesics. This reduces spasm.*
- *Apply general supportive measures to optimize heart and lung function.*
- *Make sure that the haemoglobin is normal, administer oxygen and cardiac support if necessary.*
- *Treat heart failure actively to ensure a good blood pressure.*
- *Heparinize the patient to prevent extension of the thrombus. A thrombus which enlarges can block collateral vessels.*
- *Elevate the head of the bed to improve blood flow to the legs by gravity.*
- *Expose the limb to room temperature and remove all constricting objects such as socks and bandages.*
- *Re-evaluate the condition of the limb regularly. If the collateral flow becomes adequate and symptoms and signs improve, there is no indication for emergency intervention. One can wait, persist with conservative treatment and re-evaluate the patient at a later stage.*
- *If the collateral flow appears to be inadequate, in that symptoms and signs worsen, especially if the calf muscles swell and motor function is affected, the patient is developing an acute threatened limb and limb loss will occur if the blood supply is not restored.*

Questions that must precede arterial surgery

Is there an indication for surgery?

An acutely threatened limb is an absolute indication for surgery.

Is the patient fit for surgery?

Atherosclerosis is a disease which affects all the blood vessels to a greater or lesser extent. To determine fitness in a patient with peripheral arterial insufficiency, the blood supply and hence the function of the vital organs can be evaluated.

Cerebral function and the carotid arteries must be examined. Renal functions must be measured. Lung and cardiac functions play an especially important role in the patient's fitness. Because these patients are usually smokers, their lung functions are poor. The coronary vessels are often affected by the underlying disease.

A skilled physician and anaesthetist can be consulted to help determine the patient's level of fitness. Emergency treatment to improve inadequate organ function rapidly is an extremely important factor in the treatment.

Is the proposed operation possible?

An indication exists and the patient is fit for surgery; it must now be determined whether an operation is possible. This is usually done by performing arteriography to determine whether there is a patent inflow tract proximal to the obstruction and, very importantly, whether there is a patent outflow tract distal to the obstruction. Arterial reconstruction can only be done if there are good patent vessels distal to the obstruction.

An arteriogram must be performed to show the aorta, the iliac vessels, the femoral vessels, the popliteal artery and its three branches, the posterior tibial artery, anterior tibial artery and peroneal artery. Two methods are available:

- **Translumbar aortogram**

A long needle is inserted from behind alongside the spinal column, at an angle of 45 degrees, into the abdominal aorta and a bolus of radio-opaque solution (urografin) must be injected while X-rays are taken of the entire arterial tree.

- **Percutaneous transfemoral catheter arteriography (Seldinger technique)**

A catheter is threaded over a guidewire in the femoral artery into the aorta and a bolus of urografin is injected. X-rays are taken of the whole arterial tree.

Aorto-iliac occlusion

This is a less common cause of acute vascular insufficiency, because the collateral flow via the internal iliac vessels and their branches is usually good. Extensive bilateral thrombosis is sometimes the cause of acute insufficiency.

Femoropopliteal thrombosis

This is a common cause of acute vascular insufficiency. If the common femoral artery is occluded, the distal outflow tract can consist of the superficial femoral artery and profunda femoris artery. This is a good outflow tract and collateral vessels via the profunda femoris are so good that an acutely threatened limb is a rare occurrence.

More often, one finds a combination of occlusions of the common femoral artery and the superficial femoral artery, with a patent *profunda femoris*. If the popliteal artery is occluded, surgery is less likely to be possible, as the outflow tract is inadequate.

Bypasses to the following outflow tracts are possible:

- *Profunda femoris artery. A small endarteriectomy is usually performed at its origin to make the bypass possible.*
- *To the popliteal artery and its branches. The arteriogram can show that a bypass is impossible, because the outflow tract is not patent. If the arteriogram shows pronounced stenosis proximally, the bypass must not be performed, unless the stenosis in the inflow tract is also corrected.*

Choice of operation

Arterial bypass

It is preferable to use the patient's reversed greater saphenous vein. If this is not available an artificial prosthesis can be used, especially in the aortofemoral region.

A dacron prosthesis is used for aortofemoral bypasses. Below the inguinal ligament and for femoropopliteal bypasses, PTFE (Goretex) prostheses are preferred.

Prognosis

The results of reconstruction are not very satisfactory in cases with acutely threatened limbs. The threat exists because collateral flow is poor which usually implies that the outflow tract is inadequate. Thrombosis often takes place in smaller branches, weakening the prognosis. The muscles have often been ischaemic for too long and a compartment syndrome develops, with ischaemic necrosis of the muscle, especially in the anterior compartment. If ischaemia has been present for some time, fasciotomies must be performed to bring about decompression of the compartments.

If reconstruction is not possible because there is no outflow tract, amputation of the totally ischaemic limb cannot be delayed, as the patient can develop renal failure and the mortality is high.

Chronically threatened limb

The limb is viable, but there is constant rest pain. Patients often develop gangrene of the tips of the toes and ischaemic ulceration can also develop.

There is therefore an absolute indication for surgery; and if the patient is fit for surgery and reconstruction appears to be possible on arteriography, an operation must be performed.

If an operation is not possible, or if the patient is unfit for a major procedure, one must treat conservatively in the hope that collateral flow will improve in time. Eventually these patients request amputation due to unbearable, constant pain.

Acute arterial occlusion by embolization

The source of the embolus is usually a fibrillating heart. The embolus moves to the periphery in the arteries and lodges at a bifurcation, as the embolus is too large to move through the next smaller branch of the blood vessel.

A large embolus will lodge in the bifurcation of the aorta - a saddle embolus. It is so named because it lies like a saddle over the two legs of the bifurcation. The next common site where emboli lodge is at the bifurcation of the common femoral artery into superficial femoral and profunda femoris arteries. If the embolus is small enough to move even further, it will lodge at the trifurcation of the popliteal artery.

Patients must undergo emergency surgery. If they are unfit due to their cardiac condition, the embolectomy can be done under local anaesthetic.

The femoral artery is opened in the inguinal region. If the embolus is lodged here, it is removed under direct vision. If it is situated higher up or lower down, it is pulled out with a Fogarty catheter. The catheter resembles a Foley catheter, but is a more delicate instrument made of plastic material. The catheter is pushed past the embolus, the balloon inflated and the embolus pulled out by the inflated balloon. Any fresh clot that has formed in the blood vessel due to stasis is also removed using the Fogarty catheter.

Acute traumatic arterial occlusion

The management of arterial trauma will be discussed in the chapter dealing with trauma.

Chronic vascular insufficiency

This condition is mainly found in the lower limbs. The collateral vessels in the upper limbs are so good that the condition rarely presents, except in patients with diabetes mellitus. Chronic insufficiency in the arm is also found in patients with thoracic outlet syndrome. Chronic vascular insufficiency in the lower limbs is caused by atherosclerosis in 90% of cases. Rare arterial diseases such as Buerger disease and collagen diseases are responsible for the rest.

Chronic insufficiency follows acute occlusion if the collateral vessels are adequate, or develops gradually as stenosis of the vessels increases. By the time the vessel is eventually occluded by clot, the collateral vessels have already developed gradually so that the patient's limb is not acutely threatened.

Clinical presentation

Claudication

This is pain which arises in muscle groups on exercise, and is relieved by rest. The muscle groups involved will depend on the site of the occlusion.

Occlusion of the aorto-iliac vessels causes claudication in the buttocks. Impotence is associated with this. It is known as the Le Riche syndrome.

Claudication is more commonly found in the calves, with stenoses or occlusions elsewhere in the blood vessels.

Rest pain

This pain comes on without exercise, e g at night in bed, and is not found in muscle groups, but in the toes and feet. If rest pain becomes continuous and nagging, it means that the blood supply has become so inadequate that a chronic threat to the limb is developing.

Abnormalities of sensation

Patients complain of a numb feeling in their feet, but sensation is intact on testing.

Impotence

Patients complain of inability to develop or maintain erection. In such cases, there is usually occlusion of both iliac vessels.

Clinical presentation

Pulses

Pulses may be absent on palpation or only a weak pulsation may be palpable. If pulses disappear after exercise, this usually means that there is a critical stenosis above the weak pulse.

Bruits

A murmur will be audible over the blood vessel at the site of the weak pulse if a stenosis is present. The bruit will become louder on exercise.

The skin

The skin may be pale, or pallor may be elicited by elevating the feet and asking the patient to flex the soles of his feet continuously. The sole on the side of the worst insufficiency will become deadly pale.

If the foot is now suspended, it will assume a dark red colour (rubor). This is caused by accumulated metabolites dilating the arterioles and because excessive oxygen is withdrawn from the blood that does keep flowing in.

The time required for the development of rubor can be measured. It should normally happen within twenty seconds, otherwise there is a suggestion of vascular insufficiency. The skin feels cold.

If the leg above and below the knee feels cold, but the knee itself feels warm, the popliteal artery is occluded and the blood flows closer to the skin through the collateral vessels, thus warming the skin (Gaylis sign). The area of the transition from warm to cold gives an indication of the site of occlusion.

Subcutaneous tissue

This may be oedematous. If atrophy of the subcutaneous tissue develops, the skin indents on pressure like a table-tennis ball (ping-pong sign).

Skin appendages

The nails are brittle and grow slowly. Hair falls out and is absent on the foot on the affected side.

Muscles

Atrophy of the calves and interosseus muscles may be present. Muscle weakness and even paralysis can occur.

Venous filling time

The feet are elevated to empty the veins. Allow the feet to hang free and measure the filling time. Normally, the veins will within seven seconds.

Special investigations

Claudication distance on a treadmill

A treadmill can be used to measure the distance taken for the patient to develop claudication. This can give an indication of the degree of vascular insufficiency and can be used to measure improvement following treatment.

Doppler studies

The ankle-brachial artery pressure index can be measured. The pressure, as measured by the Doppler apparatus at the posterior tibial artery, can be divided by the brachial artery pressure. Normally, the index is one or more. Values of less than one indicate vascular insufficiency. Rest pain usually starts developing if the index is less than 0,3.

Duplex-Doppler

This method can be used to measure the arterial wave profile, pressures and ultrasound appearance of the arteries. It is a useful screening test.

Arteriography

This is an invasive and dangerous investigation and must be performed only if surgery is planned. Digital subtraction angiography (DGA) or computer angiography, with venous bolus injection, can also be used for a screening test, but these do not provide sufficient definition for planning of operations.

Management

Chronic vascular insufficiency can remain constant for long periods, without deterioration. Claudication as such is not an indication for arterial reconstruction. As arterial reconstruction can merely be regarded as palliation, the risks of the operation must be weighed against the patient's functional limitation. Atherosclerosis is a disease which affects all the blood vessels and usually, the blood supply to vital organs such as the heart, brain and kidneys is also insufficient, thereby increasing the operative risk.

The natural course of the disease is not influenced by surgery. In time, the disease process will develop further and cause additional arterial insufficiency.

Only claudication which restricts the patient to such an extent that he cannot do his work or even fulfil his normal daily functions, is an indication for reconstruction. This is called incapacitating claudication.

Conservative management

Conservative management is aimed at minimizing risk factors, improving collateral flow and protecting the feet.

- *Patients must stop smoking.*
- *They must adjust their diets to limit obesity and dietary fat intake.*
- *Hypertension must be treated.*
- *Collateral circulation must be improved. Patients must try to walk further every day within the limits of their claudication. As collateral flow improves, they will be able to walk further every day.*
- *It is probably advisable to give aspirin prophylaxis against platelet clots.*
- *There is no support for the use of vasodilators. They work better on healthy vessels, thus further reducing the flow through the diseased vessels.*
- *The feet must be kept clean and dry.*
- *Fungal diseases of the feet must be avoided.*
- *Good, soft socks and strong, protective shoes must be worn.*
- *Injuries must be avoided.*
- *If small injuries or infections arise, the patient must see a doctor immediately.*

Surgery

If the claudication is seriously limiting and the patient is fit, an arteriogram must be done and arterial reconstruction planned.

Thrombo-endarteriectomy

This is seldom done. Patients with a short, local occlusion in the larger vessels (aorta or iliac vessels) may be considered. It is also useful for resolving local stenosis in the origin of the profunda femoris artery in older, unfit patients. Meaningful improvement in the blood supply to the limb can be achieved.

Thrombo-endarteriectomy often forms part of the preparation of an artery on which a bypass is to be carried out.

Arterial bypass

In aortofemoral occlusion, an aortobifemoral bypass is done, using a dacron bifurcation prosthesis. Below the inguinal ligament, an autotransplant is done, using the patient's own greater saphenous vein. If a prosthesis must be used, PTFE (Goretex) is preferred.

Extra-anatomical bypasses

In unfit patients, a bypass can be made from the subclavian artery to both femoral arteries. This is a minor operation, because the prosthesis is inserted via a subcutaneous tunnel and an abdominal operation is thus avoided. In unilateral disease, a femoro-femoral bypass can be done. A prosthesis is fed subcutaneously from one femoral artery to the other. Patients tolerate this procedure well.

Distal arterial reconstruction

If the popliteal artery is occluded, a bypass, using a vein to one of its branches, must be considered. Most surgeons would do such an operation only if the limb is threatened.

Percutaneous transluminal angioplasty

Dilatation of the stenosis by means of a Gruntzig catheter can be considered in unfit patients with a localized stenosis. This is especially indicated in the iliac or femoral arteries. It is also useful intraoperatively to dilate a stenosis above an occlusion so that a bypass can be done more distally.

Lumbar sympathectomy

This operation does not improve claudication. However, it is useful in patients with a cold limb and skin ulceration, whose lesions are not suitable for reconstruction. It is done in conjunction with aortofemoral bypasses to dilate the outflow tract.

Prognosis

Aortofemoral reconstruction

The operative mortality is 5%. The five year patency is 80%.

Femoropopliteal reconstruction

The operative mortality is 2%. If a venous bypass is done, the five year patency is 60%. If a PTFE prosthesis is used, this figure is lower than 50%. The five year survival of patients with extensive arterial disease is 60%. The main cause of death is coronary vessel disease.

Thrombo-angiitis obliterans (Buerger disease)

This disease is characterized by multiple occlusions of smaller arteries of the limbs distal to the brachial or popliteal arteries. Thrombophlebitis of vessels on the limb often occurs in association with arterial occlusions. The disease in an angiitis, i e there is round cell infiltration of the walls of the affected artery. The artery becomes occluded due to fibrosis, which is part of the healing process of the angiitis. The disease is found almost exclusively in cigarette-smoking young men.

Aetiology

The precise role of cigarette smoke is not clear. All these patients smoke and the disease improves dramatically and progresses at a slower rate if the patient stops smoking. Humoral antibodies to arterial wall antigens can be demonstrated in these patients. They can also be differentiated using HLA typing. It therefore seems highly probable that there is a genetic predisposition; and that it is triggered by cigarette smoking.

Clinical presentation

A young or middle-aged man who usually smokes heavily, develops pain in his fingertips or claudication in the foot muscles. The toes are cold and cyanotic and develop necrosis and gangrene.

On examination, the larger vessels are patent and the pulses e g the popliteal pulse, are palpable. The occlusion is segmental and the posterior tibial artery may be occluded, while the dorsalis pedis is palpable. In the hands, only certain arteries of the fingers may be affected.

Special investigation

On arteriography, there are no signs of atherosclerosis in the large vessels. Distally, these vessels typically narrow down and further on, the vessel is completely occluded.

Histology

The diagnosis is made on biopsy. Sometimes a segment of vein can be removed to show the typical lesion of fibrotic strangulation of the artery, vein and nerve.

Management

Arterial reconstruction is not possible, because the disease affects the smaller vessels. If the patient stops smoking, the disease process arrests. Usually, patients continue to smoke and the segmental occlusion advances with serial losses of fingers or toes and eventual distal limb loss.

Sympathectomy is very useful if the patient stops smoking.

Amputation usually succeeds if the incision is made just proximal to the area of gangrene, as the larger vessels are still patent.

Popliteal artery entrapment syndrome

This occurs when the popliteal artery does not follow its usual course through the heads of gastrocnemius. Four different anomalies have been described. The most common of these is when the artery runs medial to the head of gastrocnemius. It can also run through the head if the head has an abnormal origin. There is sometimes a fibrous band proximal to the medial head, which entraps the artery and lastly, it can run deep to the popliteal muscle.

The artery is compressed every time the knee is fully extended. This causes chronic recurrent injury to the wall, with fibrosis. Dilatation develops distal to the stenosis and is complicated by thrombosis.

Clinical presentation

The condition is usually found in young men. They either present with claudication or develop an acutely threatened limb. If the patient is examined during the claudication phase, a weak ankle pulse is palpable, and disappears completely on extension of the knee.

Arteriography shows the abnormal course of the artery. The management is splitting of the restricting muscle and excision of the stenotic artery, with replacement by a vein. If technically possible, a bypass must be done, using a vein. This condition is fortunately rare.

Cystic degeneration of the popliteal artery

Mucoid cysts sometimes develop in the adventitia of the popliteal artery. These cause stenosis, with claudication. Diagnosis is confirmed on ultrasound or CT.

Excision and replacement by a vein is indicated.

Chronic vascular insufficiency and diabetes

Atherosclerosis is more common in diabetics. About 30% of such patients have occlusion of peripheral vessels. This atherosclerosis involves large, medium-sized and small arteries. In diabetics, occlusions are typically not restricted to the popliteal artery and the origin of its branches, but extend to the ankles.

These patients have micro-angiopathy, characterized by degenerative changes in the arterioles and thickening of the capillary basal membranes. They also have neuropathy, with reduction in, or loss of, sensation and loss of foot muscle tone. This leads to collapse of the arch. The combination of sensory disturbances and abnormal foot architecture leads to pressure necrosis and ulceration.

There are also abnormalities in normal white cell function, making patients more susceptible to infection.

Clinical presentation

Patients with diabetes can present with thrombosis and an acutely or chronically threatened limb. Patients can also present with claudication.

Diabetic foot

A very important clinical presentation is the patient with foot lesions. Usually the patient is a middle-aged woman, who has one of the following lesions:

- Atrophy of foot muscles with unstable arch.
- Patients present with very painful feet, or with pain and cyanosis in some toes.
- They present with superficial sepsis of the foot or toes.
- They present with a very painful foot, which has redness and tenderness on its dorsum or sole. This is an indication of deep sepsis in the compartments of the sole, which spreads along the tendon sheaths.
- Dry or wet gangrene of the forefoot or toes.

Special investigation

Urine or serum glucose measurements can be used to diagnose diabetes mellitus. X-rays of the feet show calcification of the small blood vessels. One must also be on the lookout for osteitis.

Management of the diabetic foot

The key to management is the status of the blood supply to the foot. The ankle pulses are usually absent, but may be present, implying that occlusion is confined to the smaller vessels of the foot. If the popliteal pulse is also absent, there is a combination of small- and large vessel disease. If the popliteal pulse and ankle pulses are present, a good prognosis can be expected with adequate local surgery.

If the popliteal pulse is palpable, but not the ankle pulses, the prognosis for local surgery is not good. If the popliteal pulse is absent, reconstruction of the larger vessels must be attempted before local procedures can be carried out on the foot. If reconstruction is not possible because the outflow tract (branches of the popliteal artery) are occluded by clot, it is highly unlikely that local surgery will succeed.

General measures

- *Control the diabetes with insulin.*
- *Administer antibiotics.*

Superficial sepsis of the foot

Saucerize the abscess. Beware of the tip-of-the-iceberg phenomenon. What sometimes resembles superficial sepsis can reach deep down into the tendon sheaths, or underlying osteitis may be present.

Deep sepsis of the foot

Once the diabetes has been treated and antibiotics have been given, the foot must be operated on as an emergency procedure. The principles are as follows:

- *All septic and necrotic material must be mercilessly excised.*
- *If the sepsis runs along tendon sheaths in the sole, the toe and its metacarpal must be cut out, so that the foot is split open (ray excision).*
- *After excision of septic necrotic tissue, the wound must be left open.*
- *After forty-eight hours, the wound must be inspected in theatre under anaesthetic. Once again, all necrotic tissue must be removed.*
- *This must continue until no more necrotic tissue forms.*

- *If it becomes clear that sepsis and necrosis has spread inexorably each time, lower leg amputation is preferable. Local procedures are often unsuccessful if the popliteal pulse is impalpable and reconstruction of larger vessels is not possible.*
- *If necrotic toes are amputated, the wound must be left open to granulate. It may not be sutured, otherwise necrosis of the skin flaps develops.*
- *Amputations higher up are managed according to the blood supply. The skin flaps are closed primarily and must therefore have a good blood supply.*
- *It is unfortunately necessary to do amputations above the knee in about 40% of these cases.*

Idiopathic neurotrophic foot

This is a condition which is found almost exclusively in black patients. Patients present with pigmentation, deformity of the feet with collapse of the arches, distortion of the toes and trophic ulcers, which become infected. The ankle pulses are usually palpable. The nerves and small vessels are affected. The arterioles show thickening of the intima with hyperplasia of smooth muscle of the media. The nerves show demyelinization, with axonal degeneration. The cause is unknown, but at present there is consensus that it can be ascribed to alcoholism and malnutrition.

Diabetes, syphilis, tuberculosis and leprosy must be considered in the differential diagnosis. The management is conservative: improvement of nutrition, particularly administration of B-group vitamins. Conservative surgical procedures, such as excision of necrotic tissue and amputations of toes with septic arthritis and osteitis, must be done.

Chronic vascular insufficiency of the upper limbs

Atherosclerosis is relatively common in the arch of the aorta and its main branches. Because the collateral circulation is so good, patients seldom present with an acutely threatened limb. Emboli to more distal vessels of the arm can present as an acutely threatened limb.

Raynaud syndrome

Primary Raynaud phenomenon

This is a disease of young women and is precipitated by cold or emotional stress. The hands are usually affected, but sometimes also the feet. The condition occurs bilaterally.

The disease presents with an attack of pallor, followed by cyanosis, coldness and a numb feeling in the fingers. If the hands are warmed, the fingers become bright red, with a burning pain. This colour change disappears gradually and normal skin colour returns.

In time, these patients develop atrophy of the skin and subcutaneous tissues (pulp spaces) and ulcers develop, with secondary infection. They eventually develop gangrene of the fingertips.

On examination, the radial pulse is palpable. Arteriography shows patent arteries, with occlusion of the peripheral digital arteries.

Management

- *Patients must avoid cold.*
- *They must wear gloves and avoid injuries or infections.*
- *They may not smoke, use the "pill", or use beta blockers.*
- *Alpha blockers, such as guanethidine, may be useful.*
- *Calcium channel blockers and prostaglandins may also be tried.*
- *Sympathectomy sometimes yields good results.*

Secondary Raynaud phenomenon

Attacks of this phonemenon result from a number of known causes, including frostbite, collagen diseases and the use of vibrating tools.

Patients with frostbite must be treated with rapid rewarming, heparinization and Rheomacrodex. Sympathectomy can be considered. The collagen diseases, such as scleroderma, lupus erythematosus, polymyositis and drug- induced vasculitis, cause degeneration of the walls of the arterioles, with fragmentation of the elastic fibres and fibrinoid necrosis of the media and intima. These diseases are treated with steroids and anticoagulants.

Vibrating tools cause vasoconstriction via the autonomic nervous system.

The causes of secondary Raynaud phenomenon must be differentiated from the thoracic outlet syndrome, Buerger disease and atherosclerosis.

Acrocyanosis

This is a condition found in young women. It is characterized by continuous cyanosis of the hands and feet, a numb sensation and pain. The cyanosis is also found on the thighs and arms and has a reticular pattern.

Management

Patients must keep their limbs warm.

Thoracic outlet syndrome

This term is used for a variety of conditions which cause compression of arteries, nerves and veins behind the clavicle. Mechanisms which can play a role include a cervical rib, abnormal ligaments, hypertrophy or abnormal insertion of the scalenus anterior muscle, or pressures on structures where they run over the first rib, between the rib and clavicle, during certain arm movements. It is now generally accepted that this syndrome is most often caused by nerve compression, with secondary spastic vascular changes, rather than by direct compression of the blood vessels themselves. Despite this, stenoses of the artery do occur, with poststenotic dilatation in the region of the first rib. Thrombus forms in such a dilatation and small emboli block distal vessels. The artery can sometimes be totally occluded by a clot.

Clinical presentation

Patients present with pain, paraesthesia and a dull feeling, particularly in the section of the hand supplied by the ulnar nerve. The symptoms are provoked when the patient carries out certain shoulder movements for a long time, especially working with his hands above his head. Others complain of onset of symptoms if they carry heavy objects with their shoulders dropped.

On examination, neurological deficit or arterial signs can usually not be detected. The radial pulse sometimes disappears if the arm is abducted and the head is rotated and pulled to the opposite side (Adson test). This phenomenon is also found in normal people. A bruit is sometimes palpable in the supraclavicular fossa.

Special investigations

X-rays may show a cervical rib. Arteriography is often completely normal. Sometimes compression of the artery on the first rib can be demonstrated by using the Adson test. In rare cases, a stenosis and poststenotic dilatation can be seen.

Differential diagnosis

This condition must be differentiated from cervical disc lesions and carpal tunnel syndrome. Underlying atherosclerosis with stenosis or thrombosis must be excluded on angiography.

Management

Initially, patients must be treated conservatively with physiotherapy. If they do not respond to conservative treatment, surgery must be considered. If the patient has a cervical rib on X-ray, the neck must be explored via a supraclavicular approach. The cervical rib must be removed and the scalenus anterior muscle cut during such an operation. If there is no rib, but an indication for surgery does exist, the first rib must be removed via a transaxillary approach (Roos approach). The scalenus anterior muscle musts also be cut at the site where it inserts into the rib during this operation. Good results are achieved in 90% of cases.

Axillary vein thrombosis

Patients present with oedema, cyanosis and a heavy feeling in the arm.

On examination, prominent collateral veins can be seen around the shoulder. This condition arises after strenuous sport and work with the arms elevated above the head. It may form part of the thoracic outlet syndrome. There are sometimes underlying reasons, such as hypercoagulability or the use of the "pill".

Patients must be treated conservatively, and will improve as collateral vessels develop.

Takayasu arteritis

This is a disease which is particularly common in young black women in South Africa. An arteritis, particularly of the branches of the aortic arch, arises. It is characterised by obliteration of the *vasa vasorum* and round cell inflammation, with breakdown of the elastic and muscle fibres of the media and fibrotic thickening of the wall. This leads to stenosis, followed by thrombosis. Some patients develop aneurysms.

The cause is unknown. Most of these patients have tuberculosis. Complement-fixing immune complexes have also been described.

Clinical presentation

There is an initial inflammatory phase. Patients present with an influenza-like illness. Later they present with progressive arterial obliteration. The disease spreads and affects multiple vessels.

Patients may present with claudication of the arms and legs, transient ischaemic attacks (small strokes), renal hypertension and cardiac failure.

Differential diagnosis

The disease must be differentiated from the collagen arteritises and syphilis. Atherosclerosis must also be considered.

Management

In the early stages, patients must be treated conservatively, using steroids. If occlusions are already present, arterial bypasses must be considered.

Prognosis

The prognosis varies considerably. About 30% of these patients will die within five years.

Insufficiency of cerebral blood flow

Atherosclerosis of the large blood vessels which supply the brain with blood, is very common. Endarteriectomy of the internal carotid artery is the most common vascular operation in the USA. In other countries, including South Africa, it is far less common than operations on the blood vessels of the lower limb, but this could be ascribed to differing interpretations of the indications for surgery.

The symptoms and signs are usually caused by micro-emboli which break free from atherosclerotic plaques and ulceration of the intima on the lateral wall at the origin of the internal carotid artery. They can also be caused by diminished blood flow due to a critical stenosis or a total occlusion. The brain is supplied by four vessels, two internal carotid arteries and two vertebral arteries. Even a total occlusion of one artery will not necessarily cause symptoms. About 80% of symptomatic patients will have a lesion in an artery which can be reached surgically. The micro-emboli can lodge in the first branch of the internal carotid artery, namely the ophthalmic artery, and cause a temporary loss of vision known as *Amaurosis fugax*. The emboli can move more distally and cause small occlusions in the area supplied by the internal carotid, leading to transient attacks of paresis and a numb feeling in the arm or leg. These phenomena are known as transient ischaemic attacks (TIA). About 30% of patients with TIA will, in time, develop a stroke with permanent neurological damage. The stenotic, ulcerated blood vessel may become occluded by a clot, or a large embolus may dislodge and cause total obstruction of the blood vessel.

Clinical presentation

Patients may be divided into five main groups:

- **Asymptomatic patients**

Patients present with another condition, e g vascular insufficiency of the lower limb, and chance discovery of a bruit in the neck.

- **Transient ischaemic attacks**

These attacks of visual disturbance or paresis and a numb feeling in a limb usually last for only a few minutes. All neurological signs must disappear within twenty-four hours for it to be a TIA, by definition. If the retina is examined, the emboli can sometimes be seen as small spots in the arterial bifurcation of the retina.

- **Acute unstable neurological deficit**

The ischaemic attack starts as a small attack, becomes worse and lasts longer than twenty-four hours. The prognosis is not good and the patient often develops a full-scale stroke.

- **Full-scale stroke**

Patients develop a full-scale stroke and then recover partially with permanent neurological damage.

- **Vertebrobasillar disease**

Diminished blood supply via the vertebral arteries or emboli cause a combination of symptoms and signs which usually manifest bilaterally. Patients are clumsy, drop things, complain of dizziness, double vision and even dysphagia.

On examination, a bruit can usually be heard, depending on where the lesion is situated.

- A bruit high up in the neck is usually from stenosis of the internal carotid artery.
- Bruits lower down in the neck, especially those audible posterior to the trapezius muscle, usually come from the vertebral artery.
- A bruit at the midpoint of the clavicle comes from a subclavian artery stenosis.
- A difference in blood pressure between the two arms indicates a subclavian artery stenosis.

Special investigations

Non-invasive tests

- Duplex Doppler scanning can give a good indication of the appearance of the artery and the nature of the stenosis; and also of the appearance of the pulse wave and the degree of impairment of blood flow.
- Ocular plethysmography. This measures the pressures in the ophthalmic artery and gives a good indication of blood flow through the internal carotid artery.

Invasive tests

Cerebral arteriography: Digital subtraction angiography (DSA) is useful to determine the nature of the stenosis and can be done with small catheters and small volumes of dye, making it a safe investigation. Unfortunately, it does not always provide enough definition.

Most surgeons prefer direct arteriography before reconstructive surgery can be attempted. It is advisable to obtain an image of all four arteries that supply the brain as well as the arch of the aorta.

Management

The aim of management is to prevent further TIA's by preventing micro-emboli. The blood supply must then be improved by relieving the stenosis.

Medical management

There are two possible options, anticoagulant therapy and antiplatelet coagulation therapy, with e g aspirin. Prospective trials with anticoagulant therapy showed that it did not reduce the complications of stroke significantly. A high risk of bleeding exists. What trials have shown is that aspirin does improve the prognosis.

Surgical management

A symptomatic patient (TIA) must undergo an operation. A thrombo-endarteriectomy of the internal carotid artery must be done. During the operation, the cerebral blood pressure must be maintained and it is advisable to improvise a temporary bypass to maintain blood flow during the clamping of the artery.

Patients who have recently survived a full-scale stroke, must not be operated on. If the blood supply is restored at this stage, a severe bleed can arise at the site of infarction in the brain.

Patients who have recovered from a stroke must be operated on later, as they run a high risk of developing further strokes.

Asymptomatic patients with an internal carotid artery stenosis

This is a controversial condition. Some physicians prefer to treat such patients with antiplatelet coagulation drugs. Others believe that if the stenosis involves more than 80% of the lumen, or if duplex Doppler shows severe ulceration, an endarteriectomy must preferably be performed. If a patient has to undergo any other major operation, e g a resection of a large abdominal aortic aneurysm, and he has an asymptomatic internal carotid artery stenosis, it is probably wiser to treat the stenosis before tackling the aneurysm. Should the blood pressure fall during aneurysmectomy, the patient runs the risk of developing a stroke.

Vertebral insufficiency

If there is stenosis at the origin of the right vertebral artery, an endarteriectomy must be done. The origin of the left artery is difficult to reach through the neck and it must preferably be transected and sutured end-to-side to the left common carotid artery.

The subclavian artery steal syndrome

There is a critical stenosis or occlusion of the subclavian artery proximal to the vertebral artery's origin. When the patient exercises his arm, he develops neurological symptoms, because blood from the vertebral artery flows in a retrograde direction to the area of lower pressure in the subclavian artery distal to the stenosis. The condition is treated with a bypass from the common carotid artery to the subclavian artery.

Other conditions which can impair blood flow in the great vessels of the brain

- Dissections of the aortic arch or the internal carotid artery.
- Fibromuscular dysplasia. This is a disease which is found mainly in young women. It is usually bilateral. There is overgrowth of the media of the internal carotid artery in a segmental pattern, with stenoses. The arteriogram shows a "string of beads" appearance. Patients begin with TIA's and may develop stroke. The disease may also occur in the renal vessels, causing hypertension. Patients must be operated on and the stenoses must be dilated. Percutaneous transluminal angioplasty is used by some researchers, but it has a higher incidence of complications than direct open dilatation.
- Takayasu arteritis. This can also cause impairment of cerebral blood flow. It has already been discussed.

Prognosis of surgical management of TIA

The operative mortality is lower than 1%. Permanent neurological damage occurs in 2%. Recurrence of disease is rare.

RENOVASCULAR HYPERTENSION

Stenosis of the renal arteries is responsible for about 3% of cases of hypertension. Eighty per cent of renal stenoses are caused by atherosclerosis, 15% by fibromuscular dysplasia and the rest by conditions such as emboli and injuries.

Atherosclerosis is common in men over forty and occurs bilaterally in 90%. It mainly affects the openings of the renal vessels. Fibromuscular dysplasia is found mainly in women under forty, occurs bilaterally in 50% and affects the middle third and branches of the renal artery.

The mechanism of renal stenotic hypertension can be explained as follows:

- Reduced perfusion stimulates the juxtaglomerular apparatus to increase its renin secretion.
- This stimulates angiotensinogen to form angiotensin I, which is then converted to angiotensin II.
- This causes constriction of arterioles, raised aldosterone secretion and sodium retention.
- The blood pressure rises.
- After a while, secondary changes occur in the kidneys.

Clinical presentation

Patients are often asymptomatic, but may present with headaches. The diastolic pressure is consistently raised and a bruit is audible in the lumbar area. If there is no family history of hypertension, especially in young women, renal hypertension must be considered. The severity of the hypertension worsens and it does not respond well to medication.

Special investigations

Measuring sodium levels in urine obtained separately from each kidney is unreliable, as bilateral disease often occurs. Selective renin measurements in the renal veins are useful. Once again, these are not very reliable due to bilateral disease.

Captopril inhibits the conversion of angiotensin I to angiotensin II. In renal stenotic hypertension, the blood pressure drops sharply when this drug is given. It is also used to provoke differences in radionuclide flow studies in the kidneys.

Intravenous urography may be useful in unilateral disease. There is a delay in excretion on the side with hypoperfusion, with eventual high density of dye in the pelvis, due to water extraction by the tubuli.

The most important special investigation is arteriography. This shows the stenosis of atherosclerosis and the "string of beads" appearance of firbromuscular dysplasia. Oblique views are needed to show lesions in the aorta. Digital subtraction angiography is often used as a screening test.

Management

If the stenosis is caused by atherosclerosis, it is safer and easier to do an aortic bypass, using dacron or a vein. Sometimes a nephrectomy is indicated in proven unilateral cases. If there is a short stenosis, confined to the osteum of the artery, an endarteriectomy can be considered, but this is more difficult than a bypass.

If fibromuscular dysplasia is confined to the main renal artery, it is excised and replaced with a vein or an artery. The patient's own internal iliac artery is often used. If the disease involves the branches, the stenoses can be dilated under direct vision, or the kidney can be cooled down and operated on outside the body (workbench surgery). The branches can be excised and replaced by the internal iliac artery and its branches or by multiple veins. After this, the kidney is replaced and the main vessel is sutured to the iliac artery and the vein to the iliac vein, as an autorenal transplant.

Percutaneous luminal balloon angioplasty can be considered in suitable cases.

Prognosis

Only 60% of patients with atherosclerosis have a good result. Most of the rest are better controlled on medication. About 90% of fibromuscular dysplasia patients have a good result.

ANEURYSMS

Aneurysms can be divided into true aneurysms and false aneurysms. A true aneurysm is dilatation of a blood vessel which involves all three layers of the arterial wall. The dilatation can be fusiform or saccular.

Aneurysms follow degeneration of the media and lamina elastica and are usually caused by atherorsclerosis or syphilis.

A false aneurysm is a pulsatile haematoma which is enclosed in a fibrous capsule. It follows an injury to an artery or disruption of the anastomosis between a prosthesis and the artery and the blood that leaks becomes confined by the surrounding tissues.

Aneurysms are most commonly found in the aorta below the renal vessels. Less common sites are in the popliteal artery, the common femoral artery and the thoracic aorta. Rarely, they can be found in the common carotid artery and blood vessels of the viscera.

Aneurysms of the abdominal aorta

These aneurysms usually arise below the renal arteries. In only 5% of patients, the aneurysm involves the renal artery. The reasons for this are not completely clear, but there are differences in the metabolic rate of the arterial wall. There is a rich vasa vasorum supply to this part of the aorta and this may play a role.

Clinical presentation

This condition occurs in older patients. The patient is usually only conscious of a pulsatile mass in the abdomen, which is found by chance. Sometimes the patient complains of pain, especially backache. If the aneurysm enlarges rapidly, or causes erosion of the vertebral column, there may be considerable pain. On examination, expansive pulsations are palpable in the abdomen. Pulsation palpated in the midline just below the umbilicus strongly favours an aneurysm which has lengthened this aorta (Gaylis sign).

Special investigations

X-rays

Abdominal X-rays show calcification of the aorta; and widening of the vessel is visible. This is particularly clear on the lateral X-ray.

Ultrasound

This is the most useful way of determining the length and size of the aneurysm.

CT

This yields similar information to ultrasound but is perhaps a little more reliable for determining whether the renal vessels are involved in the aneurysm.

Arteriography

This is not usually necessary. It is often misleading, because when the aneurysm is filled with clot, the lumen can look normal. Arteriography must be considered if doubt exists as to whether the renal vessels are involved, or whether there is distal arterial insufficiency, in order to evaluate the outflow tract.

Differential diagnosis

- **Unfolded aorta:** In elderly people, there is often lengthening of the aorta with tortuosity which may feel like an aneurysm on palpation. Ultrasound will confirm the diagnosis.

- **Horseshoe kidney:** This can sometimes present as a pulsatile mass (transmitted pulsation). The diagnosis is made on ultrasound or intravenous urogram.

- **Other abdominal masses** with transmitted pulsation can feel like aneurysms.

Management

The presence of an aneurysm is an indication for surgical excision and replacement with a prosthesis, provided the patient is a standard operative risk for his age. The reason for this is that such patients develop complications. The aneurysm can also become occluded by clot, with ischaemia, or emboli can break off and cause obstruction in distal vessels.

During surgery, if possible, a tube is inserted just below the renal vessels up to just above the bifurcation. If the aneurysm involves the bifurcation, a Y-shaped dacron prosthesis is inserted, with anastomosis to the iliac vessels, or the femoral vessels in the groins.

If the patient is not a standard operative risk, the following factors must be considered:

- **Symptoms**

Pain is an indication that the aneurysm is enlarging and that there is thus a greater risk of rupture.

- **The size of the aneurysm**

Six centimetres is the arbitrary cutoff point. It has been found that if the aneurysm is larger than 6 cm, the patient's average survival time is eighteen months, while if it is smaller than 6 cm, the survival time is twice as long. If a patient's aneurysm is asymptomatic, but larger than 6 cm in diameter, surgery is probably preferable, even if he is relatively unfit. If he is asymptomatic, the aneurysm is less than 6 cm in diameter, and the patient is unfit, the operative mortality is greater than the risk of rupture. The mortality for elective aneurysmectomy is lower than 5%.

Complications of aneurysmectomy

Major complications, such as bleeding, renal failure, limb loss due to clotting or embolization of the distal vessels, bowel ischaemia and infection of the prosthesis occur in 10% of cases.

Aortic aneurysm which involves the renal vessels

This is found in less than 5% of cases. The risk in aneurysmectomy is probably greater than the risk of rupture if the aneurysm is smaller than 8 cm. It is safer to follow the patient up with regular measurement of the size of the aneurysm. One must operate only if its size increases by more than 0,5 cm per year.

The aneurysm must then be operated on, using a thoraco-abdominal approach, with implantation of the renal arteries into the prosthesis. It may also be necessary to implant the superior mesenteric artery.

Complications such as renal failure, bowel ischaemia and even paraplegia are more common than in infrarenal aneurysms.

Rupture of an abdominal aortic aneurysm

The larger the aneurysm, the greater the chance of rupture. All aneurysms can rupture, regardless of their size. An aneurysm can rupture in various ways and the prognosis is directly related to the nature of the rupture. If the aorta ruptures into the abdominal cavity, i e free rupture, the prognosis is poor. The aneurysm can leak and form a small retroperitoneal haematoma, or a large tear can form a growing retroperitoneal haematoma, which eventually breaks through to the abdominal cavity. If there is just leakage or a retroperitoneal haematoma, without free rupture into the abdominal cavity, the prognosis is much more favourable, as long as an operation is performed immediately.

Clinical presentation

Rupture can take place without the patient ever having been aware of the aneurysm, or an aneurysm which has already been diagnosed can rupture suddenly. There are sometimes warning symptoms of pain or signs of a growing aneurysm. Patients present with sudden, severe abdominal pain which radiates to the back. They are shocked, pale and cold. They develop anuria. On examination, there is an enlarging, painful, pusatile mass in the abdomen, especially in the left flank. Femoral pulses are usually impalpable.

Management

- *The patient must be resuscitated as rapidly as possible and operated on as soon as possible. Surgery must not be delayed in an attempt to resuscitate the patient fully before operating. It is better to take the patient directly from the emergency room to the theatre.*
- *While resuscitation is continued actively in theatre, the abdomen is opened and immediate control of the aorta above the rupture is achieved.*
- *It is sometimes even necessary to clamp the aorta temporarily above the renal vessels until a clamp can be placed below these vessels. The prognosis depends on the nature of the rupture which, in turn, determines the patient's general condition.*

The mortality is higher than 50%. If the bleeding remains confined to the retroperitoneal tissues, the prognosis is far more favourable (mortality 10%). The mortality is about 80% in cases with free rupture into the peritoneal cavity.

The complications of renal failure and clotting in peripheral vessels, with ischaemia of the lower limbs, are found more commonly in cases with rupture.

Aneurysms of the peripheral blood vessels

The popliteal artery

This is the most common type of peripheral aneurysm. Rupture is seldom a complication. The danger is clotting or embolization, with acute arterial insufficiency.

Clinical presentation

The condition is often bilateral. A patient may be unaware of the aneurysm and may notice a pulsatile mass in the popliteal fossa quite by chance. Sometimes patients present with claudication, usually due to embolization to peripheral vessels. If the popliteal artery is occluded by clot, the patient presents with a threatened limb.

Special investigations

Ultrasound is extremely useful for confirming the diagnosis. Before operation, arteriography is indicated, especially to demonstrate the distal outflow tract.

Management

If the limb is threatened, an emergency operation must be performed. The aneurysm can be ligated and a bypass done, using a vein. There is still a danger that the aneurysm may persist if fed by collateral vessels.

If technically possible, it is better to resect the aneurysm and replace it with a vein.

Common femoral artery

These are not as common as aneurysms of the popliteal artery. They seldom rupture or clot, but there is a danger of embolization. If the patient is a standard operative risk, the aneurysm must be resected and replaced by a vein or dacron prosthesis.

False aneurysms

The management of false aneurysms secondary to injuries will be discussed in the chapter dealing with "Trauma". False aneurysms also sometimes arise at anastomoses between prostheses and arteries.

Anastomotic aneurysms (AA)

False aneurysms arise at suturing sites in about 3% of arterial operations. The most common site is in the groin at an aortofemoral bypass. Fortunately, false aneurysms at the upper anastomosis between the prosthesis and the aorta are rare, since this is a very dangerous complication.

Various factors are responsible for the breakdown of an anastomosis: disintegration of the arterial wall, breakdown of suturing material or the prosthesis secondary to infection. Infection of the anastomosis occurs particularly in the groin and is life-threatening.

Clinical presentation

Femoral false aneurysms

Non-infective false aneurysms usually take between one and twelve years to develop. A pulsatile mass gradually develops in the groin. It is often bilateral.

If the aneurysm is associated with sepsis, it usually arises in the month following the operation. At first it presents as a haematoma, which later starts bleeding and secretes pus. There is considerable danger that the patient can develop fatal secondary bleeding.

False aneurysms at the aortic anastomosis

Breakdown of the anastomosis with false aneurysm formation can occur without any obvious clinical symptoms or signs. If a patient has had an aorta replacement and develops any symptoms, this complication must be borne in mind and ultrasound or CT must be performed. Breakdown with haematoma formation can be discovered by means of these investigations. If the diagnosis is delayed, the aneurysm can erode into the duodenum and patients then present with gastrointestinal tract bleeding. The condition has a high mortality rate.

Management of false aneurysms

The patient must be operated on and the anastomosis must be revised. If there is sepsis, the anastomosis cannot be redone at the same site, because sepsis will develop again in the prosthesis. The prosthesis must be removed and, if possible a bypass must be made to a more distal artery. If this is not possible, it is sometimes necessary to sacrifice the limb to save the patient's life.

Exceptional cases of mild sepsis, especially where a vein has been used for the bypass, will resolve on antibiotics and good drainage.

If a septic false aneurysm develops at the aortic anastomosis, the prosthesis must be removed, the aorta ligated below the renal vessels, and a bilateral axillofemoral bypass done.

THE VENOUS SYSTEM

The venous drainage of the lower limb comprises three groups of veins:

The superficial veins

There are two systems. The greater saphenous system drains the superficial tissues of the anteromedial lower leg. The greater saphenous vein runs from the anterior aspect of the medial malleolus, behind the medial condyle of the knee and then at an angle anteromedially to pierce the *fossa ovalis* of the deep fascia and join the femoral vein (deep system).

The lesser saphenous vein drains the superficial tissues of the posterior aspect of the lower leg. It pierces the deep fascia a handbreadth below the popliteal fossa and then joins the popliteal vein (deep system). The two superficial systems communicate freely with each other.

The deep veins

These veins accompany the arteries in the muscle compartments of the leg. There are usually two veins accompanying each artery.

The communicating veins (perforators)

The superficial veins join the deep venous system via veins which perforate the fascia and join the veins in the muscle compartments. There are certain relatively consistent perforators. In the lower leg, four or five perforating veins are situated every few centimetres above the medial malleolus, just posterior to the posterior edge of the tibia. Usually there are also three perforators just anterior to the fibula on the lateral side of the lower leg.

The origin of the lesser saphenous vein can also be regarded as a large posterior perforator. In the upper limb, there is a large perforator just above the knee, in the adductor canal.

The junction of the greater saphenous and femoral veins can also be regarded as a large perforator.

The valves

A vein contains valves which allow blood flow in the direction of the heart, but prevent retrograde flow in the direction of the feet. There are also constant valves in the perforating veins, which allow flow from the superficial veins to the deep veins. There is a constant valve at the junctions of the two saphenous systems with the deep veins.

The pump system

The muscles of the lower leg are covered by a fascial compartment. When these muscles contract, the muscle groups work as a pump. Blood moves in the direction of the heart and is prevented by the valves, from flowing backwards. When the muscles relax, the pressure in the deep veins falls and blood moves from the superficial system, through the communicating veins, to the deep system. When the muscle pump contracts, blood is pumped towards the heart and the valves in the communicating veins prevent blood being pumped to the superficial veins.

Competent valves are therefore the key to the success of this system.

The valve mechanisms can be damaged in the following ways:

- The veins can stretch excessively so that the cusps of the valves no longer close tightly.
- The valves can be occluded by clot and when they recanalize the valve is damaged and consequently incompetent.
- Valves may also be congenitally absent.

Varicose veins

This is a very common condition, found mainly in women, especially in certain families.

Primary varicose veins

There is no clear underlying cause for the valvular incompetence.

Aetiology

This is unknown, but the following factors play a role:

- The underlying mechanism is stretching of the superficial veins, leading to serial valvular incompetence with further stretching of the superficial veins.
- Absence of the veins of the junction of the saphenous veins may be the primary abnormality. The other valves then become incompetent as the veins gradually stretch further.
- Pregnancy plays a double role. The disturbance in hormonal balance causes relaxation of the smooth muscle, also in the wall of the veins. The enlarged uterus and rich blood supply in the pelvis may cause venous congestion in the veins of the lower limb.
- Other factors playing a role are obesity and occupations which require the patient to stand for long periods.

Secondary varicose veins

These are caused by deep venous thrombosis, with recanalization of valves, which are then incompetent. The high pressure in the deep system stretches the communicating veins, making their valves incompetent. Eventually the superficial veins also dilate secondary to the raised pressure which is transmitted to them. Congenital or acquired arteriovenous fistulae also cause secondary varicose veins by the same mechanism.

Clinical presentation

Primary varicose veins are often completely asymptomatic and patients are often worried about their cosmetic effect. They sometimes complain of a heavy feeling which becomes aggravated through the day and is painful in the evenings. All symptoms disappear when the patient is in bed. Patients also provide a history of aggravation of symptoms before menstruation.

A small percentage may present with a severe bleed due to an injury to a superficial varicose vein.

Patients can also present with severe pain, redness, tenderness and a hard swelling of the varicose veins, all signs of inflammation (thrombophlebitis).

On examination, prominent, dilated, tortuous veins can be seen in the distribution of the saphenous system. The condition is far more common in the greater saphenous vein, but often both systems are involved.

Clinical tests

Trendellenburg test

Allow the patient to lie down. Lift the leg to empty the veins. Apply a tourniquet around the upper thigh, just below the point where the greater saphenous joins the deep veins. Ask the patient to stand. A normal patient's veins will fill slowly from below. If the veins fill rapidly from below, there must be incompetent communicating veins below the tourniquet.

If the veins do not fill rapidly, remove the tourniquet. If the greater saphenous fills rapidly from above (i e retrograde flow), the valve at the origin of the greater saphenous is incompetent. This is a positive Trendellenburg test.

The Perthe test

This test determines the status of the communicating and deep veins. This is adjusted to obtain maximum information. The patient lies down and the leg is lifted to empty the veins. Three tourniquets are applied, one around the upper thigh, one just above the knee and the third just below the knee. If the veins between two tourniquets fill, there are incompetent veins in the area.

Allow the patient to rock up and down on his toes to contract the muscle pump. If the valves in the deep veins are incompetent, the veins will enlarge still further. If they are competent, the superficial veins will empty. If the deep veins are clotted due to DVT, the veins will dilate and the leg will become painful.

Differential diagnosis

If there is pigmentation or ulceration on the medial side of the lower leg, the varicose veins are secondary to deep venous thrombosis.

Management of primary varicose veins

Mild asymptomatic varicose veins require no treatment. Cosmesis is not usually a consideration in men who wear long trousers, but it may be important in young women.

Conservative management

Patients must avoid long periods of standing upright. They must elevate the leg as often as possible to reduce pressure in the veins. Elastic stockings are recommended.

Compression sclerotherapy

The principle of this treatment is to obliterate the veins by sclerosing their walls and allowing them to grow together. Thrombosis must not be caused, since the vessels will then simply recanalize.

While the patient is lying down and the veins are empty, 0,5 to 1 ml of sclerosant, usually sodium tetradecylsulphate (STD), is injected into the lumen, while the vein is compressed on either side by the fingers. After various areas have been injected, tight elastic bandages are applied around the legs and left on for six weeks. In the meantime, the damaged intima will grow together, thus obliterating the varicose veins.

One must take care that the STD does not leak out into the subcutaneous tissue, as this will cause a necrotic ulcer, followed by pigmentation.

Surgery

The operation which is performed is known as a Trendellenburg- and strip procedure. An incision is made in the thigh just overlying the junc-

tion of the greater saphenous vein with the deep veins. One must take care to locate and ligate the five branches that enter directly into the greater saphenous or the femoral vein, otherwise varicose veins will recur.

After this, the greater saphenous vein must be found where it runs over the medial malleolus and ligated. A long stripper is pushed up into the vein until it appears at the junction with the femoral vein. The vein is secured to the stripper and a pressure bandage is wound around the leg while the vein is stripped upwards and out. Remaining varicose veins which are not stripped out, must be ligated individually.

It is very important to start the pressure bandage at the toes, to prevent swelling of the feet.

The lesser saphenous can be stripped out with a short stripper and ligated at its junction with the popliteal vein.

Prognosis

Varicose veins tend to recur. A few can be treated effectively with sclerotherapy. If there is a strong family history, it is advisable that elastic stockings be worn postoperatively.

Deep venous thrombosis (DVT)

Postoperative thrombosis is an important complication. It is more common after major orthopaedic surgery, such as hip replacement, where it occurs in 2% of cases. It is less common after major general surgical procedures, where it occurs in fewer than 1% of cases. There is a considerably higher incidence following major trauma. It is found, for example, in 10% of elderly patients with hip fractures.

The following are regarded as risk factors for an increased incidence of DVT:

- elderly people with obesity
- a patient with a previous history of DVT
- patients with varicose veins
- patients who have undergone a major operation for carcinoma
- a patient who has fractured a hip
- a patient who has undergone an operation and is immobilized in bed
- women on the "pill" and young women who are pregnant also have an increased incidence.

Pathogenesis of DVT

Virchow's postulation that thrombosis occurs due to stasis, changes in the intima and hypercoagulability, is still the triad on which the management of this condition is based. Stasis increases the contact time between the clotting factors and the vessel wall; and delays dilution of the activated factors by clotting inhibitors. Immobilization of a patient leads to stasis and clotting usually develops in the venous sinuses of the calves and the valves of the deep veins, which are areas of relative stasis.

Hypercoagulability is perhaps the most important factor. In postoperative patients, clotting factors increase and clotting is most frequently found at the peak of these changes. In the postpartum period, there is a rise in fibrinogen, prothrombin and other factors and a drop in fibrinolysin. The "pill" also causes a hypercoagulable state.

DVT is much more common in the above conditions. Thrombosis may also be brought about by the absence of certain proteins which inhibit thrombosis, such as antithrombin III, protein C and others.

Thrombosis often seems to occur in the presence of an ostensibly intact epithelium. On scanning electron microscopy, it has been found that the endothelium is damaged by trauma or chemical factors such as endotoxins. The intimal defect leads to breakdown of the basal membrane and exposure of the subendothelial collagen, with formation of a primary platelet thrombus and secondary deposit of fibrin.

Clinical presentation

There is a wide spectrum of symptoms and signs, depending on the primary site and the extent of the thrombosis.

Sometimes this condition is completely asymptomatic and the patient presents with a sudden, unexpected complication such as pulmonary embolism.

Thrombosis most commonly occurs in the venous sinuses of the soleus muscle and the other calf muscles. Patients may either complain of pain in the calves, or not experience any pain. Oedema posterior to the medial malleolus is an early sign. The calves are tender on palpation and patients experience pain on dorsiflexion of the foot (Homan's sign). The lower leg is swollen and warm and there is sometimes erythema. **It is very important to bear DVT in mind in the postoperative period, especially if the patient develops a fever and slight oedema posterior to the medial malleolus.**

If the thrombus extends higher up to the popliteal and femoral veins, the swelling exacerbates dramatically. If the iliac veins are also involved, the entire leg will become severely swollen and oedematous. It can impair venous drainage to the extent that cyanosis develops *(phlegmasia caerulea dolens)*. Sometimes thrombi form in the arterioles and patients present with a swollen, cold, pale leg *(phelgmasia alba dolens)*. Both these conditions can lead to gangrene.

The diagnosis of DVT is often missed because many patients have no symptoms or signs. The diagnosis should be confirmed before the patient is put onto anticoagulants. The following diagnostic special investigations are available:

- **Venography**

The contrast medium is injected into a vein on the surface of the foot, with the leg in a 40° dependent position and a tourniquet applied just above the medial malleolus, so that the contrast medium is forced into the deep system. Good venography of the calf veins, the popliteal and femoral veins is obtained. The iliac veins are not always clearly visible. Filling defects and abnormal collateral vessels indicate thrombosis.

- **Radionuclide venography**

Venography can be done using Technesium ^{99}-marked albumin. This is not quite as reliable as contrast venography.

- **I^{125}-marked fibrinogen scanning**

This is a very sensitive way of detecting thrombi which are forming. It is not reliable in the iliac veins and hyperaemia caused by injury or infection yields false positive findings.

- **Ultrasound**

This is operator-dependent. It is useful in total occlusion of larger vessels, but less reliable in calf vessel disease.

- **Blood tests**

The presence of breakdown products in fibrin indicates fibrinolysis, which is an indirect indication of clotting. These tests are non-specific.

Complications

The complications of DVT will determine the further clinical course. Most patients have relatively mild thrombosis. This may be completely asymptomatic and may cause no significant complications. There may be temporary oedema, which resolves spontaneously as collateral vessels develop or thrombosed veins recanalize.

- **Pulmonary embolus**

A thrombus may break off and occlude the pulmonary arteries distally. Pulmonary embolus is the third most common cause of death in developed communities. It is the most common cause of maternal death during pregnancy.

The diagnosis is often missed. Patients present with dyspnoea, pleural pain, haemoptysis and discomfort. On examination, one finds tachypnoea, ràle, tachycardia, fever and sweating.

Special investigations

- **Chest X-rays**

These show consolidation with a pleural effusion. There is usually atelectasis, with prominent pulmonary vessels visible in the lung. The diaphragmatic domes are elevated.

The chest X-ray, in conjunction with perfusion lung scans and radionuclide venography, is the best screening test. The diagnosis is confirmed by selective arteriography of the pulmonary arteries.

Management

Anticoagulant therapy is the most important measure. Heparin must be given as soon as the diagnosis is suspected and while special investigations are being done.

- *Give an IV bolus of 7500 units. As soon as the diagnosis has been confirmed, full heparinization can be commenced.*

- *Thrombolytic therapy with urokinase did not, unfortunately, come up to expectations. Although it speeds up the dissolution of clots, it does not significantly improve the mortality and lung functions in a prospective trial.*
- *Open embolectomy must be considered if patients do not respond to full heparinization and deteriorate, despite intensive supportive therapy; and there is persistent hypotension. Temporary partial heart-lung bypass is converted to a total bypass and open embolectomy is performed. The mortality is 30%.*
- *Removal of the embolus by suction, using a large catheter inserted transfemorally, holds promise.*

Prevention of pulmonary embolus

If patients have DVT which involves the large vessels, or if small warning emboli have already broken loose, steps must be taken to prevent embolization or further embolization.

Anticoagulant therapy

Heparin

A bolus of 100 units per kilogram is given. This is followed by

$$\frac{1000\ \text{U} \times \text{body mass (kg)}}{2}$$

over the next twenty-four hours. The dose is adjusted to keep the activated partial thromboplastin time (APTT) between 50 and 80 seconds. The thromboelastogram is useful. The r-time must be prolonged by between one and a half and twice the normal time. Heparin is given for ten days.

Oral anticoagulants

On the fifth day, administration of oral drugs is commenced. The ratio between the prothrombin time of the patient's plasma in seconds, divided by the prothrombin time of control plasma, is measured. A ratio between 2,0 and 3,0 must be sustained.

Thrombolytic therapy

Urokinase and streptokinase can dissolve clots, but complications from haemorrhages are common. At present these drugs do not really appear to offer any substantial advantage, because of the price and complications.

Thrombectomy

In theory, it would be useful to remove a large thrombus because this:

- would prevent embolization
- would prevent the postphlebitic syndrome
- could save the limb in *phlegmasia caerulea dolens.*

In practice, it has been found that the majority clot again after thrombectomy, even when it is done within twenty-four hours. If anticoagulant or thombolytic therapy are given as adjuncts to this, haemorrhage is often a serious complication. The operation should perhaps be considered only in a case of *phlegmasia caerulea dolens* or *alba dolens,* if the patient is seen within forty-eight hours of the onset of the condition.

Interruption of venous drainage

The aim is to prevent recurrent emboli, which would occur in spite of adequate anticoagulant therapy. Because fatal emboli usually arise in the iliac veins, it is advisable to interrupt the venous return in the *vena cava.* If the vena cava is ligated below the renal veins, pulmonary embolus will be prevented. Sometimes patients develop severe swelling of the legs, especially if there has been extensive thrombosis from the veins in the legs. To prevent this, various methods have been developed to trap emboli, while still permitting venous drainage.

There is a variety of filters, of which one can be inserted into the vena cava transvenously under local anaesthetic. The Greenfield filter is the most popular.

The indications for venous interruption are:

- Recurrent emboli despite adequate anticoagulant therapy.
- Multiple small emboli, which cause pulmonary hypertension.
- Septic emboli, which do not respond to anticoagulant therapy and antibiotics.
- Postpulmonary artery embolectomy.
- If there is a contraindication to anticoagulant therapy.

Prophylaxis against postoperative DVT

Physical measures

Active exercise, elevation of the legs and elastic stockings, increase venous flow and reduce the incidence of postoperative DVT. Sitting still in chairs must be avoided and early ambulation encouraged.

Anticoagulant therapy

Heparin

Prospective trials indicate that prophylactic heparin reduces the incidence of DVT and fatal emboli. The method which is most commonly used is subcutaneous heparin in low dosage. Five thousand units are given twelve-hourly for seven days, until the patient is ambulant.

Warfarin

The two-stage administration low-dose warfarin is more effective in high-risk groups (hip fractures and hip replacements). The drug is given for a few days before the operation and is continued for a few days postoperatively. Haemorrhage is a problem.

Dextran

Dextran reduces blood viscosity and platelet aggregation and makes fibrin more susceptible to fibrinolysis. In prospective trials, it reduced the incidence of pulmonary embolism. It is especially useful after orthopaedic operations. Disadvantages are overload of the circulating blood volume and anaphylaxis, which sometimes occurs.

In summary, it can be said that low dosages of heparin should be used for the majority of general surgical operations. Combine heparin and dextran if there are high-risk factors, especially a recent DVT. Use warfarin for elderly patients undergoing hip surgery.

Postphlebitic limb

Chronic deep venous inadequacy or postphlebitic syndrome, also known as venous hypertension, is the most common complication of DVT. The veins are occluded by clot and then recanalize, with resultant partial obstruction, destruction of the valvular system and reflux of blood from the high-pressure deep veins to the lower pressure superficial veins. The pressure in the superficial veins is normal if the patient stands still, but does not drop on exercise. There is thus continuous venous hypertension.

Clinical presentation

The patient complains of a constant, pressing pain. The pain is relieved if the patient lies down with the leg elevated.

The leg swells. This starts as mild oedema and becomes progressively worse. At first, it disappears at night when the patient lies down, but later the oedema is continuously present. Subcutaneous fibrosis arises and the skin and subcutaneous vessels become congested and hard. The red cells move out of the capillaries and are taken up by macrophages; and haemosiderin is deposited in the tissues. The melanocytes react and pigmentation occurs. Eczema and pruritis develop. Minor trauma, such as a skin scratch, leads to breakdown and ulceration. Low-grade infection contributes to further swelling and fibrosis. The ulcer usually arises because of an incompetent perforator on the medial side, just above the medial malleolus.

The clinical presentation is determined by the extent of the thrombus and the degree of reflux in the communicating veins. If there is relatively poor outflow of venous blood from the lower leg, the patient develops a large, swollen, indurated leg.

If reflux through incompetent perforators is the prominent problem and the deep veins are patent, the leg can be relatively soft, with large venous ulcers. These two components are often found in conjunction.

Special investigations

The status of the deep veins and the communicating perforators can be determined by using Perthes' test. A venogram will provide the most information on the pathological anatomy of the venous system.

After recurrent episodes of infection and ulceration, the lymphatic system also sometimes becomes involved and thus contributes to the swollen leg. A lymphangiogram may show occlusion of the lymphatics.

Differential diagnosis

Other causes of ulceration of the lower leg which must always be considered include:

- Ischaemic ulceration due to arterial insufficiency
- Infective ulcers, such as tuberculosis, syphilis and fungal infections
- Malignant ulcers, such as squamous cell carcinoma, melanoma or Kaposi disease.
- Traumatic ulcers: insect bites, burns and irridation
- Neurotrophic ulcers due to diabetes, alcoholism and *tabes dorsalis*
- Metabolic diseases: ulcers occur in ulcerative colitis, sickle-cell anaemia and avitaminosis.

Management

The aim of management is to neutralize the high venous pressure which is transferred to the superficial veins via incompetent perforators, to reduce oedema and to prevent further development of oedema and infection in the ulcer.

Conservative management

If the patient is put to bed with the foot of the bed elevated, this aim is achieved. The pressure in the superficial system is low and the oedema improves due to improved lymph drainage. Bedrest heals venous ulcers.

Alternatively, tight elastic bandages can be wrapped around the lower legs to achieve the same goal. This prevents the raised pressure from the deep system from being transmitted by the incompetent system. They also improve lymphatic drainage and reduce oedema. Elastic bandages heal venous ulcers. Once the ulcers have healed, the patient must wear well-fitted elastic stockings permanently.

Surgical management

It is seldom possible to effect healing, especially permanent healing, of venous ulceration by simple ligation of incompetent perforators. This is only possible if the deep veins are patent and their valvular action has been at least partially preserved.

If the condition has developed fully and conservative means cannot keep the ulcer healed, an operation can be combined with pressure bandages. The perforators are ligated deep to the fascia, via a long posterior midline incision. After the operation, the patient must wear elastic stockings permanently, because the underlying venous hypertension is naturally still present.

Prognosis

To a large extent this depends on the patient's motivation and cooperation. If elastic stockings are worn properly and regularly and the legs elevated regularly if the slightest oedema arises, the ulcers will probably remain healed.

If ulcers do not heal in spite of adequate treatment, a biopsy must be taken to exclude possible malignant transformation (Marjolin ulcer).

The severely injured patient 10

Injuries are very common, but fortunately the majority of them are minor, such as lacerations, abrasions and sprains. Nevertheless, major injuries are the third most common cause of death. They are the most common cause of death in patients under forty.

Motor accidents are the most important cause of serious, multiple injuries. Violence is the second most important cause, followed by household injuries, including burns. Sports injuries are lowest on the list.

In a study done in the USA, it was found that half the deaths related to injury could probably have been prevented by optimal management in a well-equipped trauma unit manned by skilled personnel. In the same study, time-consuming attempts by paramedics to establish intravenous infusions at the scene of the accident were deplored. Most life-threatening injuries require skilled surgery in a well-equipped trauma unit, to save lives.

The main causes of death in severely injured patients are head injuries (50%), massive haemorrhages (30%) and airway and ventilation problems.

At the scene of the accident, the priorities are the following:

- Establish an open airway. Clean the mouth, pull the tongue out and ventilate, using a face mask and ambu-bag. This is much safer than unsuccessful time-consuming intubation attempts by the inexperienced.
- Support respiration with an ambu-bag.
- Control external bleeding with pressure dressings. The MAST suit, if available, may play a rôle in controlling internal bleeding. Whether or not an intravenous line should be established at the scene of the accident is controversial. It is better to get the patient to expert care in a well-equipped unit than to waste time on an infusion, which will in any case provide less than a litre of fluid during transit to the hospital.
- Splint fractures to prevent further injuries. Be especially careful of neck injuries.

It is far better to take a patient to a recognized trauma unit as rapidly as possible than to the nearest hospital, where skilled surgical help is seldom available. The first hour following the injury, the so-called "golden hour", is a critical period for the severely injured patient.

The trauma unit

The first five minutes

The priorities are airway, breathing and circulation. Suction debris from the mouth and throat, pull the tongue forward and apply a face mask and ambu-bag. Skills are now available and in-

tubation can be performed. Beware of neck fractures, because transection of the spinal cord can occur during attempts to intubate. Tense neck muscles and a haematoma in the occipital area are warning signs.

Once the airway has been established, good ventilation must be ensured. Multiple rib fractures with an unstable segment, pneumohaemothorax or tension pneumothorax can impair adequate filling of the lungs and alveolar ventilation to such an extent that respiratory distress ensues. Open thoracic wounds must be closed immediately, thoracocentesis performed and thoracic drains inserted.

Urgent attention must now be devoted to the circulation. The vital signs, pulse and blood pressure, must be determined. In a severely injured, shocked patient, one must immediately attempt to distinguish between hypovolaemia due to massive blood loss and impairment of venous return to the heart due to pericardial tamponade or tension pneumothorax. If the patient's jugular veins are distended, consider tamponade. Rapid insertion of thoracic drains and pericardiocentesis can help to differentiate these two very important conditions. It is much more likely that a large haemorrhage has taken place.

Multiple lines to provide intravenous access are urgently necessary. If the expertise is available, central lines must be inserted via subclavian catheters. Otherwise, do multiple cutdowns of peripheral veins. Send blood for compatibility tests and infuse large volumes of Ringer lactate.

This early stage is known as the tube stage:

- *Intratracheal tube*
- *Nasogastric tube*
- *Three intravenous catheters, including a central venous pressure catheter*
- *One or two thoracic drains*
- *Bladder catheter*

The course of events during the next ten minutes is important. The patient may stabilize, or may not react to resuscitation. The question now is whether the patient is not already dead. The asystolic patient, with fixed, dilated pupils, who does not react to resuscitation, was probably dead on admission. If there is no improvement after thirty minutes, the patient must be declared dead.

The third type of presentation is the patient who initially responds well to resuscitation, but then struggles to maintain his circulation.

The next thirty minutes

The further management of the patient is best handled by a general surgeon who is skilled in the management of severely injured patients and is willing to consult his colleagues with special skills. His task is to recognize the patient who will need an emergency operation within the next half hour. If tension pneumothorax and cardiac tamponade have been excluded, patients who cannot maintain their blood pressure despite adequate resuscitation usually fall into this category. Patients who are still hypovolaemic after three litres of Ringer lactate, are bleeding actively and massively somewhere and must be operated on urgently.

The usual sources of such massive blood loss are:

- *Arterial bleeding, probably from the aorta*
- *Laceration of the liver and/or hepatic veins*
- *Laceration of the vena cava*
- *Massive fracture of the pelvis*
- *Injury to the heart and great vessels*

Although the spleen and mesentery of the small bowel can sometimes bleed massively, such patients can usually be effectively resuscitated with large volumes of Ringer lactate. It is not advisable to perform an ultra-emergency operation in the trauma unit. Only penetrating wounds of the heart or large mediastinal vessels must be operated on there. All other cases must be operated on formally in the well-equipped operating theatre.

Although head injuries are responsible for the majority of deaths, they seldom develop so rapidly that cranial operations need to be considered within the first thirty minutes. The most important measure for these patients during this early phase is maintenance of airway and breathing and resuscitation of hypovolaemic shock.

Orthopaedic injuries are seldom life threatening and are not the priority during this early phase. External bleeding must be stopped and fractures splinted, while the life-threatening conditions enjoy first priority.

The next three hours

During the first "golden hour" following injury, the urgent decisions must be made and implemented, so that patients with life-threatening trauma can be recognized and treated expedi-

tiously. During the next three hours, all the attention must be directed at:

- *Recognition and diagnosis of continued blood loss.*
- *Diagnosis of unexpected or masked underlying injuries (central nervous system, gastrointestinal canal and urinary tract). Surgical exploration may be necessary for diagnosis and treatment.*
- *Management of orthopaedic and vascular injuries.*

During this period, it will be essential to consult specialist colleagues.

Tetanus prophylaxis and antibiotics must be administered.

A complete history and clinical examination are now carried out, once all clothing has been removed. The full clinical findings must be noted on the trauma record. This trauma record must be kept up to date continuously.

X-rays of the head and neck, vertebrae and thorax are essential. All bruised limbs or those with obvious fractures must also be X-rayed. Computer tomography, intravenous pyelography and arteriography can be very useful, but one must be careful not to perform these examinations on patients who are not resuscitated and stable. Members of the trauma unit must accompany the patient to the X-ray section, to ensure continued monitoring and resuscitation. The X-ray section personnel must concentrate on diagnostic procedures and they cannot be expected to have the skills to manage the patient's general condition as well.

HEAD AND NECK INJURIES

Consult a neurosurgeon to help with diagnosis and management of the patient with a severe head injury. The following principles apply:

- Life-threatening lesions must always enjoy priority.
- Neck injuries are often associated with severe head injuries and must always be borne in mind.
- The unconscious patient with neck muscle spasm or an occipital haematoma must be regarded as having a cervical vertebral fracture and urgent X-rays are essential to confirm the diagnosis. Until they can be taken, the head must be immobilized with sandbags and pillows.
- The next life-threatening condition is rising intracranial pressure due to intracranial haemorrhage.
- The neurological status, especially the level of consciousness, must be monitored continuously to detect development of a neurological deficit and deterioration of the level of consciousness.
- Haemorrhage can be extradural, subdural, subarachnoid, intracerebral or intraventricular.
- Remember that it is impossible to determine the level of consciousness properly in a patient who is anoxic or shocked.
- The respiratory tract and circulation thus always enjoy priority.
- Commence a monitoring chart for the patient. This chart will usually include a Glasgow coma scale and other neurological observations.

Glasgow coma scale

Eyes open	**Score**
• *Spontaneously*	*4*
• *On command*	*3*
• *On pain stimulus*	*2*
• *None*	*1*
Best verbal response	
• *Orientated*	*5*
• *Confused*	*4*
• *Inappropriate speech*	*3*
• *Incomprehensible sounds*	*2*
• *None*	*1*
Best motor response	
• *Obeys commands*	*6*
• *Localizes pain stimulus*	*5*
• *Withdraws limbs*	*4*
• *Abnormal flexion*	*3*
• *Extensor response*	*2*
• *None*	*1*

Maximum achievable score 15.

Minimum score 3.

The lower the score, the poorer the prognosis. Ninety-five per cent of those with a score of less than 5 die and 95% of those with a score of more than 7 survive.

Observations must be made on pupillary size and reactions, movements, muscle tone and reflex status. The pulse, blood pressure, respiration and temperature are also monitored. The skull must be examined thoroughly to diagnose open and compression fractures. CSF exuding from the nose and preorbital ecchymosis are indicative of a fracture of the anterior orbital roof and cribriform plate. The ears must be examined for blood or CSF, the presence of which would suggest a fracture of the base of the skull. Such cases must receive prophylactic antibiotics to prevent meningitis.

Clinical presentation of raised intracranial pressure

- The level of consciousness deteriorates gradually and signs of tentorial herniation are found, such as contralateral paresis and extensor or decerebrate rigidity.
- The pulse and respiratory rate fall and the blood pressure rises.
- Paralysis of the third cranial nerve on the same side as the lesion is common.
- There is paralysis of the medial rectus muscle of the eye; and the pupil on the side of the lesion temporarily constricts and then dilates, with loss of light reflex. As the pressure rises, both pupils become involved.
- Bilateral, small, fixed pupils suggest brainstem damage.
- Intracranial pressure can be monitored continuously, using a pressure screw, which is inserted through a small burrhole in the skull.

Principles of management of severe head injuries

The patient must be treated with anticonvulsants. Some neurosurgeons use barbiturates. The patient must be nursed on sheepskins and turned regularly to protect pressure points. Hyperpyrexia is common and must be treated with cooling by fans and wet sheets. A Foley catheter must be inserted into the bladder. A nasogastric tube must be introduced for suction in the early stages and feeding in the later stages. Intravenous fluids must be provided and overhydration must be prevented.

Management of specific injuries

Laceration of the skull

These wounds can bleed a lot. The wound must be cleaned and sutured.

Fractures

Simple hairline fractures do not require treatment.

Open fractures

These must be debrided, and loose pieces of bone and brain removed. If possible, the dura must be sutured.

Compression fractures

Slight compression (a few millimetres) is left as it is. Compression fractures overlying venous sinuses are treated conservatively. Other compressions are lifted out. CSF leakage from the nose or ear due to fractures of the base of the skull must be treated conservatively with prophylactic antibiotics. If it is a large leak, or if it continues for more than a week, the leak should be repaired operatively to prevent the possible complications of meningitis or abscess.

Raised intracranial pressure

If the intracranial pressure rises, the cause must be diagnosed. At present, the investigation of choice is computer tomography. If this is not available, carotid angiography is used.

Haematomas must be operated on. If the raised pressure is caused by cerebral oedema, the patient must be treated conservatively. Hyperventilation reduces the intracranial blood volume and intracranial pressure. Mannitol administered in a dose of 1,5 g/kg IV, dehydrates the brain and reduces cerebral oedema and pressure. The use of barbiturates and steroids is controversial.

Prognosis of severe head injuries

The mortality is higher than 40%. The prognosis is much better in children.

PENETRATING NECK WOUNDS

These are divided into three groups:

- Wounds below the clavicle
- Wounds between the clavicle and the angle of the mandible
- Wounds above the angle of the mandible

Wounds between the clavicle and the angle of the mandible can be treated conservatively, on condition that the following danger signs are absent:

- Difficulty with swallowing or respiration
- Subcutaneous emphysema
- Voice changes
- Active bleeding
- Haematemesis or haemoptysis
- A murmur over the carotid artery
- Neurological deficit
- Haemothorax with persistent bleeding

If any of these signs are present, the carotid artery and jugular vein must be explored, after an oesophagogram has been performed. In injuries which cause dysphagia or respiratory difficulty, an oesophagogram and arteriography of the carotid artery must be performed and if these are normal, conservative treatment can be applied.

FACIAL INJURIES

Lacerations must be sutured as quickly as possible, with due consideration of the cosmetic result. It is advisable to consult a plastic surgeon. Fractures of the nose are not urgent and can be treated a few days later. Mandible fractures are best treated by a maxillofacial surgeon. Remember that an open airway must always enjoy priority over reduction or fixation of a mandibular fracture.

THORACIC OR DIAPHRAGMATIC INJURIES

Blunt trauma

Two types of blunt trauma are found in motor vehicle accidents:

- Compression force of the steering wheel against the driver's chest, leading to multiple fractures of the ribs and sternum. The unstable segment of the thoracic wall moves paradoxically on respiration and causes a flail chest. The indented sternum causes cardiac contusion.
- Deceleration injury: This causes laceration of the fixed structures in the thorax. Laceration of the aortic arch is a particularly life-threatening injury. The bronchus, oesophagus and thoracic duct can also tear.

Blunt trauma also causes haemopneumothorax, because rib fractures penetrate the lung and intercostal blood vessels tear. A tension pneumothorax can also develop.

Penetrating trauma

Stab wounds and gunshot wounds of the thorax are common. Central penetrating wounds are often responsible for cardiac injury, with resulting pericardial tamponade. Penetrating injuries of the great vessels cause massive bleeds with haemopneumothorax.

Life-threatening situations

Penetrating injuries of the heart and great vessels

A patient with a penetrating wound in the cardiac region presents with lowered blood pressure, a barely audible heartbeat and dilated neck veins. Diagnose pericardial tamponade. Insert a needle at the junction of the costal cartilage and the xiphisternum, at an angle of 45°, in the direction of the lower end of the right scapula. Aspirate the blood from the pericardium. If the patient does not improve immediately, do an emergency thoracotomy in the trauma unit via the fourth and fifth anterior intercostal spaces. Use a finger to occlude the hole in the ventricle, or position a vascular clamp on the hole in the aorta. Call a cardiac surgeon. If he is not immediately available, close the hole with nonabsorbable sutures.

Massive intrathoracic bleeding

The patient has a penetrating or blunt thoracic injury with a lowered blood pressure and respiratory distress. Respiratory sounds are inaudible. A large needle must immediately be inserted into the second intercostal space below the clavicle to relieve the tension pneumothorax. If air under pressure does not escape, insert a large thoracic drain to drain the haemothorax. If the patient bleeds more than 200 ml per hour, a thoracotomy is essential.

Tension pneumothorax

This occurs if air builds up in the pleural cavity, but cannot escape because a ball valve has formed. The lung collapses and the mediastinum shifts to the opposite side. The patient presents with respiratory distress. Respiratory sounds are absent and the trachea is displaced laterally. Surgical emphysema is often present.

Tension pneumothorax and pericardial tamponade both cause distended neck veins. Haemothorax often causes collapsed neck veins due to blood loss.

A needle must be inserted into the second intercostal space immediately, to allow the air under pressure to escape. The needle must be replaced by a thoracic drain, with underwater drainage. Open sucking wounds of the thoracic wall must be sutured and an intrathoracic underwater drain must be inserted.

Injuries to mediastinal structures

Deceleration injuries, such as those which result from motor vehicle accidents and falls from high buildings, cause laceration of the aorta just distal to the origin of the left subclavian artery. Usually the adventitia remains intact and a large false aneurysm arises, and can rupture at any minute. X-rays show widening of the mediastinum.

A thoracic surgeon must be consulted urgently. The diagnosis can be confirmed on arteriography and an emergency operation must be performed.

Unstable thoracic wall

This occurs after severe blunt injuries to the thoracic wall, and several ribs sustain double fractures. The segment moves paradoxically on respiration and respiratory distress arises. A haemothorax is also often present. Insert an underwater drain. Perform tracheal intubation and support the patient with positive pressure ventilation when necessary, but discontinue as soon as it is considered feasible. After a few weeks, the fractures will heal and the thoracic wall will regain stability.

Oesophageal injuries

Oesophageal injuries present with haemoptysis, dyspnoea, hoarseness and emphysema in the neck and mediastinum. A contrast study, using gastrografin, will confirm the diagnosis. The defect in the oesophagus must be repaired surgically. Patches of pleura or the fundus of the stomach can be used to strengthen the repair.

Important principles in the management of thoracic injuries

- *Establish a patent airway. Perform tracheal intubation.*
- *Urgently insert a thoracic underwater drain.*
- *Resuscitate the patient with intravenous fluids.*
- *Consult a thoracic surgeon.*

Diaphragm injuries

Traumatic hernia of the diaphragm occurs more commonly after penetrating injuries than after blunt injuries. Any stab wound or bullet wound below the seventh rib space must arouse suspicion of thoraco-abdominal penetration. X-rays usually show a haemopneumothorax; and bowel can sometimes be seen in the thoracic cavity. The hernia itself is not life threatening, but it is often associated with injuries to other organs, which dominate the clinical presentation. The diagnosis is often made weeks or months later. In the acute situation, the hernia must be operated on via an abdominal approach, so that other organ injuries can be dealt with simultaneously. A thoracic approach can only be used if there are indications of thoracic organ injuries.

In late cases, presenting weeks or months later, it is probably better to operate via the thorax, because adhesions can be loosened with a greater degree of safety, and abdominal organ injuries are no longer a concern.

ABDOMINAL INJURIES

Abdominal injuries can be divided into:

- Blunt injuries, which mainly cause injuries to solid organs; the spleen, the liver, the pancreas and the kidneys. Less commonly they can lead to injuries of the gastrointestinal canal, especially the fixed parts of the bowel, the duodenum and the colon.
- Penetrating injuries:
  - *Stab wounds.* These cause penetration of the large organs, with less serious bleeding and holes in the gastrointestinal canal, leading to peritonitis.
  - *Gunshot wounds.* These cause graver damage to the solid organs and the great intra-abdominal vessels, with life threatening bleeding. They also cause more extensive holes in the gastrointestinal canal, with peritonitis.

Blunt injuries

The severely injured patient is often unconscious and diagnosis of abdominal organ injuries can be difficult. If the patient has rib fractures and fractures of the pelvis, vertebrae and lower limbs, it is highly probable that there is also an abdominal injury.

If all external bleeding has stopped and chest X-rays are normal, but the patient is struggling to maintain his blood pressure in spite of fluid administration, a haemorrhage in the abdominal cavity is probably the cause.

Special investigations

Peritoneal lavage

A peritoneal lavage catheter is inserted into the peritoneal cavity under local anaesthetic, via a short midline incision just below the umbilicus. If more than 10 ml of blood is found during catheter placement, the test is positive. Allow one litre of Ringer lactate to drain into the abdominal cavity and then to drain out again. If the fluid is bloodstained to the extent that a newspaper cannot be read through the fluid, the test is positive. If there are more than 100 000 red cells or more than 500 leucocytes per cubic millilitre of fluid, the test is also positive. Such patients must undergo surgery. Peritoneal lavage is not effective in diagnosing injuries to the retroperitoneal organs such as the duodenum, pancreas and kidneys.

Computer tomography

CT is very useful, not only in diagnosing injuries of the liver and spleen, but also those of the pancreas and kidneys. It must be emphasized that an unstable patient must not be sent for CT.

Penetrating injuries of the abdomen

All abdominal gunshot wounds must be urgently explored. The majority of penetrating stab wounds also warrant exploration. If the stab wound is directed away from the diaphragm and the patient is stable, without any signs of peritoneal irritation, the patient can be kept under careful observation. About 40% of patients can be spared an unnecessary operation. Only 3% of patients observed in this manner will develop signs which will necessitate laparotomy. If prophylactic antibiotics are given and one operates as soon as signs develop, this is a safe policy.

Principles of management of injuries to the abdominal organs

Retroperitoneal haematoma

Haematomas can be caused by penetrating or blunt injuries.

Special risks are posed by haematomas caused by gunshot wounds. These haematomas can be divided into:

- *Central haematomas*
- *Lateral haematomas*
- *Pelvic haematomas*

• Central haematomas

These haematomas lie in relation to the duodenum, pancreas, vena cava and aorta. All such haematomas, regardless of their cause, must be explored. If the haematoma has been caused by a gunshot wound, injury to the great vessels can be expected and these vessels must be controlled proximal and distal to the haematoma before it is explored. In blunt injuries, rupture of the duodenum and pancreas must be expected.

• Lateral haematomas

A stable haematoma around the kidney which is found at operation must preferably not be explored. If a haematoma is found preoperatively, CT or arteriography must be done first, to evaluate the status of the renal vessels before exploration. If crepitus is present in the haematoma, the colon must be mobilized to exclude colonic injury.

• Haematomas of the pelvis

The cause of the haematoma is of critical importance. If the haematoma has been caused by blunt trauma, with pelvic fracture, it must not be explored. If it has been caused by a gunshot wound, it must be explored to exclude vascular injuries and pelvic organ injuries (rectum, ureter).

Hepatic injuries

The vast majority of hepatic injuries (70%) are so mild that no treatment is necessary. Blunt or crushing injuries cause lacerations in the liver tissue or hepatic veins.

- The most important requirement is to stop the bleeding. It is better to ligate bleeders individually than to insert large, deep sutures.

- In large liver lacerations it is necessary to ligate blood vessels and bile ducts and to fill the cracks with omentum.
- In large lacerations which involve the hepatic veins, it is better to compress liver tissue bimanually to control bleeding, and then to open the thorax by sternal splitting. While an assistant stems the bleeding with direct pressure and temporary clamping of the portal tract (Pringle manoeuvre), the bleeders must be ligated with individual sutures.
- Currently, large liver lobe resections are seldom performed. The only indication is removal of a severely injured liver lobe in order to expose the hepatic vein.
- Drainage of the bile ducts, which was recommended in the past, is contraindicated. Mortality is high in blunt injuries and in high-velocity gunshot wounds, especially if other organs, e g colon, have also sustained injury.

Splenic injury

Splenic injury is the most common type of abdominal injury found in the severely injured patient. Currently, peritoneal lavage and CT play an important rôle in the diagnosis. CT also plays a rôle in the conservative management of subcapsular splenic haematoma. Because of the gram positive infections which have been described following splenectomy, most surgeons try to preserve the spleen.

- Splenorrhaphy with omental patching, hemisplenectomy, or direct repair by means of sutures, are commonly performed. In the severely injured patient, a splenectomy is preferable if a repair cannot be done rapidly and safely.
- Subcapsular haematoma can be managed conservatively, using CT monitoring. Ninety per cent resolve spontaneously. Such patients must be kept under observation in hospital.

Pancreas and duodenum

Diagnosing injuries to these two organs is sometimes difficult. In penetrating and blunt injuries of the upper abdomen the possibility of injuries to the retroperitoneal structures must always be borne in mind. Abdominal X-rays sometimes show gas bubbles in the retroperitoneal tissues. Peritoneal lavage is not of much use. Computer tomography is the most reliable investigation. This may show a large haematoma in the area being explored. If there is a pancreatic fracture, it can usually be seen on CT.

- Perforations of the duodenum can be closed and strengthened with a jejunal patch. If there is any doubt as to the security of the repair, a tube duodenostomy must be performed.
- In combined duodenal and pancreatic injuries, it is safer to close the pylorus temporarily and to perform a gastrojejunostomy as a short-circuit procedure.
- Pancreatic injuries are managed by means of control of bleeding and good drainage.
- If the pancreas has been fractured by kinking over the vertebral column, the distal pancreas must be resected.
- If the head has been crushed, bleeding must be controlled and good drainage implemented. Fistulae often develop, but the majority close spontaneously.
- A pancreaticoduodenectomy must be performed only if the injury is so extensive that there is no other alternative.

The gastrointestinal canal

Holes in the stomach and small intestine must be closed, or a partial bowel resection must be performed. Stab wounds of the colon and even clean gunshot wounds from civilian, small-calibre handguns can be sutured and drained. The majority of colonic wounds, especially gunshot wounds and blunt injuries, must always be brought out as a colostomy. **Rectal injuries are very dangerous and are sometimes missed, with very serious consequences.** Rectal injuries are treated by means of a proximal colostomy, thorough lavage of the rectum, closure of the perforation (if possible), presacral drainage and broad spectrum antibiotics, which must include aminoglycosides.

Pelvic fractures

The majority of pelvic fractures do not bleed so massively that they are life threatening. If they do bleed massively, they can be very difficult to treat effectively. The following principles apply:

- Try to avoid exploration.
- Stabilize the fractures (with external apparatus).
- Give adequate blood transfusions.
- The MAST suit must also be tried.
- If massive bleeding persists, perform arteriography and try to embolize the bleeding points.
- Ultimately, it may be necessary to explore.
- Control the proximal aorta temporarily when the haematoma is opened.
- Ligate the internal iliac artery, and, if this does not control the bleeding adequately, pack the pelvis with swabs. The mortality in these severe injuries exceeds 30%.

Injuries to the urinary tract

The urine of all severely injured patients should be examined after a catheter has been inserted into the bladder. If the urine is normal, nothing further need be done.

- If there is a pelvic fracture, or blood at the tip of the penis, a urethrogram must be done to exclude urethral injury before a catheter is passed.
- If there is blood in the urine, a cystogram and an IV urogram must be done.
- If only one kidney is functional, consider a vascular injury.
- CT or arteriography must then be done urgently.

Principles of management of injuries to the urinary tract

Consult a urologist.

The kidneys

- *Blood in the urine with a normal cystogram and urogram – observe.*
- *Both kidneys are excreting on the urogram, with mild extravasation of dye and the patient is stable – observe.*
- *Extensive extravasation of dye in an unstable patient indicates a crushed kidney – operate.*
- *A nonfunctioning kidney with vascular injury on CT or arteriogram – operate urgently.*

The renal pedicle is often injured in penetrating trauma such as a gunshot wound. At operation, one must always attempt to preserve as much renal parenchyma as possible. An arteriogram is useful for showing whether part of the damaged kidney still has a good blood supply and can thus be spared.

The ureters

Ureteric injuries are diagnosed by means of a retrograde ureterogram.

Principles of management

- *Remove all damaged ureter, and anastomose over a catheter splint.*
- *Remember to consider a nephrostomy tube, to divert urine away from the anastomosis, if one suspects that the anastomosis is insecure.*

The bladder

Bladder injuries are found in fifteen percent of patients with pelvic fractures. Bladder rupture is often associated with urethral injuries. In blunt injuries, a full bladder can rupture into the peritoneal cavity. The diagnosis is made by means of a cystogram.

Management

- *Do a suprapubic cystostomy.*
- *Suture the bladder.*
- *Drain the perivesical tissues thoroughly.*
- *Drain the bladder by means of a transurethral catheter.*

Urethral injuries

If there is blood at the tip of the penis or there is a pelvic fracture, urethral injuries must be considered.

Principles of management

- *Do a urethrogram.*
- *There is controversy concerning the management of urethral injuries.*
- *Some urologists believe that the injury should be repaired immediately.*
- *In the severely injured patient, it is better to do a suprapubic cystostomy and repair the urethral injury later.*

Fractures and dislocations with associated vascular injuries

Although orthopaedic injuries are commonly found in severely injured patients, they are seldom life-threatening and normal splinting, covering of open fractures and prophylactic antibiotics are usually all that is required, while other more serious injuries are being attended to. If vascular injuries are associated with fractures or dislocations, the limb, or even the patient's life, are endangered. In orthopaedic injuries, blunt trauma plays an important rôle and the arterial injury is often overlooked because it is not obvious, occlusion is not total and the circulation is maintained by collateral flow. Vascular injuries which can occur include penetrating injuries (stab wounds), lacerations caused by low or high velocity missiles, occlusion by an intimal flap, injury to the intima with thrombosis, intramural haematoma, with thrombosis, and spasm. Although spasm does occur, it is a diagnosis that must not be made without arteriographic proof.

Arterial injuries usually occur at points where the blood vessels are relatively well fixed by branches. The elbow and knee joints are classic sites for arterial injuries associated with dislocations. The artery is damaged by stretching, compression, or laceration caused by bone fragments. Blunt trauma causes intimal injuries followed by thrombosis. Penetrating trauma causes bleeding and haematoma formation.

The complications of vascular injuries include:

- Bleeding, with hypovolaemic shock
- Haematoma with sepsis
- Thrombosis
- False aneurysm
- Arteriovenous fistulae
- Arterial ischaemia

Principles of management

It has already been emphasized that fractures are not a priority in the severely injured patient.

- *Splint the fractures, reduce dislocations, assess the vascular status of the patient.*
- *Active bleeding requires exploration.*
- *Ischaemia is an indication for arteriography.*
- *Once life threatening injuries have been attended to and the patient has been resuscitated, the arterial injuries must be operated on and repaired, using a suitable method. The arterial repair is done first, followed by fixing of the fracture.*
- *Four-compartment decompression is essential after vascular repairs associated with fractures and soft tissue injuries.*
- *The suture line of the artery must be covered by muscle, especially if the wound is to be left open because of extensive injury and contamination.*
- *Once any life threatening crisis has been dealt with, the orthopaedic surgeons must be called in to treat the fractures.*

BURNS

Where burns involve more than 25% of the body surface, skin destruction leads to increased permeability of capillaries in that area of the skin, and also in other tissues. There is thus a massive loss of fluids from the circulation, especially in the first twelve hours after the burn, decreasing gradually over the next forty-eight hours. The second important problem is that the skin's resistance to bacterial invasion is radically impaired. The management of burns must thus be aimed at the two major problems of fluid loss and bacterial infection of the wound. Mortality is largely dependent on the measure of success in managing these problems. The mortality is directly related to the amount of skin destroyed (and thus fluid loss). The mortality is 50% for a 50% burn and 80% for an 80% burn. Half the deaths in patients who survive the early stages are due to sepsis.

Causes of burns

- Thermal – flames, boiling water, hot objects, hot gases, smoke- or air-inhalation burns.
- Electrical burns – high tension electrical current, lightning.
- Chemical burns – acids, alkalis and other irritants such as phosphorus.

Depth of burns

- First-degree burns: Only the epidermis is involved. Sunburn and mild steam or hot water burns.
- Second-degree burns: These involve the epidermis and parts of the dermis.
- Third-degree burns: These comprise full thickness destruction of the skin, epidermis

and dermis, and even subcutaneous tissues and structures.

For practical purposes, it suffices to divide the burns into partial thickness and full thickness burns. Partial thickness burns can heal spontaneously. Full thickness burns always require skin grafts.

Classification according to severity of the burns

Mild burns

- *Second-degree burns which involve less than 15% of the body surface area.*
- *Third degree burns which involve less than 2% of the body surface area.*
- *Hospitalization is not essential.*

Moderate burns

- *Second-degree burns which involve between 15 and 25% of the body surface area.*
- *Third-degree burns which involve less than 10% of the body surface area.*
- *Such patients must be hospitalized, but a low mortality can be expected.*

Severe burns

- *Second-degree burns, involving more than 25% of the body surface area.*
- *Third-degree burns, involving more than 10% of the body surface area.*
- *Burns involving the hands, face, eyes, ears, feet and perineum.*
- *Inhalation burns.*
- *Electrical burns.*
- *Burns in the severly injured patient.*
- *Burns in patients with underlying medical risk factors.*
- *Burns involving more than 20% of the body surface area in children.*
- *The mortality is high and local complications are common in this group of patients.*

Resuscitation

An adequate IV line must be established immediately. It is preferable that cannulae be placed in large veins in the arm, through normal skin. If the arms are not available, a central venous catheter must be inserted percutaneously subclavicularly, or, if this is not possible, a cutdown must be done through normal or burnt skin.

A variety of formulae are used to replace fluids. The one which is most favoured is the Brooke revised formula.

Fluid is administered in the form of Ringer lactate, at a rate of 2 ml/kg/% burn. The percentage burn must be calculated using the rule of nines or with special body surface area charts, especially in children.

Each arm forms 9%, each leg 18%, the anterior torso 18% and posterior torso 18%, the head and neck 9% and the perineum 1%. Half the calculated fluid must be administered within the first eight hours and the rest during the next sixteen hours. Fluid administration must be adjusted according to the clinical response of the patient. The urine output must be maintained at more than 50 to 70 ml per hour. In children, 1 ml/kg/hour.

If fluids are administered aggressively, renal failure is rare. Patients with electrical burns, extensive burns involving muscle, and severely injured patients with burns must be given special attention. A larger urine output must be ensured, between 70 to 100 ml per hour. This may require additional fluids and diuretics. It is now relatively generally accepted that, during the first twenty-four hours, colloids do not remain in the circulation any longer than crystalloids. For this reason, only crystalloids are used. During the second twenty-four hours, colloids can be given in the form of plasma or albumin (albumin is very expensive). **It must be emphasized that these formulae are only guidelines and fluids must be adjusted according to the patient's response.**

The well-resuscitated patient

- Urine output 50–70 ml/hour.
- The patient is awake and well orientated. Control pain with small doses of IV morphine.
- Blood pressure, pulse and temperature must be satisfactory.
- The haematocrit drops and the electrolytes are normal.
- Central venous pressure is 5 – 14 cm water.

Management of burns

- *Resuscitation enjoys priority and, during this period, wounds must be covered by sterile cloths only. As soon as resuscitation is well under way and the patient is stable, the wounds must be attended to.*
- *Tetanus prophylaxis must be administered, depending on the immune status of the patient. As a routine, antibiotics are not given prophylactically.*
- *The wounds must be cleaned with surgical soap.*
- *All dead loose skin and debris must be removed.*
- *Bullae must be opened and removed.*
- *Hair around the wound is shaved.*

Partial thickness burns will heal spontaneously after a few weeks if severe infection can be avoided. Wounds can be left open, or covered with dressings. Facial wounds do very well when left open. Other wounds are more comfortable when bandaged.

At present, such wounds are covered with an antimicrobial substance and cleaned and rebandaged every few hours. The substances which are available include:

- **Silver nitrate 0,5% solution.** *This colours everything black. It must be reapplied frequently, because the silver ion is inactivated by proteins. This hypotonic substance leaches Na, K and Cl from the wound surface. This is the reason for frequent reapplication.*
- **Sulfamylon.** *This is painful. It is a strong carbonic anhydrase inhibitor and respiratory acid-base adjustments are necessary. Patients develop a tachypnoea.*
- **Povidine iodine (Betadine).** *This is very effective against gram negative bacteria. It is inclined to harden the eschar, which makes débridement more difficult.*
- **Silver sulphadiazine (1%) cream (Flammazine).** *This is painless, but does not penetrate the eschar very well.*

In third-degree burns, the aim is to prepare the wound as soon as possible for coverage by skin graft. Infection must be controlled. An attractive approach is surgical excision of the dead tissue followed by skin grafts. This is particular successful in small, full thickness wounds. In large third-degree wounds, it is impractical, except in first class burn units. There is extensive blood loss and usually inadequate amounts of skin available to cover the large, raw wound.

Some surgeons regard tangential excision as a compromise. The dead skin is cut away in layers until punctate bleeding is visible. Skin grafts are then placed on these areas. This reduces blood loss, but the lack of adequate skin for grafts remains a problem.

The usual technique comprises the following:

- *An antimicrobial agent (Flammazine) is applied.*
- *When the eschar begins to soften, the patient must be placed in a bath every day and pieces of eschar must be removed.*
- *When a raw, clean, granulating surface develops, skin grafts must be done, using the postage stamp method.*
- *Before the skin graft, care must be taken that the patient's serum proteins and haemoglobin status are optimal.*

Prevention of infection

The following principles apply:

- *Previous active débridement of all dead tissue.*
- *Protect and cover all open and healing wounds with an antibacterial agent.*
- *Prevention of cross-infection by isolation.*
- *Speedy coverage of the wound with skin.*

Use of antibiotics

It is almost impossible to keep a third-degree burn free of all infection. Systemic antibiotics must be used if penetrating infection is present.

Indications for antibiotics

- *A positive blood culture, especially in the absence of IV catheters.*
- *Exacerbation of any mild wound infection to a severe infection associated with clinical signs of sepsis.*
- *Signs of skin necrosis, with colour changes and blistering. A biopsy must be taken immediately. The biopsy must be divided into two. One part must be sent to microbiology for quantitative cultures. If there are 10^5 or more bacteria per gram of tissue cultured, this is a strong indication of penetrating infection.*

The other part must be examined histologically for signs of invasion of adjacent normal tissue. The management comprises general supportive measures and suitable antibiotics. Currently, Enterobacteriacea and the Klebsiella species are the most common causes of life threatening infections.

Important complications

Early

Inhalation burns

It has been calculated that 30% of patients with burns also have inhalation burns. This is a chemical tracheobronchitis which follows inhalation of smoke or irritating byproducts of incomplete combustion. It is usually a complication found in people who sustain burns indoors, or were unconscious or under the influence of liquor during burning. Although the majority of these patients have burns of the head and neck area, the presence of such burns is not diagnostic of the condition.

Clinical presentation

Patients present with gasping respiration, hoarseness and secretion of discoloured sputum. Symptoms usually begin twenty-four to forty-eight hours after inhalation. Bronchoscopy shows inflammation and oedema. Lung functions show airway resistance with suppression of the maximal expiratory flow volume.

Management

- *Provide humidified respiratory gases and stimulate coughing.*
- *In severe tracheobronchitis, hypoxia and bronchospasm, intubation, with intermittent positive pressure ventilation, is necessary.*
- *Bronchoscopy may be necessary to keep the trachea and bronchi clean.*
- *Bronchial cultures must be done regularly and appropriate antibiotics administered.*

The use of steroids is controversial. They should perhaps be administered to patients with severe bronchospasm and oedema. Decadron is the steroid of choice.

Impairment of circulation or respiration by circumferential eschars

It may be essential to split eschars around the arms and legs, as the circulation may become impaired by the oedema which builds up in the enclosed space. If the circulation does not improve immediately, a fasciotomy of the particular compartment must also be done. A circumferential eschar of the thoracic wall can sometimes impair respiration. The eschar can be split in the ward, without anaesthetic, as it has no sensation and does not really bleed.

Ileus

An ileus may arise, and the patient will then have to be treated with nasogastric suction and will not be allowed to take food by mouth.

Late complications

Suppurative thrombophlebitis

If cannulae are left in veins for too long without being changed, especially if the cannula was inserted through the burn into the vein, severe, even life-threatening, septic thrombophlebitis can arise. The bacteria involved are the same as those found in the burn. Such septic veins must be excised.

Gastrointestinal haemorrhage

If the stomach and duodenal mucosa of patients with burns of more than 30% of body surface area are examined, 80% will have erosions. About 25% of these erosions become ulcers (Curling ulcer). About 13% of these patients develop bleeding or perforation. They must be surgically treated.

Patients with severe burns must be treated with prophylactic antacids.

Metabolic disturbances and nutrition of patients with severe burns

The natural human reaction to massive burns is hypermetabolism, resulting in a negative nitrogen balance and weight loss. The nitrogen losses are directly proportional to the size of the burn and may be as much as 30 g per day in large burns. Large amounts of exogenous proteins and nonprotein calories can prevent this to a certain extent. Patients with 40% burns will lose 20% of their body mass unless large amounts of calories are provided.

Management

Patients with burns exceeding 30% will require more than 2000 kcal and 15 g nitrogen per square metre of body surface area to maintain a positive nitrogen balance. If enteral feeding, which is preferred, is not adequate, parenteral hyperalimentation must be administered. A diet must be planned to exceed the caloric and nitrogen requirements by 25%. Vitamins, trace elements and polyunsaturated fats must also be provided.

Longterm scar complications

The most important factor preventing scar contractures is early, effective skin grafting. The extensive scarring which often follows burns can lead to contractures. These can be prevented by using splints, physiotherapy and elastic pressure bandages, all of which must be used for months. Plastic surgical intervention is sometimes necessary, especially round the neck and other joints.

Bites 11

HUMAN BITES

Three main types of human bites can be identified:

- **Deliberate bites** – these are bites inflicted by an attacker or in self-defence.
- **Nondeliberate bites** – these are wounds caused by the teeth of a victim on the knuckles of an attacker.
- **Selfinflicted bites** – these occur in the mentally disturbed, or during grand mal epilepsy.

Human bites are mainly found on the upper limbs or neck and face. The most important complication is secondary infection. The large variety of bacteria which are found in the mouth include: streptococci, staphylococci, Spirochaetes, fusiform bacilli, proteus vulgaris, ps. pyocyaneus, *Actinomyces, Haemophilus* species, *Neisseria-, Corynebacterium* and *Nocardia* species. Anaerobes, such as the bacteroid species, are also found.

Management

The following principles apply:

- *Prevent infection and loss of function.*
- *Clean the wound thoroughly.*
- *Administer prophylactic broad spectrum antibiotics; a cephalosporin is probably the best.*
- *Facial and knuckle wounds can usually be sutured if there has been no delay and infection has not already set in.*
- *Other human bites must preferably first be left open and then sutured secondarily.*

DOG BITES

These are the most common bites. They are more frequently found in children. The most common site is the lower limb.

The dangers related to dog bites include secondary infection and rabies. The depth of a dog bite must never be underestimated. There may be penetration of bone, joints and tendon sheaths.

Tetanus can follow a dog bite. A dog's mouth has rich flora, including pseudomonas and Pasteurella species. Staphylococcus aureus and streptococcus viridans are common.

Management

The following principles apply in the management of dog bites:

- *Relieve pain and calm the patient.*
- *The local wound must be treated to promote maintenance of good function and appearance.*
- *Secondary infection, including* Cl. tetani. *must be prevented.*
- *If there is a risk of rabies, prophylaxis must be applied.*

The wound must be carefully inspected, with specific attention to underlying injuries to nerves, tendons, bones or joints. The wound must be cleaned thoroughly and débrided.

Because of the excellent blood supply, facial wounds can usually be sutured. Other wounds should preferably be left open and sutured secondarily.

Give prophylactic antibiotics – a cephalosporin is a good choice. Also give tetanus prophylaxis.

Approach to rabies prophylaxis

Rabies is rarely found in pets. It is not usually necessary to apply rabies prophylaxis if the patient has been bitten by an urban pet. If the patient has been bitten by a wild animal, or by a dog where circumstances suggest a possibility of rabies, active immunization with human diploid cell vaccine is indicated. The patient must also be given human rabies immunoglobulin. The allergic reactions seen with duck embryo vaccines and horse serum are less frequently seen with the human products.

SNAKE BITES

In South Africa, snake bites occur in about 24 per 100 000 of the population. More than 80% of these bites are found in men, more than 80% on the hand and arm; and more than 50% in snake handlers (snake park attendants or snake catchers). The mortality rate is low.

The majority of snakes are harmless. The poisonous snakes of importance in South Africa can be divided into three groups:

Colubidrae

Snakes with poisonous fangs situated in the posterior part of the mouth.

The boomslang and the bird-snake (twig snake)

These snakes fall into this group. Bites are rare. The venom has a haemolytic effect. The patient develops bleeding tendencies with bruising, subcutaneous haemorrhage, epistaxis, haemoptysis, haematemesis and haematuria. Patients become anaemic and develop hypovolaemic shock. They develop consumption coagulopathy.

Atractaspis bibronii

This is a subspecies of the group. The snake is usually known as a mole adder, and also as the stiletto snake. Its poison fangs are very long and it often uses a sideward motion of the head to bite. These snakes are dug up and, if handled, bite the handler's thumb with a sideward motion of the head. The venom is mainly neurotoxic, but it causes local pain, swelling and necrosis of tissue.

Viperidae

The most important snake in this group is the puffadder, which is found throughout South Africa. The Gaboon viper is very dangerous, but fortunately rare. It is found only in KwaZulu in South Africa. The nightadder is also fairly common.

Puffadder venom is cytotoxic. It causes severe pain, swelling, ecchymosis and blood blisters. Most bites are found on the lower limbs. The swelling can be so severe that patients develop compartment syndrome.

Systemic symptoms include nausea, vomiting and dizziness. Patients can also become shocked and die.

The Gaboon viper is large and its venom is also cytotoxic. The nightadder causes local necrosis, but no deaths.

The mountain viper is an exception in this group. Its venom is neurotoxic and affects the eye muscles particularly. Deaths are very rare.

Elapidae

This group includes many dangerous snakes. The green and black mamba, the cobras (Cape cobra and Egyptian or bushveld cobra), the rinkhals and the spitting cobras. The mambas and cobras have neurotoxic and cardiotoxic venom and the spitting cobras have mainly cytotoxic venom.

The venom of mambas and cobras is fast-acting and can cause death between ten minutes and eight hours. If the patient is still alive after twenty-four hours, subsequent death is unlikely. There is motor paralysis of the cranial and spinal nerves, as well as a central effect, which manifests as vertigo, convulsions and coma. Respiratory paralysis is the usual cause of death. The local reaction varies widely. Cobra bites are very painful, swell severely and develop necrosis.

The rinkhals tends to spit for the eyes. The venom causes a transient ophthalmia. Conjunctivitis can sometimes occur and blindness can result.

Mamba venom works extremely rapidly and causes respiratory failure within the first hour. Cardiac failure can also arise.

Management of snake bite

First aid

- *Reassure the patient.*
- *Wipe the wound with an antiseptic.*
- *Do not make incisions; this only causes bleeding and damages underlying structures.*
- *Apply a crepe pressure bandage around the limb and over the bite.*
- *Transport the patient to hospital as quickly as possible.*
- *A tourniquet must be considered only in cases of black mamba bite.*
- *Do not use the tourniquet for adder or viper bites, as it exacerbates tissue damage.*
- *Pressure bandages are much safer than tourniquets.*
- *Try to bring the dead snake to hospital for identification.*

A few points to consider

- *In more than 50% of snake bites, no venom is injected.*
- *If two hours have elapsed after an alleged snake bite, without manifestation of any local or systemic signs, treatment will probably not be necessary.*
- *Ptosis and glossopharyngeal paralysis are important early signs of systemic venomation.*

Hospital management

General measures

- *Put the patient to bed.*
- *Take a careful history and try to identify the snake. Examine the wound carefully.*
- *Clean the wound.*
- *Administer tetanus prophylaxis.*
- *Keep the patient under careful observation.*

If the snake is definitely identified as being harmless and there are no symptoms, the patient can be discharged. If the snake is identified as being dangerous and bite marks are present, but the patient has no symptoms or signs, observe the patient and do not administer antiserum. If there are still no signs or symptoms after four hours, the snake was probably harmless. Keep the patient under observation, as respiratory failure can arise later and haemotoxic manifestations can be delayed for twenty-four hours. If there are no signs or symptoms after thirty-six hours, the patient can be discharged.

If symptoms and signs develop, such as pain, swelling and systemic signs such as tachycardia, sweating, dysphagia and a drop in blood pressure, specific measures must be applied.

Specific measures

- **Administration of antiserum:** *Polyvalent antiserum, 6 ampoules (60 ml) must be administered IV. An hour later, a further 2 ampoules must be given. Sometimes there is time to do a skin sensitivity test beforehand. A subcutaneous injection of a 1:10 dilution of serum is administered. If there is a positive reaction, hydrocortisone (200 mg) must be given IV, as well as adrenaline 1:1000 (0,5 ml) subcutaneously, before commencing the serum infusion.*
- *Commence IV fluid administration.*
- *If there is respiratory distress, patients must be intubated and ventilated.*
- *If signs of compartment syndrome develop, the fascia must be split. Later, débridement and skin grafts may be necessary.*

Boomslang bite

Specific boomslang antiserum is available at the SA Institute for Medical Research in Johannesburg. It must be administered as soon as possible. Fresh blood, platelet concentrate, fresh frozen plasma and cryoprecipitate must be used to treat the consumption coagulopathy. Where special skills are available, heparin can be used, but only with very careful monitoring. Under normal circumstances, it should be avoided.

SCORPION STINGS

The broad-tailed scorpions (*Buthidae*) can be dangerous. Their venom is neurotoxic. Cases of death have been reported.

Apply a pressure bandage to the limb and treat symptomatically. Do not administer morphine derivatives or barbiturates, as they can exacerbate the condition.

SPIDER BITES

There are four important groups:

Latrodectus species

Commonly known as the button spider. There are two types which are of importance in South Africa. The one has red marks on its body and the other an hourglass pattern. Their venom is neurotoxic. Cases of death have been reported.

Management

- *A firm pressure bandage on the limb is useful.*
- *Ten per cent Calcium gluconate (10 ml) IV relieves pain.*
- *Antiserum is available.*

Loxosceles (violin spider)

Two types have been described, the cave dwellers and the savannah dwellers. Bites usually occur at night.

Churacanthum (sac-forming spider)

These are fastmoving, strawcoloured spiders with black pincers. They are aggressive and bites usually occur at night in bed and comprise two bite marks.

Sicarius (six-eyed crab spider)

These are found in dry areas under the sand. They are very poisonous and their bites can cause death.

These cytotoxic spiders cause a haemorrhagic, swollen lesion. Later, the bite undergoes necrosis and secondary infection. It takes a long time to heal. Excision, followed by a skin graft, is sometimes preferable.

Patients can also develop diffuse intravascular coagulation and renal failure.

BEE STINGS

Some people are sensitive to bee stings. They develop an anaphylactic reaction characterized by urticaria, oedema, vomiting, dysphagia, respiratory problems, cyanosis, hypotension and coma.

Adrenaline and hydrocortisone must be administered and respiration supported.

Index

E

F

G

Q

R

S

T